Endovascular and Neurovascular Surgery for Spinal Vascular Malformations

Xianli Lv
Editor

Endovascular and Neurovascular Surgery for Spinal Vascular Malformations

Springer

Editor
Xianli Lv
Department of Neurosurgery
Beijing Tsinghua Changgung Hospital
School of Clinical Medicine, Tsinghua University
Beijing, China

ISBN 978-981-97-4660-6 ISBN 978-981-97-4661-3 (eBook)
https://doi.org/10.1007/978-981-97-4661-3

This Springer imprint is published by the registered company Springer Nature Singapore Pte Ltd.
The registered company address is: 152 Beach Road, #21-01/04 Gateway East, Singapore 189721, Singapore

Preface

Spinal vascular malformations have a complex anatomical structure. Since their low incidence, it is generally well known to scholars. Their natural courses often lead to hemiplegia, bowel and bladder dysfunction, and a high disability rate. If treated properly, the patient's prognosis can be significantly improved. There has been a significant breakthrough in the surgical treatment and endovascular treatment of spinal vascular malformations. This made me think of editing a monograph on spinal vascular malformations, bringing together clinical and basic research on spinal vascular malformations. It is hoped that the research progress of spinal vascular malformations can be promoted, and breakthroughs can be made in basic and clinical aspects after appearance of this book. As far as I know, this is a monograph on *Endovascular and Neurovascular Surgery for Spinal Vascular Malformations*. Previously, there was a monograph on *Vascular Anatomy of the Spinal Cord*, which was published by Springer, editor-in-chief of Armin K. Thron. Together with this book on spinal vascular malformations, Springer Press will become more complete in spinal vascular anatomy and lesions. I thank all experts and scholars who have contributed to spinal vascular malformations to complete this monograph together. This will be a very interesting monograph because their contribution is rich and diverse, and their viewpoints are diverse.

Beijing, China
March 6, 2023

Xianli Lv

Commemorative of Academician Zhongcheng Wang

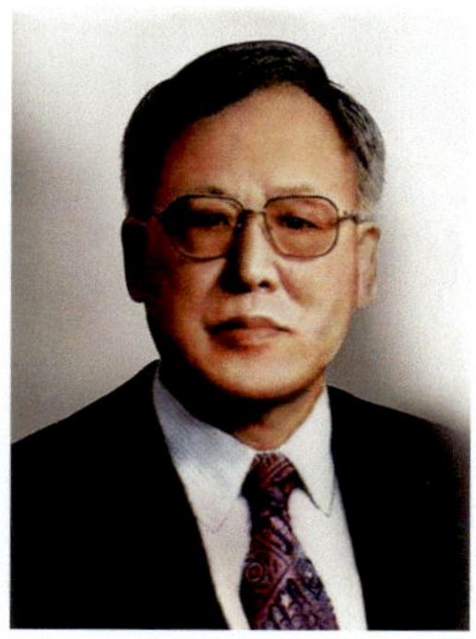

Prof. Zhongcheng Wang (20th, Dec, 1925 – 3 0th, Sep, 2012), Academician of Chinese Academy of Engineering

Acknowledgment

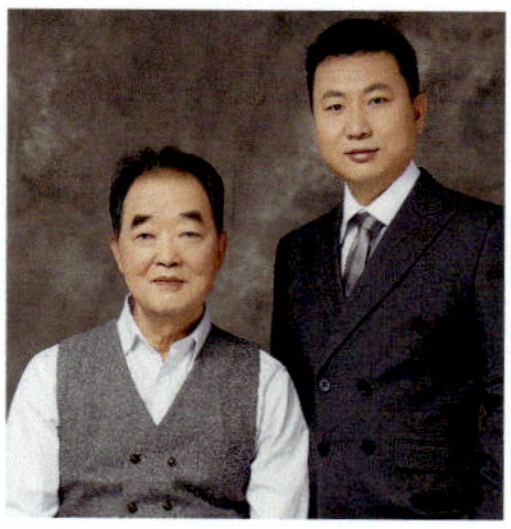

Thanks to Prof. Zhongxue Wu for his great contribution to Chinese Endovascular Neurosurgery, my great teacher, who is a human being of immense qualities, a man of incredible energy, and an extraordinary individual whom we will always love and admire.

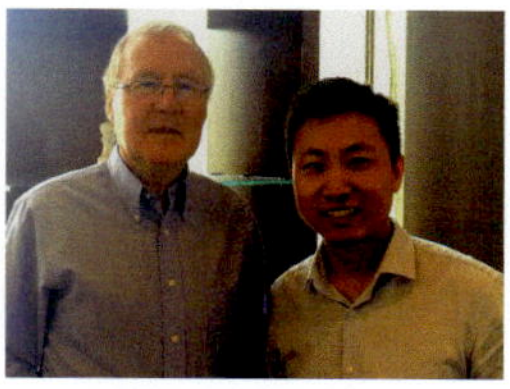

Dr. Karel terBrugge (on the left), former Head of the Division of Neuroradiology and Site Chief of Medical Imaging at Toronto Western Hospital, and Dr. Xianli Lv (on the right) in 2012, Beijing, China

Contents

About the Editor

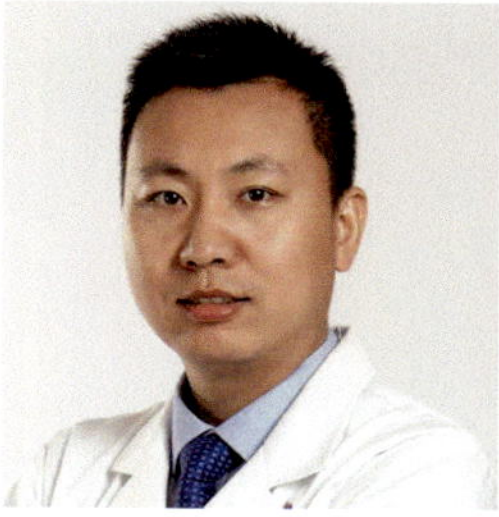

Xianli Lv MD, is an associate professor of endovascular neurosurgery, at the Department of Neurosurgery, Beijing Tsinghua Changgung Hospital, School of Clinical Medicine, Tsinghua University, Beijing, China. He is selected for the "2023 Career-long and yearly Top 2% Global Scientists List" released by Stanford University in the United States. His research focuses on neuroendovascular therapy of intracranial aneurysm, cerebral arteriovenous malformation, intracranial dural arteriovenous fistula, spinal vascular malformation, and pediatric cerebrospinal vascular malformation. He has one national invention patent and one utility model patent to his credit and has authored 195 peer-reviewed scientific articles and edited 10 books. His h-index is 31 in 2024 (Scopus). He is an editorial member of *Interventional Neuroradiology*, *Stroke and Vascular Neurology*, *Journal of Neuroradiology*, *The Neuroradiology Journal*, and *World Journal of Radiology*. He is also a deputy editor of Neuroscience Informatics and Frontiers in Neurology. Dr. Lv is a member of the World Stroke Organization (WSO) and the World Federation of Interventional and Therapeutic Neuroradiology (WFITN). He was featured on the cover of World Journal of Radiology in April 2022 and in June 2024, and journal of *China Science and Technology Achievements* in August 2023.

Vascular Anatomy of the Spine and Spinal Cord

1

Eilat Sapirstein, David Felzensztein, Eyal Hendler, and Eyal Itshayek

Abstract

This chapter reviews the arterial and venous anatomy of the spine and spinal cord, notably the intersegmental artery and its cranial and caudal derivatives: the vertebral, supreme intercostal, and sacral arteries.

Keywords

Artery · Vein · Anatomy · Spinal cord · Spine · Embryology

1.1 Introduction

The blood supply of the spine and spinal cord is highly complex and variable. Therefore, thorough knowledge of vascular anatomy and embryology is critical for understanding the pathophysiology of spinal vascular lesions and diseases. In addition, it serves as an essential tool for planning safe surgical and endovascular interventions.

Variability in the vasculature is frequently encountered; thus, the spine surgeon and endovascular interventionalist must be familiar with the possible anatomic variations before undergoing extensive diagnostic or therapeutic spinal procedure. Understanding the vascular supply to the spinal cord is especially important when considering different surgical approaches to avoiding devastating complications such as spinal cord ischemia or infarction.

This chapter provides a detailed description of the standard anatomical arterial supply and venous drainage of the spine and spinal cord, as well as embryological background and anatomic variations one must consider while considering surgical and endovascular interventions.

1.2 Embryology of the Spinal Vasculature

1.2.1 Embryology of Arterial Supply of the Spine and Spinal Cord

The embryological development of the arterial and venous system of the spine and spinal cord consists of four stages. The vascular system is fully established before 6 months of age, and there are no significant changes after that in the spinal cord vasculature.

The first stage, "the primitive segmental stage," occurs between 2 and 3 weeks of gestation. During this stage, 31 pairs of segmental vessels arise from the paired primitive dorsal aorta to supply 31 somites (segmental masses of the

E. Sapirstein · D. Felzensztein · E. Hendler · E. Itshayek (✉)
Department of Neurosurgery, Rabin Medical Center, Petah Tikva, Israel
e-mail: eyalhe1@clalit.org.il

X. Lv (ed.), *Endovascular and Neurovascular Surgery for Spinal Vascular Malformations*,
https://doi.org/10.1007/978-981-97-4661-3_1

mesoderm) [1]. The primitive segmental artery divides into dorsomedial and dorsolateral branches and forms a capillary network on the surface of the developing neural tube. Each segmental artery supplies blood to the corresponding ipsilateral metamer—consisting of the future skin, muscle, bone, spinal nerve, and spinal cord [2, 3].

In the second stage, which occurs during 3–6 weeks of gestation, known as the "initial stage," arterial anastomoses continue to develop, as well as the formation of venous channels. This stage of development is susceptible to maldevelopment and malformations, and it is the stage in which the genesis of vascular malformation occurs and persists to adulthood [1].

From the sixth week to the fourth month of uterine life, the "transitional stage" occurs, in which the classic adult pattern of vascular supply will progressively form. Each longitudinal ventral neural axis provides several arterial branches, which run longitudinally and deep within the ventral sulcus and supply the anterior two-thirds of the spinal cord; these vessels are perforators that will become a part of the intrinsic arterial supply. The primitive ventral longitudinal arteries eventually fuse into a single ventral longitudinal vessel, the future anterior spinal artery. Posteriorly, two channels coalesce from a pial network on the lateral and dorsal surfaces to form the posterior spinal arteries. This process's alteration can lead to duplication and fenestration of the developing ASA [4].

During vasculogenesis, the future segmental arteries give rise to the radicular artery, which initially contributes to the anterior and posterior spinal arteries. By the end of the fourth embryological month, variable regressions of the segmental vessels take place, leaving about 4 to 8 anterior branches of the radicular arteries to supply the entire axis via the anterior spinal artery and from 10 to 20 posterior branches that supply the posterior spinal cord via posterior spinal arteries [5]. Variable segmental artery regression also leads to the formation of the vertebral arteries, thyrocervical trunks, and costocervical trunks in the cervical region and the iliac arteries and median sacral artery in the lumbar region. Regression is more prominent in the caudal region, leaving a single ARA at the lower thoracic and three upper lumbar regions that enlarge to supply the cord at this level—this artery is known as arteria radicularis magna or "artery of Adamkiewicz."

The last stage, the "terminal stage," occurs after 4 months of development in which the blood vessels mature and become more tortuous [1].

1.2.2 Embryology of the Venous Supply of the Spine and Spinal Cord

The first stage of venous development begins at the fourth gestational week. During this stage, two paired longitudinal veins, the anterior and posterior cardinal veins, are formed as the common cardinal vein. Concurrently, paired supracardinal and subcardinal veins develop inferior to the common cardinal vein and connect via transverse channels (the azygos, renal, and iliac veins). Simultaneously, the paravertebral plexus forms around the developing spinal cord, and the cardinal veins connect to the paravertebral plexus via transverse intersegmental veins [6, 7].

As the fetus matures and develops, the vertebral vein develops from the transverse intersegmental veins. The right supracardinal vein persists as the azygos vein, and the left supracardinal becomes the hemiazygos and accessory hemiazygos veins. The future internal and external jugular veins arise from the anterior cardinal veins, and the remnant of the right posterior cardinal vein becomes the arch of the azygos.

The azygos, hemiazygos, and accessory hemiazygos veins drain into the superior vena cava through the arch of the azygos vein [6, 7].

When compared to the arterial system, the venous system demonstrates high variability, especially concerning location and distribution.

1.3 Vascular Anatomy

1.3.1 Arterial Blood Supply

1.3.1.1 Arterial Supply to the Spine and Spinal Cord

Arterial blood to the spine and spinal cord can be divided into extrinsic and intrinsic or macrocirculation and microcirculation. Each spinal level has its unique vessel anatomy, with normal anatomic variations depending on the spinal level [5].

The branching anatomy of the arterial blood supply can be schematically considered as follows: a central arterial trunk (vertebral artery, aorta) gives rise to a spinal/segmental artery, which branches into radiculomedullary artery (ventral radicular artery) and radiculopial artery (ventral or dorsal artery) that give rise to a pial network, which connects the paired posterior or single anterior spinal arteries (Fig. 1.1).

Macrocirculation

The arterial supply to the spinal column derives mainly from the segmental arteries. The origin of the segmental arteries depends upon the spinal level. In the cervical region, they arise from the vertebral arteries, the ascending cervical arteries, the deep cervical arteries, and the occipital and ascending pharyngeal branches of the external carotid artery. The thoracic and upper lumbar spines originate in pairs from the posterior aspect of the descending aorta via intercostal and subcostal branches, from branches of the costocervical trunk, and from the internal thoracic artery of the subclavian artery. In the lumbosacral region, they arise from branches of the internal iliac artery (mainly the iliolumbar and lateral sacral arteries) and the median sacral artery (a branch of the aorta at the level of the bifurcation) [8]. There are extensive anastomoses between the segmental arteries providing collateral flow [9].

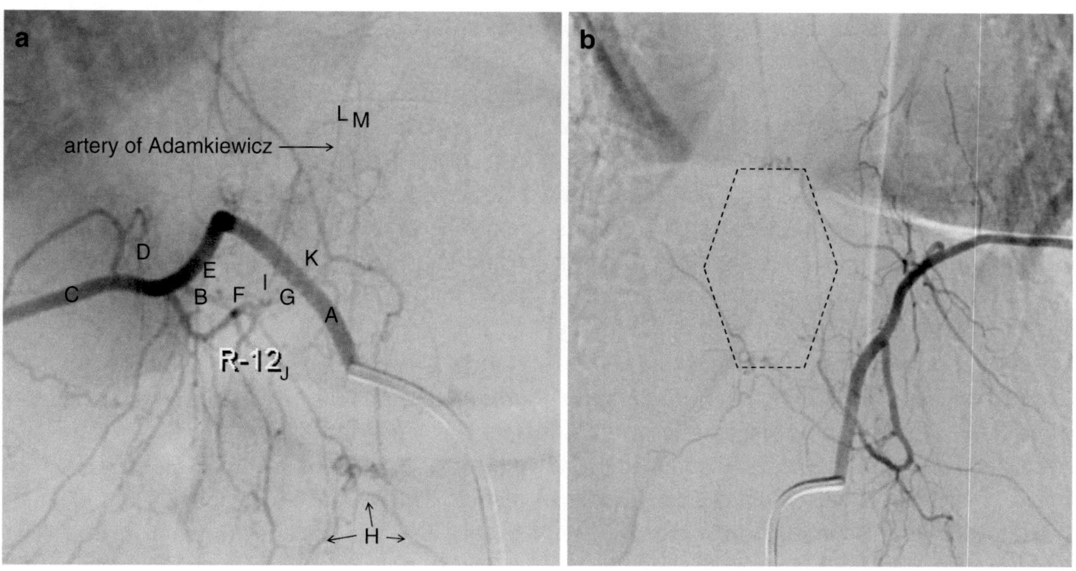

Fig. 1.1 (**a**) Right T12 segmental artery injection. (A) Segmental artery. (B) Dorsal spinal artery. (C) Intercostal/muscular artery. (D) Pretransverse anastomotic network. (E) Dorsal division of the dorsal spinal artery. (F) Ventral division of the dorsal spinal artery. (G) Radicular artery. (H) Ventral epidural arcade. (I) Nerve root sleeve dural branch of the ventral division dorsal spinal artery. (J) Dural branch of the ventral division dorsal spinal artery. (K) Radiculopial artery. (L) Radiculomedullary artery. (M) Anterior spinal artery. The artery of Adamkiewicz arising from the right radiculomedullary artery at T12 level. Notice the characteristic hairpin turn as the artery of Adamkiewicz joins the anterior spinal artery (M). (**b**) The catheter in the left T6 segmental artery and a hexagon-shaped multilevel anterior epidural arcade (retrocorporeal artery)

The segmental arteries continue their course posteriorly and laterally along the vertebral body, dividing into three significant trunks—lateral or ventral trunk, middle or dorsal trunk, and medial or spinal trunk. They enter the spinal canal via the intervertebral foramen. Each trunk further divides into anterior and posterior spinal canal arteries that supply the vertebral bony and ligamentous structures and a radicular artery that supplies the dura and nerve root at each level. The radicular arteries that supply the dura and nerve roots are called radiculoradial or radiculomeningeal arteries. At several levels but not all, the radicular artery gives branches that follow the anterior and posterior nerve roots termed radiculomedullary arteries. The radiculomedullary arteries further divide into anterior and posterior branches that supply the ASA and PSA, respectively [5].

Anterior Spinal Artery

The anterior spinal artery (ASA) arises at the level of the foramen magnum from the vertebral arteries originating from the first part of the subclavian artery. It passes along the anterior sulcus of the spinal cord and descends to the level of the conus medullaris.

Due to its long course and the significant structures it serves, additional arterial supply is required to reinforce its blood supply, which is supplied via the anterior radiculomedullary arteries. There are three major regions of blood supply to the anterior spinal artery from the radiculomedullary arteries: the cervicothoracic, midthoracic, and thoracolumbar regions. The most critical and dominant anterior radiculomedullary artery is the artery radiculomedullaris magna, also known as the artery of Adamkiewicz (AKA). This vessel almost always arises in the thoracolumbar region, between T8 and L2, and in 80% on the left side [9]. The territory of blood supply by the ASA includes the anterior two-thirds of the spinal cord [5, 10].

Posterior Spinal Artery

The two PSAs originate at the level of the foramen magnum from the ipsilateral vertebral or posterior inferior cerebellar arteries. They pass along the right and left posterolateral surfaces of the spinal cord. Around 10–20 feeders from the posterior radiculomedullary arteries supply the PSA at various levels. The anatomical distribution of the blood supply of the PSA includes the posterior third of the spinal cord [10].

Pial Plexus

The ASA and PSAs form end anastomosis at the level of the conus medullaris. Along the entire spinal cord along its surface, another extensive arterial network is found termed pial plexus or "vasocorona." It is responsible for supplying the periphery of the spinal cord [4].

Microcirculation

Microcirculation, also known as the intrinsic spinal cord supply or spinal cord perforators, consists of two groups of arteries arising from the anterior and posterior spinal arteries. These branches can be divided into centrifugal (from the center of the cord toward the surface, central) and centripetal (from the cord surface toward the center, peripheral) systems. The ASA is the main contributor to the centrifugal system, and both ASA and PSA contribute to the centripetal system. The centripetal system supplies mainly the white matter and the centrifugal gray matter of the spinal cord [4, 11].

The central system consists of about 200–400 central arteries (aka sulcal or sulcocommissural arteries) originating from the ASAs. These vessels travel in the anterior median fissure and penetrate the sulcus to enter the central gray matter. They branch centrifugally into small arteries that run toward the white matter. The sulcocommissural system supplies most of the spinal cord gray matter and the ventral half of the white matter [5].

The peripheral system consists of radial perforating arteries originating from the posterior spinal arteries and the pial plexus and penetrating the white matter. These centripetal arteries supply the posterior part of the posterior gray matter and the outer half of the white column [2].

1.4 Venous Blood Supply

The venous drainage of the spine and spinal cord can be divided, similarly to the arterial system, into an intrinsic system, which runs in proximity to the centrifugal arterial system, and an extrinsic system, which runs in proximity to the centripetal arterial system, and extradural component.

1.4.1 Intrinsic Venous System

The intrinsic system is composed of a network of radially arranged venous channels [6]. Capillaries from the medial parts of both sides of the spinal cord drain into ventral and dorsal sulcal veins. The number of ventral sulcal veins varies over the length of the spinal cord and increases over the thoracolumbar spine. Capillaries from peripheral gray matter and white matter travel toward the periphery forming radial veins; when reaching the surface, they form a venous ring that eventually drains into the external system. A longitudinally oriented intrinsic venous system is also present, interconnecting the radial veins [6, 9].

1.4.2 Extrinsic Venous System

The extrinsic system arises at the level of the spinal pia mater and includes the pial venous networks, the longitudinally oriented extrinsic venous system, and radicular veins.

The pial network, as mentioned earlier, drains the sulcal veins.

The anterior and posterior spinal veins represent the longitudinal venous system at ventral and dorsal surfaces in the midline of the spinal cord. The anterior median spinal vein accompanies the ASA and drains the sulcal veins and the veins of the ventral fissure. The posterior spinal veins (posterior median and posterolateral) accompany the PSA and receive blood supply from the radial veins of the dorsal spinal cord. Up to three ventromedial venous channels are present in the ventral cervical and upper thoracic regions. Three anterior cervical and upper thoracic longitudinal channels converge in the lower thoracic area, continue as a duplication, and unite proximal to the lumbosacral area. There is triplication in the thoracic region on the cord's dorsal surface, and the vessels converge at the cervicothoracic and thoracolumbar junctions [5, 6, 9].

The anterior and posterior median spinal veins drain into the radiculomedullary veins, which accompany the anterior or posterior spinal nerve root: the great anterior radiculomedullary vein (GARV) is the most prominent vein draining the anterior thoracolumbar spinal cord. In the intervertebral foramen, the radiculomedullary and radicular veins exit through the dura and drain into the epidural vertebral venous plexus via the spinal nerve venous channels [6].

1.4.3 Extradural Venous System

The vertebral venous plexus (Batson plexus) is divided into three divisions: the internal and external vertebral and the basivertebral plexuses [6].

The internal vertebral venous plexus (anterior and posterior) is located epidurally within the vertebral canal and continues superiorly to communicate with the cranial venous system. It includes two anterior and two posterior internal plexuses. The anterior (front of the vertebral bodies) and posterior (surrounding the posterior elements) external vertebral venous plexus surrounds the vertebral column, and the basivertebral veins run horizontally within the vertebral body [9].

Cervical, thoracic, lumbar, and sacral intervertebral veins connect the external and internal vertebral venous plexuses and communicate with various extraspinal longitudinal veins depending on the vertebral level.

Drain occurs via the vertebral, deep cervical, and jugular veins at the cervical level, ultimately into the superior vena cava. The thoracic and lumbar intervertebral veins connect to the azygos system, the ascending lumbar veins, and the superior vena cava. The ascending lumbar veins communicate with the inferior vena cava via lumbar segmental veins at the lumbosacral level. The sacral veins empty into the lateral sacral and internal iliac veins.

Valves exist only in the radicular branches draining the spinal cord. These valves prevent congestion of the spinal cord and cannot be found in other components of the venous system.

1.5 Anatomic Variations

The vasculature of the spinal cord is highly variable in size and structure due to differences in embryological development and proliferation, metabolic requirements, and blood flow demand. This section presents some of the most common anatomic variations one must consider.

Vertebral artery variants—the vertebral artery usually arises from the posterosuperior aspect of the first part of the subclavian artery. The most common variant is for the left vertebral artery to originate off the aortic arch between the left common and left subclavian artery, with a 2–5% prevalence [12]. An anomalous left VA arising directly from the aortic arch typically enters the C4 or C5 foramen transversarium, resulting in a longer course of VA in the neck. Aberrant right VA is an extremely rare anomaly.

Arterial duplication is dividing an artery into two distinct vessels with different courses. Fenestrations are a single arterial lumen that divides into two parallel channels following the same course. The frequency of duplication of the VA is around 0.72% in cadavers [12]. Other VA pathologies exist, including tortuosity, elongation, and kinking [12].

Artery of Adamkiewicz variants—75% of the time, the artery inserts into the dura and ASA at the level T9–T12. Fifteen percent inserts into the dura and ASA at the level T5–T8, and 10% of the time, the artery is inserted into the dura and ASA at the level L1–L2 [13].

Variants of ASA and AKA junction:

- Type 1: a small-caliber ASA joining a larger-caliber AKA. These vessels form a large ASA descending from that level. This variant is considered an AKA dominant circulation, and disruption of the AKA in patients with this circulation could lead to severe neurological damage.
- Type 2 variant is where the ASA and AKA are the same calibers, and when joining together, the caliber of the ASA does not increase (non-dominant AKA) [10].

Duplication of the ASA—until C5/C6 level is typical.

Variation in the number and origin of the radicular arteries.

Variations in the origin of PSAs—posterior spinal arteries can originate from either the VA or the PICA and with a symmetrical or asymmetrical configuration. The intracranial segment of the VA is the most common origin [14].

References

1. Benzel EC. Spine surgery 2-Vol set E-book: techniques, complication avoidance, and management (expert consult - online). Elsevier Health Sciences; 2012.
2. Miyasaka K, et al. Vascular anatomy of the spinal cord and classification of spinal arteriovenous malformations. Interv Neuroradiol. 2000;6(suppl 1):195–8.
3. Thron A, et al. Development of the arterial supply of the spinal cord tissue based on radioanatomical and histological studies in cattle. Clin Neuroradiol. 2022;32(2):325–43.
4. George B, Bruneau M. In: George B, Bruneau M, Spetzler RF, editors. Embryology of the vertebral artery. Pathology and surgery around the vertebral artery. Springer Paris; 2011. p. 5–24.
5. Wells-Roth D, Zonenshayn M. Vascular anatomy of the spine. Oper Tech Neurosurg. 2003;6(3):116–21.
6. Griessenauer CJ, et al. Venous drainage of the spine and spinal cord: a comprehensive review of its his-

tory, embryology, anatomy, physiology, and pathology. Clin Anat. 2015;28(1):75–87.
7. Green K, Reddy V, Hogg JP. Neuroanatomy, spinal cord veins. In: StatPearls. Treasure Island (FL): StatPearls Publishing; 2022.
8. Bosmia AN, et al. Blood supply to the human spinal cord: part I. Anatomy and hemodynamics. Clin Anat. 2015;28(1):52–64.
9. Santillan A, et al. Vascular anatomy of the spinal cord. J Neurointerv Surg. 2012;4(1):67–74.
10. Gofur EM, Singh P. Anatomy, back, vertebral canal blood supply. In: StatPearls. Treasure Island (FL): StatPearls Publishing; 2022.
11. Krauss WE. Vascular anatomy of the spinal cord. Neurosurg Clin N Am. 1999;10(1):9–15.
12. Yuan SM. Aberrant origin of vertebral artery and its clinical implications. Braz J Cardiovasc Surg. 2016;31(1):52–9.
13. N'da HA, et al. Microsurgical anatomy of the Adamkiewicz artery–anterior spinal artery junction. Surg Radiol Anat. 2016;38(5):563–7.
14. Rojas S, Ortega M, RodríGuez-Baeza A. Variable anatomic configuration of the posterior spinal arteries in humans. Clin Anat. 2018;31(8):1137.

2 Types of Spinal Vascular Malformations

Manas Panigrahi, Gudipati Ananta Ram, and Jitender Chaturvedi

Abstract

Spinal vascular malformations are often complex problems with varied clinical presentations. In this chapter, we will briefly overview common clinical presentations of patients with spinal vascular malformations after reviewing the normal vascular anatomy of the spine and then outline different types of vascular disorders, and possible treatment options. Catheter angiography remains the gold standard investigation for diagnosis and planning of treatment. Therapeutic options, treatment success rate and limitations are briefly described in particular.

Keywords

Spinal vascular malformation · Extradural · Dural · Intramedullary · Spinal dural AV fistula · Spinal angiography · Anterior spinal artery (ASA) · Posterior spinal artery (PSA) · Spinal arteries · N-Butyl cyanoacrylate · Endovascular Treatment

M. Panigrahi (✉)
Department of Neurosurgery, Krishna Institute of Medical Sciences, Secunderabad, Telangana, India

G. A. Ram
Department of Neuro-Radiology, Krishna Institute of Medical Sciences, Secunderabad, Telangana, India

J. Chaturvedi
Department of Neurosurgery, All India Institute of Medical Sciences, Rishikesh, Uttarakhand, India

2.1 Introduction

Spinal dural arteriovenous fistulae (sDAVF) are rare vascular lesions in neurovascular disease spectrum. The spine and spinal cord constitute just 1–2% of all vascular neurological disorders [1]. However, more than 80% of these spinal vascular pathologies are included within the umbrella disorder of sDAVF, making it the most common spinal vascular pathology [1]. Myelopathy is the usual presentation of this disease, though sensory and sexual symptoms are also seen. Treatment options consist of endovascular embolization, surgical disconnection, or a combination of both [2]. Surgical anatomy of arterial supply and venous drainage of the spinal cord is also discussed.

2.1.1 Endovascular Anatomy of Spinal Cord Arterial Supply and Venous Drainage

Before understanding the pathophysiology of shunting behind the origin of sDAVF, it is vital to understand the surgical anatomy of spinal cord blood supply. Various segmental arteries supply the spinal cord at multiple levels. Segmental arteries originate from the vertebral artery, thyrocervical and costocervical trunks, supreme intercostal artery in cervical and

X. Lv (ed.), *Endovascular and Neurovascular Surgery for Spinal Vascular Malformations*,
https://doi.org/10.1007/978-981-97-4661-3_2

upper thoracic region, descending aorta in lower thoracic and median sacral artery in sacral regions.

The segmental arteries are named, e.g., D10 segmental artery that supplies D10 vertebrae. Segmental arteries are not named based upon the level of origin. Segmental artery gives three branches-spinal, dorsal and ventral. Sometimes a small trunk for the dorsal and spinal branches called dorsospinal trunk is present. The dorsal branch gives medial and lateral musculocutaneous branches which supply para spinal musculature, posterior aspect of lamina and spinous process. Osseous branches from segmental artery are also known as ventral somatic branches, supply ventrolateral surface of vertebral body. Ventral branch is nothing but the intercostal or lumbar segmental arteries. Superior intercostal artery. This is the most cephalad intercostal artery arising from the aorta, ascending to supply upper thoracic vertebral levels. Supreme intercostal artery arising from the costocervical trunk providing radicular arteries to the C7 and C8 levels.

Spinal branch gives Anterior epidural, radicular, and posterior epidural (prelaminar) arteries. Anterior epidural branches (dorsal somatic) connect with opposite and adjacent arteries, and form a diamond-shaped (retrocorporeal) anastomotic network. Posterior epidural branch contributes to the prelaminar anastomosis and supplies the dura and bone of the lamina. Based upon their depth of penetration in cord, these spinal radicular arteries are named [3] as radicular (radiculomeningeal), radiculopial, and radiculomedullary. A spinal radicular branch supplying the dura and the nerve root as a radiculomeningeal artery is present at each segment. At some of these levels, the radicular artery is enlarged as it also gives supply to the spinal cord via a radiculomedullary artery (Average, 6) which has ascending course to the ASA. Similarly, it may supply the ipsilateral PSA via a radiculopial artery, with predominant pial plexus supply (range10–20). The *largest radiculomedullary artery* is the famous artery of Adamkiewicz usually originating from T9–T12 (in 75% of cases, it originates between T8 and L2 but may go as high as T3 and as low as L4 to get origin). This artery, which most commonly originates from the left side (80%), is easily identified on angiogram, with a typical hairpin loop and a large descending along with smaller ascending branch. Longitudinal arterial trunks that extend along the long axis of the spinal cord surface are Anterior spinal artery and two posterior (or posterolateral) spinal arteries. The anterior spinal artery (ASA) is typically formed at the level of the foramen magnum by the confluence of descending branches of the intracranial segments of the vertebral arteries. Due to its long course, the ASA requires additional arterial supply via anterior radiculomedullary arteries at cervicothoracic, midthoracic and thoracolumbar. The two Posterior spinal arteries (PSAs) also originate at the level of the foramen magnum by branches of the ipsilateral vertebral or posterior inferior cerebellar arteries. Multiple anastomoses exist between the ASA and PSAs; these include the circumferential vasa corona vessels (pial network), the intramedullary vessels (i.e., sulcocommissural arteries), and the basket anastomosis in the region of the conus medullaris.

In relation to the transverse process, there are two longitudinal anastomotic plexuses, i.e., *pre- and post-transverse longitudinal anastomosis.* The dorsal branch of segmental artery communicates with these pre-transverse anastomoses. Post-transverse longitudinal anastomosis communicates freely with posterior intercostal arteries and lumbar arteries. These pre- and post-transverse longitudinal anastomoses also communicate freely with each other.

In lumbar spine, only up to L4 segmental artery, the aorta is the origin. L5 segmental artery originates from iliolumbar artery and median sacral artery. Lateral sacral arteries arising from internal iliac artery supplies sacral nerve roots.

Multiple anastomoses connect the left and right PSAs across the midline (posterior plexus)-rope ladder. PSA lies on either side of posterolateral surface of cord, medial to the posterior root entry zone.

Intrinsic arterial network of spinal cord: The ASA will give sulcocommissural arteries (centrifugal) to supply mainly the spinal cord gray matter, and both the ASA and PSA will give a pial network with small perforating (centripetal) vessels, to supply the white matter.

Venous drainage of the cord runs in three types of veins: internal cord veins, longitudinal veins and radiculomedullary veins.

Radiculomedullary veins follow the anterior and posterior roots. Internal cord veins form centrifugal pattern of drainage from central to periphery.

The short peripheral veins follow a radial course ending in the coronary plexus. The perimedullary venous (coronary) network interconnects the longitudinal spinal trunks (posterior and anterior median spinal veins).

Trans-medullary veins are veins that traverse the cord parenchyma and form anastomosis between the anterior and posterior surface veins in midline.

Longitudinal veins are anterior median and posterior medial spinal veins (usually 3 in number with constant posterior median spinal vein). Interestingly, the junction of median spinal veins with the radiculomedullary veins is an obtuse angle, giving it an often quoted *"coat hook" appearance.* It is important to make sure that this "coat hook" is not mistaken with *"hairpin"* of the artery of Adamkiewicz on angiogram. Radiculomedullary veins exit the dura, usually with the nerve root, may join radicular veins and empty into the internal vertebral venous plexus of the extradural system. The radicular and bridging veins are the key link between intradural and extradural venous systems. Intervertebral (emissary/foraminal) veins link internal vertebral (epidural) and external venous plexus. Intervertebral veins via segmental veins finally drain into azygos, hemiazygos venous systems or jugular vein.

2.1.2 Pathophysiology

Shunting is the main pathophysiological mechanism leading to symptomatology of sDAVF. Direct shunting of blood from radiculomeningeal artery to radicular vein leads to venous congestion in valveless spinal cord veins. This venous hypertension causes symptom onset. Secondary to spinal arterial perfusion pressure drop, spinal cord undergoes ischemic changes, and symptoms start to appear. In the terminal stage of the disease without treatment, necrotizing myelopathy sets in, which is irreversible and devastating. Usual site seen for this shunting is the thoracolumbar region, i.e., the site of sDAVF. Etiology is idiopathic in majority of the cases, though post-surgical and post-traumatic cases have also been reported in the literature [4]. Cervical cord is an extremely rare site for sDAVF to develop.

2.2 Classification and Types

We use a classification described by Keisuke Takai as it is according to the sites (dural, intradural, and extradural) and types (AVF and AVM) of AV shunts [5].

2.2.1 Type I Dural AVF

Most commonly appearing at thoracolumbar region, type I represents the most common (~70%) type of spinal vascular malformations. Progressive compressive myelopathy is the usual presentation. When located at the level of CVJ or upper cervical spine, the lesion may present at sub arachnoid hemorrhage. These myelopathic changes occur secondary to venous hypertension and intra-medullary venous stagnation, owing to a fistula between the dural branch of segmental artery and radicular vein. Anatomically, this fistula resides at the level of dural root sleeve. More than half of the cases worsen to a level of permanent disability within 24–36 months [6], if left untreated. Treatment consists of surgically disconnecting the draining vein of the fistula, intradurally. Surgical success is around 98% if the draining vein is identified properly [6]. Other treatment option is endovascular obliteration of the draining vein at proximal location. Complete obliteration is essential to get minimal recurrence (up to 20% overall recurrence is noticed in various series) [7]. It is important to learn that endovascular treatment is contraindicated when anterior or posterior spinal artery is supplied by radicular artery.

2.2.2 Type II Intramedullary Glomus AVM

When a parenchymal or intramedullary lesion has a nidus-like cranial AVM, it is classified as type II. Intramedullary hemorrhage, in addition to more common congestive myelopathy or SAH, can also be the presenting symptom. This lesion has multiple feeders from anterior as well as posterior spinal artery.

Embolization is the first line of treatment, keeping in mind that complete obliteration may never be achieved and both complete and partial obliterations reduce the recurrences of symptoms by decreasing the re-bleed rates [8]. Usual surgical excision of the nidus is obviously too risky to be advised. In presence of inadequate obliteration after embolization or presence of angiographic high risks of embolization, a guided and planned surgical excision may be offered.

Radiosurgery is a third modality, which has been explored in these lesions. Stereotactic radiosurgery has been used by researchers with documented success in motor symptom improvement and partial obliteration of AVM nidus [8].

2.2.3 Type III Intramedullary Juvenile AVM

When lesions appear metameric, i.e., multiple vascular malformations appearing from the same spinal metameric segment, it is sine qua non for diagnosing this variant. Adolescent and young adults are the usual sufferers. Fortunately, these are rare variants. Complete obliteration is rarely observed and never a target in planning treatment of this variant. Terminating the progression of neurological deficits is considered the success of treatment as genetic mutations are involved in pathophysiology of the disease.

2.2.4 Type IV Perimedullary AVF

In the absence of intervening nidus, direct arteriovenous communication on the spinal cord pial surface is the hallmark of this variant. Perimedullary fistula form more often on ventral surface of the spinal cord and typically have a midline location.

There are three different subtypes of this variant ranging from IVa to IVc depending on the size, level of blood flow and venous drainage. Type IVa single arterial feeder to the vein with slow flow. Type IVb has multiple dilated arterial feeders of intermediate size, while type IVc has multiple dilated arteries and ectatic draining veins. Type IVc has association with HHT, i.e., hereditary hemorrhagic telangiectasia, and appear in younger patients, more often.

Type IVa perimedullary AVFs are more amenable to microsurgery. Type IVb and IVc respond favourably to endovascular treatment due to multiple feeding arteries and shunt volume. IVb may require surgery for failed endovascular treatment.

2.2.5 Type V Extradural AVF

Congestive myelopathy is the clinical presentation, often indistinguishable from type I commonly located at lumbar level with frequent bilateral epidural arterial supply. Distinction is done by angiographically proving a direct fistulous communication between an extradural artery and vein. Extradural AVFs were subdivided into Subtypes Va- with intradural venous drainage and Vb without intradural venous drainage.

Type A has a retrograde parenchymal drainage with a perimedullary vein, which goes intradural and leads to venous congestion leading to symptoms. Treatment consists of treating extradural venous lake and this intradural perimedullary vein. If the draining vein is large enough to give an access, transvenous embolization can be done, if there is single draining vein. With multiple draining veins, meticulous coagulation and separation of the epidural venous lake is advised type Vb extradural AVFs are more amenable to endovascular embolization.

2.2.6 Conus Medullaris AVM

This variant is a subtype of type II where a nidus is clearly visible, added as a separate variant since last two decades. As indicated by the name, the anatomical location at conus is obvious, and the nidus is both extra- and intramedullary. Combined approach with both surgical and endovascular treatments is recommended.

2.3 Clinical Presentation

Various case series have reported a male predominance with a M/F ratio of 4:1. A typical patient with diagnosis of sDAVF is a male in his fifth decade of life. The most common (90–95% of patients) presentation is chronic spastic motor weakness, presenting as progressive myelopathy. Sensory and sexual symptoms with sphincter disturbances and lower back pain mimicking sciatica can also be observed in these patients.

Exception to this classical presentation is always to be kept in mind because approximately 15% of the patients report in atypical fashion. Rare instances of acute deterioration of motor power due to hemorrhage or due to Foix-Alajouanine syndrome can also be seen. These acute episodes are supposed to be secondary to acute thrombosis of the pathological veins draining the fistula causing hyperacute venous hypertension, and clinical deterioration becomes erratic and acute. Episodes of remissions in between acute attacks of motor power deterioration have also been noticed.

2.4 Diagnosis

MRI and spinal angiography (both subtracted and unsubtracted) are the modalities used in diagnosing sDAVF. MRI of the spine is usually the first imaging modality that gives a clue to the diagnosis. Multiple serpiginous flow voids in the subarachnoid spaces (arterialized pial veins) seen in T1W and T2W images direct the observer toward suspecting sDAVF. Flow in dilated, tortuous vessels of the arterialized coronal venous plexus is the cause of this signal void. These pial veins may focally indent the cord surface and give a scalloped appearance on sagittal T1W images. Normal CSF flow voids also give this pattern; therefore, MRI alone with the findings mentioned above is not sufficient to conclude the diagnosis. Evidence of venous hypertensive myelopathy should be searched for and documented for sDAVF to be established as diagnosis.

This evidence comes in the form of swollen cord (usually cauda) with T2 hyper-intense signal within the cord substance associated with peripheral T2 hypo-intense signal, which indicates that the central T2 high signal is secondary to venous hypertensive myelopathy, and not due to tumor, edema, or any other cause. This peripheral hypo-intensity on T2 images of the spinal cord is a consistent and specific diagnostic feature of venous congestion associated with dural AVF.

Without doubt, the spinal angiography is the investigation of choice for diagnosing and classifying sDAVF. It gives anatomical details and angioarchitecture of the fistula with confidence; therefore, a proper management plan can be made out.

This angiographic evaluation should not only assess the fistula site but should contain thorough assessment of the whole spinal vasculature that includes vertebral arteries, thyrocervical trunk intercostal, lumbar arteries of the aorta, and the internal iliac arteries. The intercostal artery is numbered by the rib under which it runs. This helps diagnose associated lesions (missed on non-angiographic evaluation) or other feeders in compound fistulae with multiple sites of feeding vessels.

2.5 Management

The main target of treatment in sDAVF is complete elimination of venous congestion. This can be achieved only after total block of shunting, discussed in pathophysiology. Achieving this target only gives a chance for recovery of the spinal cord. Excision, obliteration, or disconnection of the fistula, which can be accomplished surgically or endovascularly. It is important to keep in mind that obliteration of this fistulous connection leads to resolution of T2 hyper-intensities seen on spinal MRI, only weeks to months after surgery or intervention.

2.5.1 Surgical Treatment: Microsurgical Technique of Pial Resection

Posterior approach is the most straightforward corridor to reach the pathology. Preferential laminectomy, laminoplasty, or hemi-laminectomy can be performed based on surgeon's selection.

The main goal in surgery is to identify the arterialized medullary vein. The most certain way (after midline dural opening) to identify this is to look for vein's dural piercing at the site of dural penetration of posterior nerve root. Confirmation of the target vein that needs to be disconnected can be done with the use of comparison between anatomy and angiography. Surgeon should always try to look for a vein that is large and arterialized and look for the vein that is crossing the subarachnoid space to join the dilated coronal venous plexus. Once the target vein is identified, it is cauterized using bipolar cautery and cut using a micro-scissors. Immediately after this, the color of venous plexus changes from red to blue after a minute or so. Use of micro-Doppler is an important aid while disconnecting the fistula, as it demonstrates a change in flow pattern in arterialized vein, before and after disconnection.

Two things should always be kept in surgeon's mind: firstly, overzealous stripping of venous plexus from the surface of cord will only exacerbate the venous hypertension in cord, thus leading to poor outcome. Secondly, change in color of the vein may not always be apparent, immediately after disconnecting. Therefore, it should not be used as a guide for surgical success per-operatively.

2.5.2 Endovascular Treatment

With the ease with which the surgical disconnection is performed, and a relatively higher recurrence rate with endovascular intervention, operative treatment has become a preferred treatment for sDAVF. Without doubt, with availability of better catheters and embolic materials, with better understanding of spinal angiography, the results of endovascular treatment are much better than the recent past. Still the usual and major causes of failure include angiographically occult fistulae, multiple feeders, and failure of microcatheter to reach fistula or failure of embolic agent to hit the target vein. The key to long-term successful endovascular treatment is a good penetration of embolization agent into draining vein. Success rates for endovascular and surgical treatment ranges between 25% to 75% and 98%, respectively. Rates of definitive embolization have wide range, depending in part on the embolic agent used and the use of variable stiffness microcatheters.

2.5.2.1 Preferred Endovascular Agent

Endovascular therapy with liquid embolic agents - N-butyl-cyanoacrylate (NBCA) and ethylene vinyl alcohol copolymer dissolved in dimethyl sulfoxide (Onyx, Medtronic, CA, USA and Squid, Balt, Montmorency, France) are preferred for treatment of sDAVF and perimedullary fistula (arteriovenous fistula). Liquid embolic should be injected super selective catheterization of the feeding artery using flow guided microcatheter. The concentration of the NBCA (glue) must be adjusted depending on the flow volume of the shunt and the distance between the tip of the catheter and the shunting zone. A slow continuous injection of much dilute glue (15% glue and 85% lipiodol) has a higher chance of reaching the draining vein and obliterating the fistula.

Ethylene vinyl alcohol copolymer can be used when a longer, more controlled injection with better penetration of the vascular bed is needed in spinal AVM.

In low flow rate glomerular AVMs, PVA particles yield a stable result if venous stagnation occurs. Obliteration of arterial or venous aneurysms which are the source of the hemorrhage in spinal AVM should also be accomplished with liquid embolic agents or coils during endovascular treatment [9].

2.5.3 Radiosurgery

Zhan et al. in a systematic review done in 2018 reported that among arteriovenous malformations, 16% showed nidus to be obliterated, decreased, and unchanged in 44.6%, and 39.3%, respectively, at an average follow-up of 46.8 months [10]. Lack of extensive research in radiosurgery in the management of spinal AVMs is the reason for its limited use.

Illustrative Cases

Case 1: Dorsal sDAVF

A 50-year-old male presented with subacute onset of progressive weakness of both lower limbs and urinary incontinence over a 9-month period. MRI and angiography are shown in Fig. 2.1. Importance of heavily weighted T2 sequence constructive interference in steady state (CISS) in better delineating the flow voids of the perimedullary vein can be seen in Fig. 2.2.

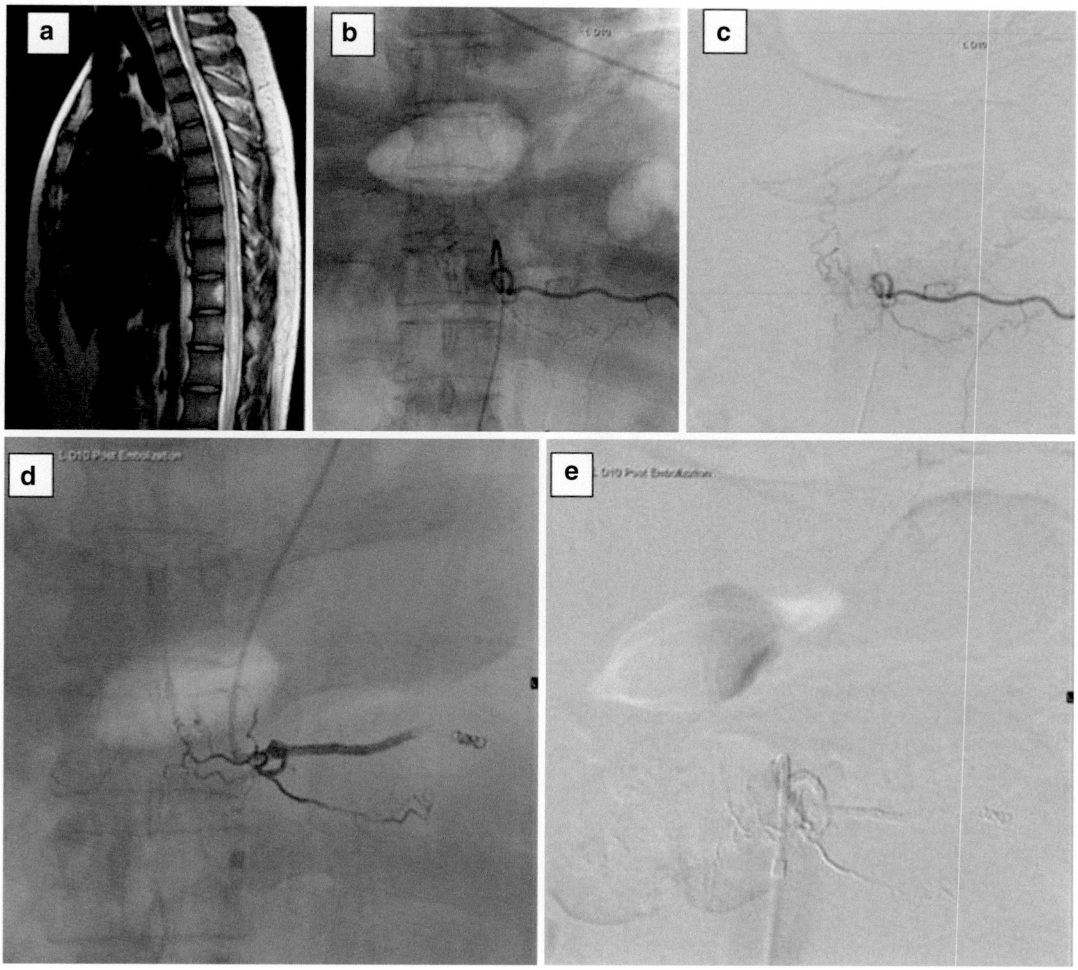

Fig. 2.1 Spinal DAVF. (**a**) Sagittal T2W image of the lumbar spine shows increased signal intensity, cord edema, and perimedullary flow voids and expansion of the lower thoracic cord and conus. (**b**) Unsubtracted AP view of the left D10 intercostal artery supplies an sDAVF beneath the left D10 pedicle and dilated radiculomedullary vein ascending to dilated perimedullary veins. (**c**) Selective left D10 distal intercostal artery injection showing the fistula. (**d**) The fistula was treated with onyx embolization and coils (coil in intercostal artery was deposited for facilitating microcatheterization of the feeding radicular artery). Onyx cast shown in unsubstracted image. (**e**) Immediate repeat angiography showed complete closure of fistula

Case 2: Role of Catheter Angiography and Advantages over MR Angiography in Spinal AVM (Fig. 2.3)

Case 3: High Cervical sDAVF (Fig. 2.4)

Case 4: Intramedullary Thoracic AVM (Fig. 2.5)

Case 5: Dorsal sDAVF (Fig. 2.6)

Case 6: Type I Perimedullary Fistula (L2) (Fig. 2.7)

Case 7: Intramedullary Glomerular AVM (Cervical) (Fig. 2.8)

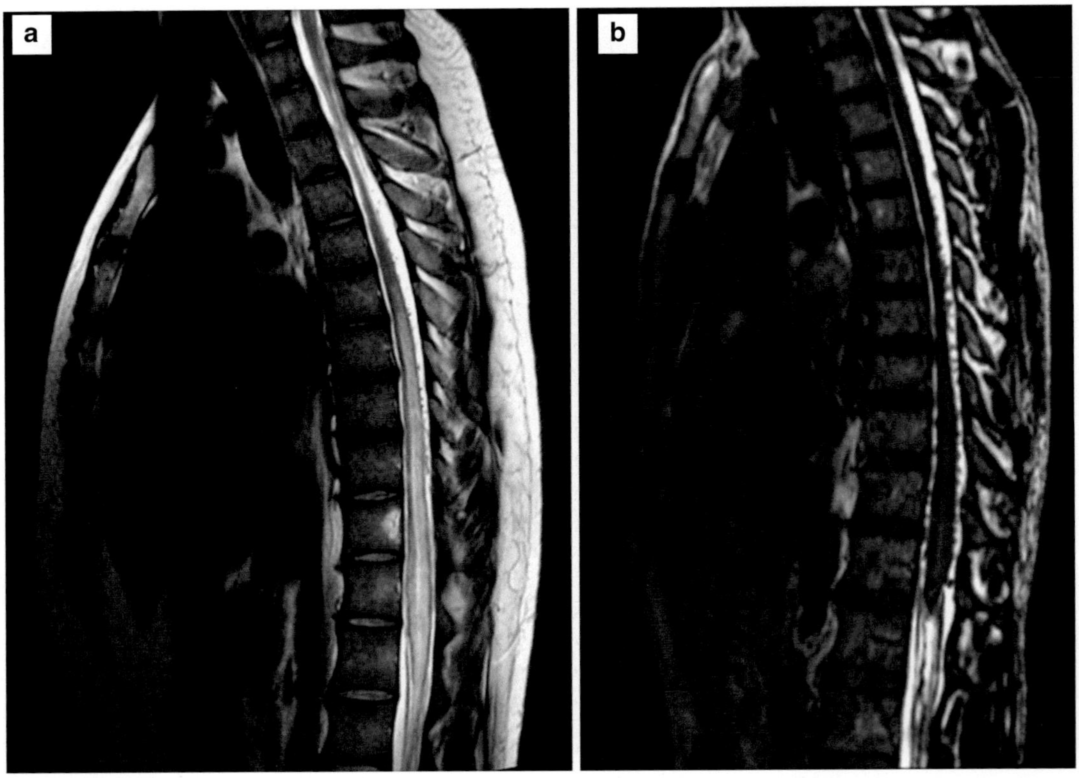

Fig. 2.2 When comparing a routine T2 TSE (**a**) sequence and a heavily T2-weighted (3D CISS) sequence (**b**), the former depicts the cord edema better, whereas the latter is better suited to demonstrate the perimedullary flow voids, as seen in this patient

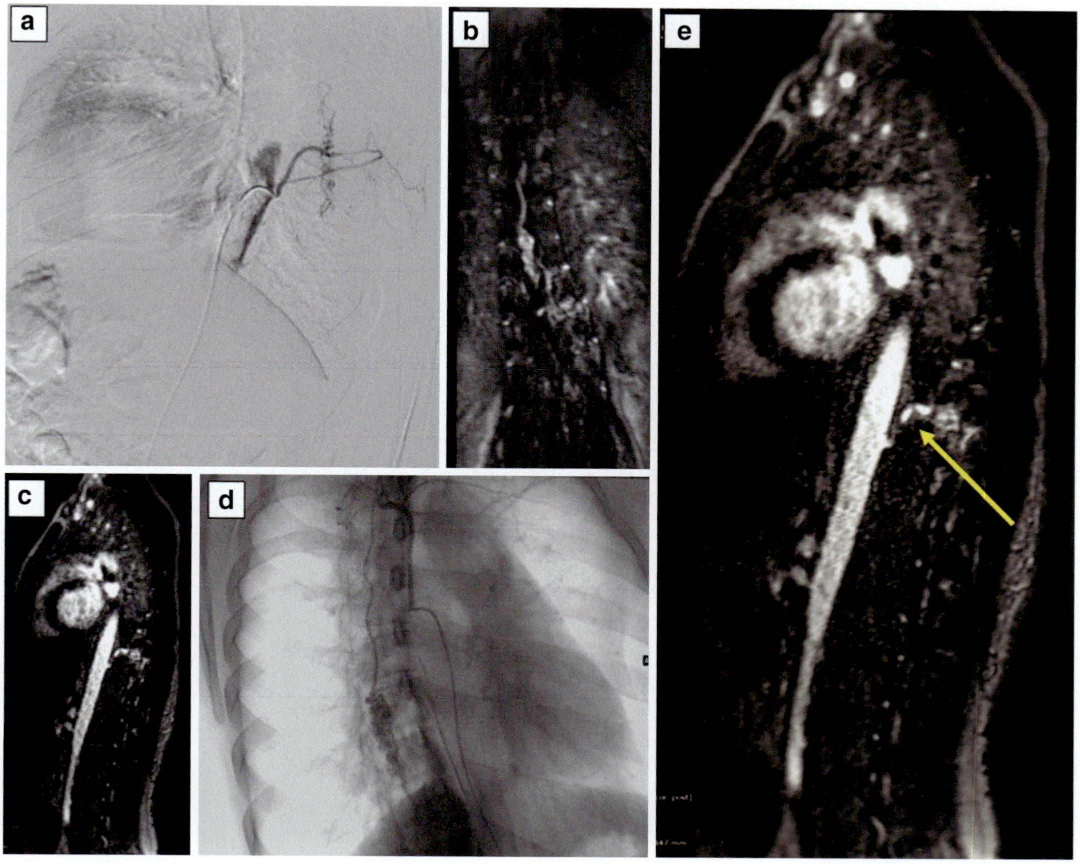

Fig. 2.3 Comparison of MR angiography with catheter angiography in a patient with spinal AVM. (**a**) Selective left D5 intercostal injection showing spinal AVM. (**b**) The coronal MIP images of contrast-enhanced MR angiography display the craniocaudal extent of the dilated perimedullary vein draining the AVM. (**c**) The magnified MR angiographic image depicts the arterial feeder of the AVM (arrow). (**d**) Early phase image of the catheter angiography examination verified the location of the AVM. Note that only the catheter angiography images can reveal the small network of vessels of the fistula (**d**) and depict the dynamic drainage pattern (**e**). (**b**) MRA helps in depicting the extent of venous drainage such that limited DSA can be obtained

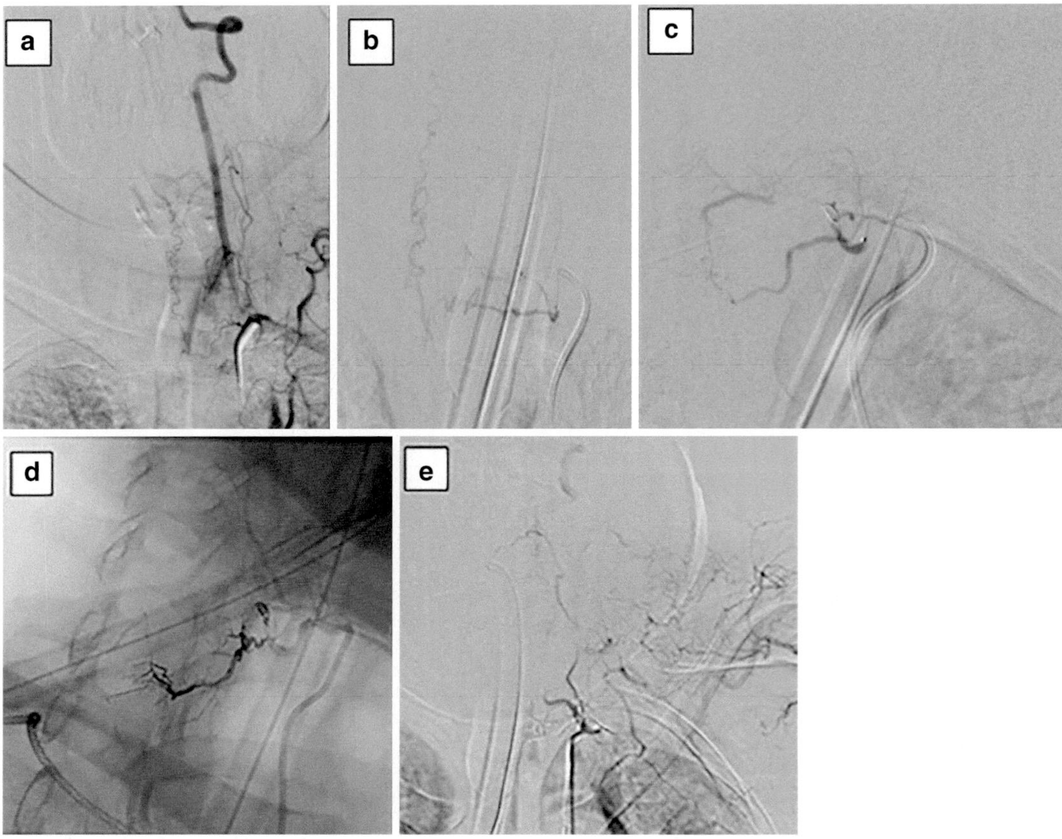

Fig. 2.4 Cervical sDAVF. (**a**) DSA showing sDAVF at C6–D1 level fed by inferior division of left costocervical trunk on left subclavian injection. (**b**) Angiogram with microcatheter positioned in costocervical trunk. (**c**) Left costocervical trunk showing coil, which was deposited for facilitating microcatheterization of the feeding radicular artery. (**d**) Unsubtracted image post-embolization showing onyx cast in the distal feeding radicular artery, spinal DAVF, and the draining radicular vein. (**e**) Post-embolization angiogram shows no filling of fistula

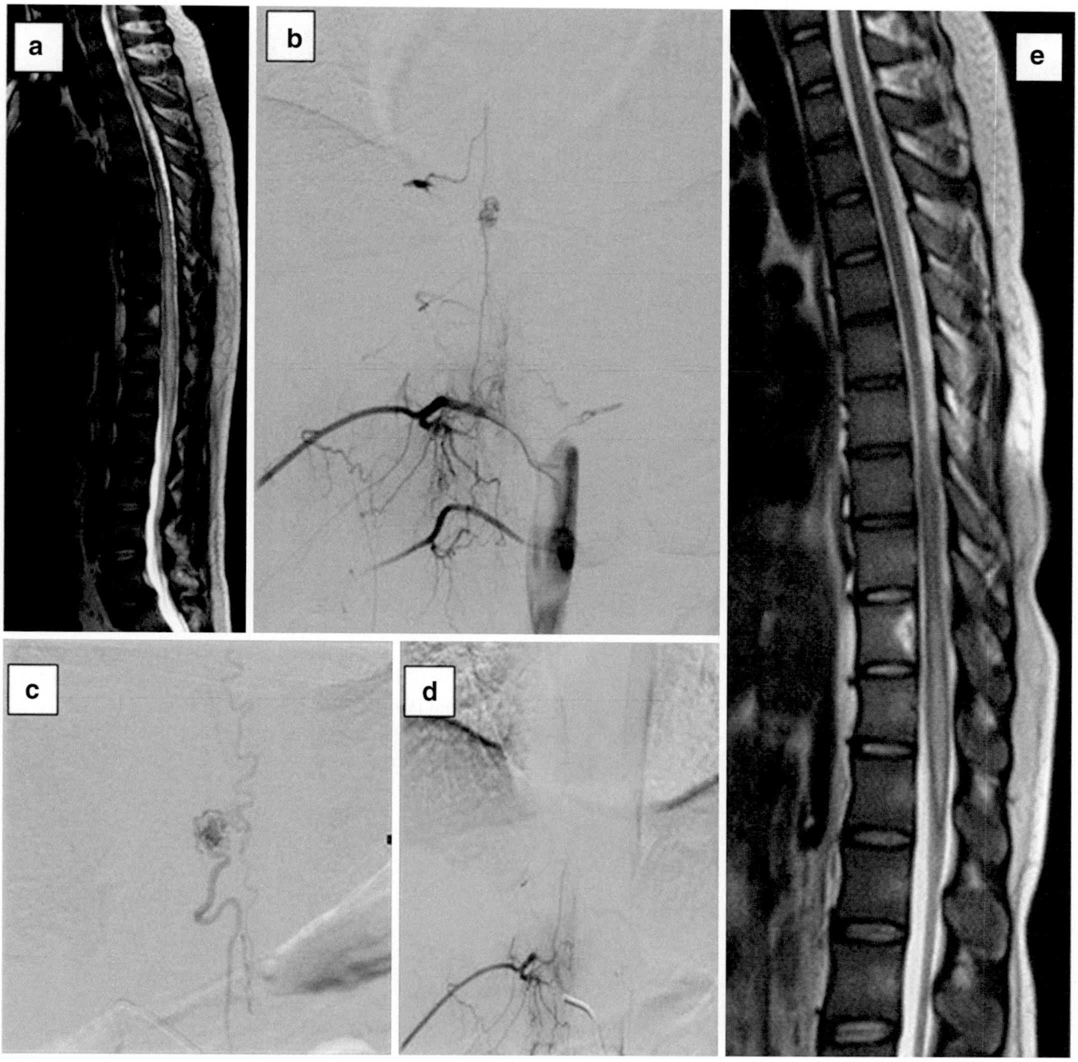

Fig. 2.5 Intramedullary thoracic AVM. (**a**) Sagittal T2-weighted MR image shows serpentine flow voids and long segment cord edema in thoracic region. (**b**) Selective angiogram of right D8 intercostal artery shows filling of the posterior spinal artery supplying the AVM. Posterior spinal artery filling noted from a vessel at different level (right T10 intercostal artery). (**c**) Angiogram with microcatheter positioned just proximal to the fistula. (**d**) Check angiogram following embolization of right D10 intercostal artery with glue shows no filling of fistula. (**e**) Sagittal T2-weighted MR image 2 months after treatment shows that the enlarged perimedullary veins and intramedullary abnormal signal intensity have reduced significantly

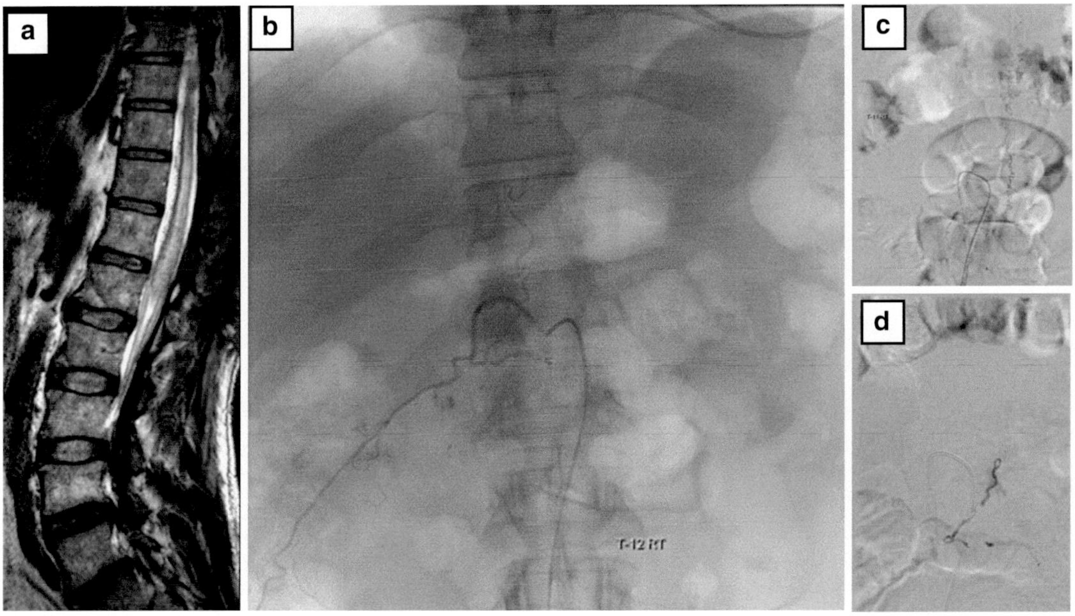

Fig. 2.6 (**a**) Sagittal T2-weighted MR image of postoperative case of right D11 sDAVF shows that the enlarged perimedullary veins and intramedullary abnormal signal intensity are persisting. (**b**) Postoperative spinal angiography with selective catheterization of the right T11 segmental artery showing residual DAVF. (**c**) Angiogram with a large FOV shows the extensive venous drainage into spinal perimedullary veins. (**d**) Right T11 intercostal artery late-phase angiogram following closure of the feeding artery with glue shows no residual fistula

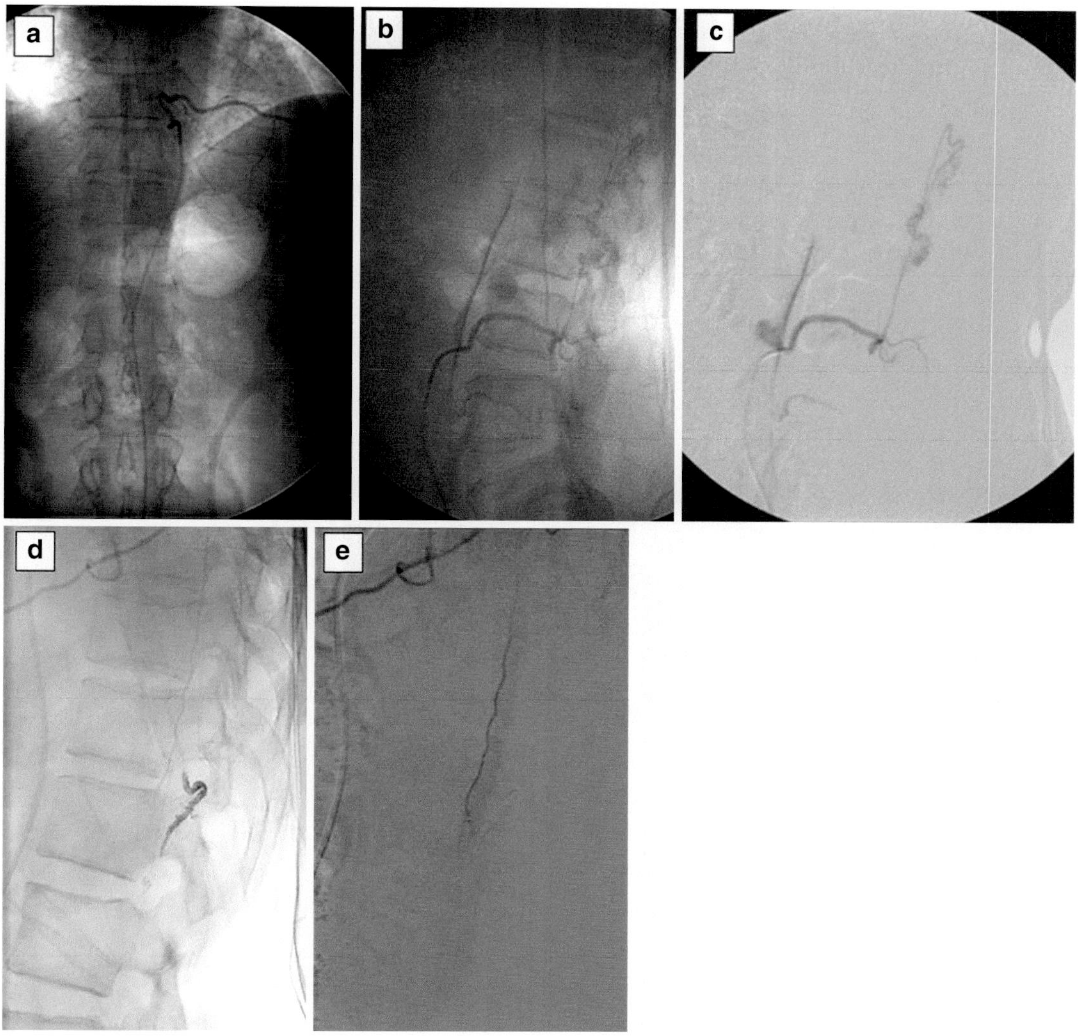

Fig. 2.7 Spinal perimedullary fistula type I at L2 level on the left side. (**a**) Selective angiogram of the left T11 intercostal artery early phase (**a**) shows slightly enlarged artery of Adamkiewicz and anterior spinal artery filling the shunt at L2 level. (**b**) Late phase, showing the serpentine perimedullary veins filling in descending fashion. (**c**) The fistula is embolized with onyx with the cast shown in the unsubtracted image. (**d**) After onyx embolization, the anterior spinal axis is still opacified, while the venous ectasia and the fistula are obliterated. (**e**) However, following procedure, patient was found to be unresponsive. CT of the brain showed diffuse subarachnoid hemorrhage

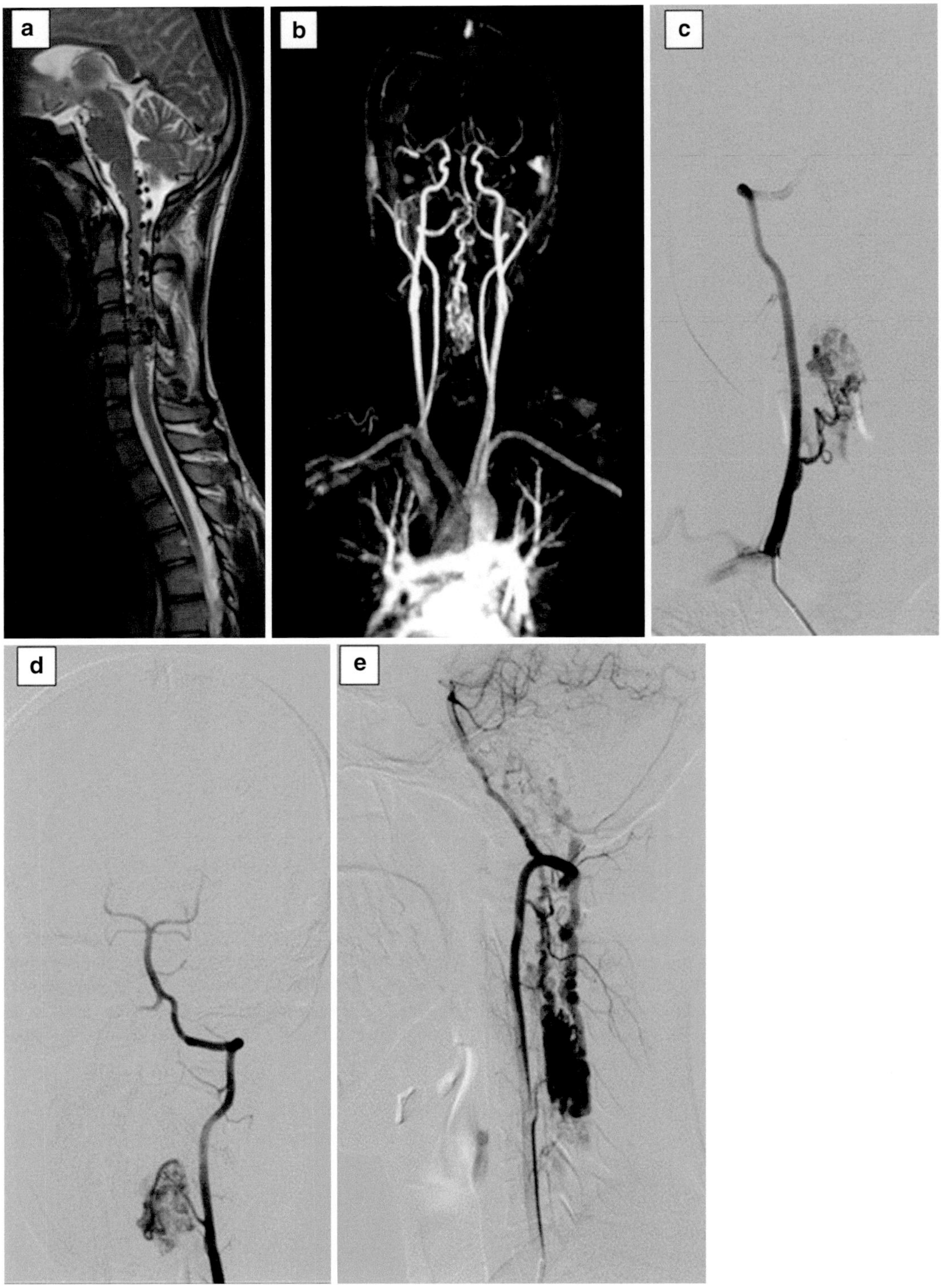

Fig. 2.8 Intramedullary glomerular cervical AVM. (**a**) Sagittal T2-weighted image shows the intramedullary position of the AVM and enlarged superficial draining veins in the cervical subarachnoid space extending intracranially to the perimedullary region. (**b**) Contrast-enhanced MR angiography revealing the nidus and spatial extent of venous drainage of AVM. Spinal AVM supplied by the feeders from bilateral vertebral arteries at C6 level on the right (**c**) and C5 level on the left (**d**). (**e**) Dilated arterialized veins extending superiorly through the foramen magnum to the level of the clivus

Key Messages

- Spinal vascular malformations are a potentially treatable cause of myelopathy.
- Spinal MRI and angiography are the main diagnostic tools.
- Patient selection after careful evaluation of angio-architecture of the spinal vascular malformation is an important factor in achieving good results, to avoid variations in treatment outcomes and to minimize complications.
- Choice of surgery or embolization depends on the type and location of lesions.
- Surgery gives outstanding results (98% success), provided draining vein is correctly identified in sDAVF.
- Endovascular treatment is getting preference over surgical obliteration.

References

1. Ferch RD, Morgan MK, Sears WR. Spinal arteriovenous malformations: a review with case illustrations. J Clin Neurosci. 2001;8(4):299–304.
2. Oldfield EH. Surgical treatment of spinal dural arteriovenous fistulas. SeminCerebrovasc Dis Stroke. 2002;2(3):209–26.
3. Thron A. Vascular anatomy of the spinal cord: radioanatomy as the key to diagnosis and treatment. 2nd ed. Springer; 2016.
4. Nishio A, Ohata K, Takami T, Nishikawa M, Hara M. Atypical spinal dural arteriovenous fistula with supply from the lateral sacral artery. J Clin Neurosci. 2007;14(1):65–8.
5. Takai K. Spinal Arteriovenous Shunts: Angioarchitecture and Historical Changes in Classification. Neurol Med Chir (Tokyo). 2017;57(7):356–65.
6. Cenzato M, Debernardi A, Stefini R, et al. Spinal dural arteriovenous fistulas: outcome and prognostic factors. Neurosurg Focus. 2012;32(5):E11.
7. Sivakumar W, Zada G, Yashar P, Giannotta SL, Teitelbaum G, Larsen DW. Endovascular management of spinal dural arteriovenous fistulas. A review Neurosurg Focus. 2009;26(5):E15.
8. Gross BA, Du R. Spinal pial (type IV) arteriovenous fistulae: a systematic pooled analysis of demographics, hemorrhage risk, and treatment results. Neurosurgery. 2013;73(1):141–51.
9. Endo T, Endo H, Sato K, Matsumoto Y, Tominaga T. Surgical and Endovascular Treatment for Spinal Arteriovenous Malformations. Neurol Med Chir (Tokyo). 2016;56(8):457–64.
10. Zhan PL, Jahromi BS, Kruser TJ, Potts MB. Stereotactic radiosurgery and fractionated radiotherapy for spinal arteriovenous malformations: a systematic review of the literature. J Clin Neurosci. 2019;62:83–7.

Current Concept of Vascular Structures of Spinal Arteriovenous Lesions

3

Kirill Yurievich Orlov and Dmitry S. Kislitsin

Abstract

Understanding of current concepts of spinal arteriovenous lesions strictly depends on understanding of spatial vascular anatomy and visualization of focal vascular structures. Most classifications up to date are based on either topical localization of fistula or arteries that form arteriovenous shunt. Regardless of the implied classification, the major point of discrimination of the pathology is the possibility to treat it weighted against certain possibility to cause neurological symptoms. Hence, understanding of angiographic findings is the most crucial skill that neurovascular specialist should develop. Multiple classification systems are proposed nowadays, but the so-called "combined effort" system is the most widely used one. According to this classification, all spinal AV lesions are divided into the following subgroups: type I, radicular arteriovenous fistulas; type II, glomus AVMs; type III, juvenile AVMs; type IV, perimedullary pial fistulas; and type V, extradural shunts. Type V comprise of heterogeneous group that is slightly out of the scope of this chapter. While established classification system somewhat lacks in risk stratification and decision-making, it is the best tool in the development of understanding of complex pathological anatomy. Despite rapid development of noninvasive imaging techniques, catheter spinal angiography is still the gold standard of spinal vascular lesion visualization. Thus, the most important skill that neurovascular specialist is ought to have is the ability to "read" spinal angiogram, to differentiate normal structures from pathology. This ability comes with a lot of diligence, as spinal angiography is more tricky and tedious than cerebral DSA. Experience in open spinal surgery is also a valuable asset.

Keywords

Spinal arteriovenous malformation · Spinal dural arteriovenous fistula · Spinal pial arteriovenous fistula · Spinal arteriovenous lesion · Spinal vascular pathology

The classification proposed by Di Chiro et al. [1] in 1967 was the first stage in the creation of complex nomenclature of spinal lesions. A lot of attempts to clarify and classify spinal lesions were made later; Borden and colleagues [2] in

K. Y. Orlov (✉)
Federal Center of Brain Research and Neurotechnologies of Federal Medical Biological Agency of Russia, Russian Federation, Moscow, Russia
e-mail: kirill.orlov@rens-russia.org

D. S. Kislitsin
E.N. Meshalkin National Medical Research Center of Ministry of Healthcare of Russia, Russian Federation, Novosibirsk, Russia

X. Lv (ed.), *Endovascular and Neurovascular Surgery for Spinal Vascular Malformations*,
https://doi.org/10.1007/978-981-97-4661-3_3

1995 proposed to stage spinal arteriovenous pathology based on the anatomy of venous drainage, and Bao et al. in 1997 proposed the nomenclature with the greatest emphasis on anatomical relation of the AVMs to the spinal cord [3]. Spetzler and colleagues, in 2002, proposed the most complex classification that would cover almost every single possible spinal lesion [4]. The result of multiple, often unrelated, scientific effort resulted in the appearance of the so-called combined effort classification [5, 6], which includes four types of lesions: radicular sleeve fistulas (type I), intramedullary glomus AVMs (type II), juvenile metameric lesions (type III), and perimedullary AVFs (type IV). There is still a lack of general consensus of definitive classification, and multiple centers propose new models of nomenclature [7], and though "modern" classifications tend to rely more on angiographic findings or allow to stratify risks precisely, for teaching purposes, in this chapter, we are going to stand with the most widespread "combined effort" system.

3.1 Type I

By far, the most common among all spinal AV lesions are radicular arteriovenous fistulas, which account for up to 60–70% of all spinal vascular conditions [8, 9]. It is presumed that the pathology is of acquired nature [10] though precise etiology is still unknown. The most prominent common feature of the lesions in this group is the anatomical relation to the dural root sleeve. The vessel of origin is always a radicular artery with the drainage into the radicular vein. That drainage is not always direct, and pathological vessel net can often be visualized (see Fig. 3.1 as an illustrative case). As most of those lesions are located posteriorly, they are a great subject for microsurgical treatment [11], though the role of endovascular methods gains much more weight with the progress of the techniques [12].

The cornerstone of endovascular embolization, for radicular fistulas, is the ability to visualize radiculomedullary artery (RMA). Those arteries are irregular and of variable origin [13], and thus, neurovascular specialist can only rely on his understanding of local spatial anatomy to discriminate them. The rule of thumb is to never embolize unless one guarantees the patency of RMA.

Although clinically most radicular fistulas appear in adult and elderly patients, the authors of this chapter have had an extremely unusual experience with high-flow thoracic radicular fistula, of highly likely congenital origin, in the 9-year-old child, who manifested with pleural effusion due to distention of the common thoracic duct. See Fig. 3.2 for an illustrative case.

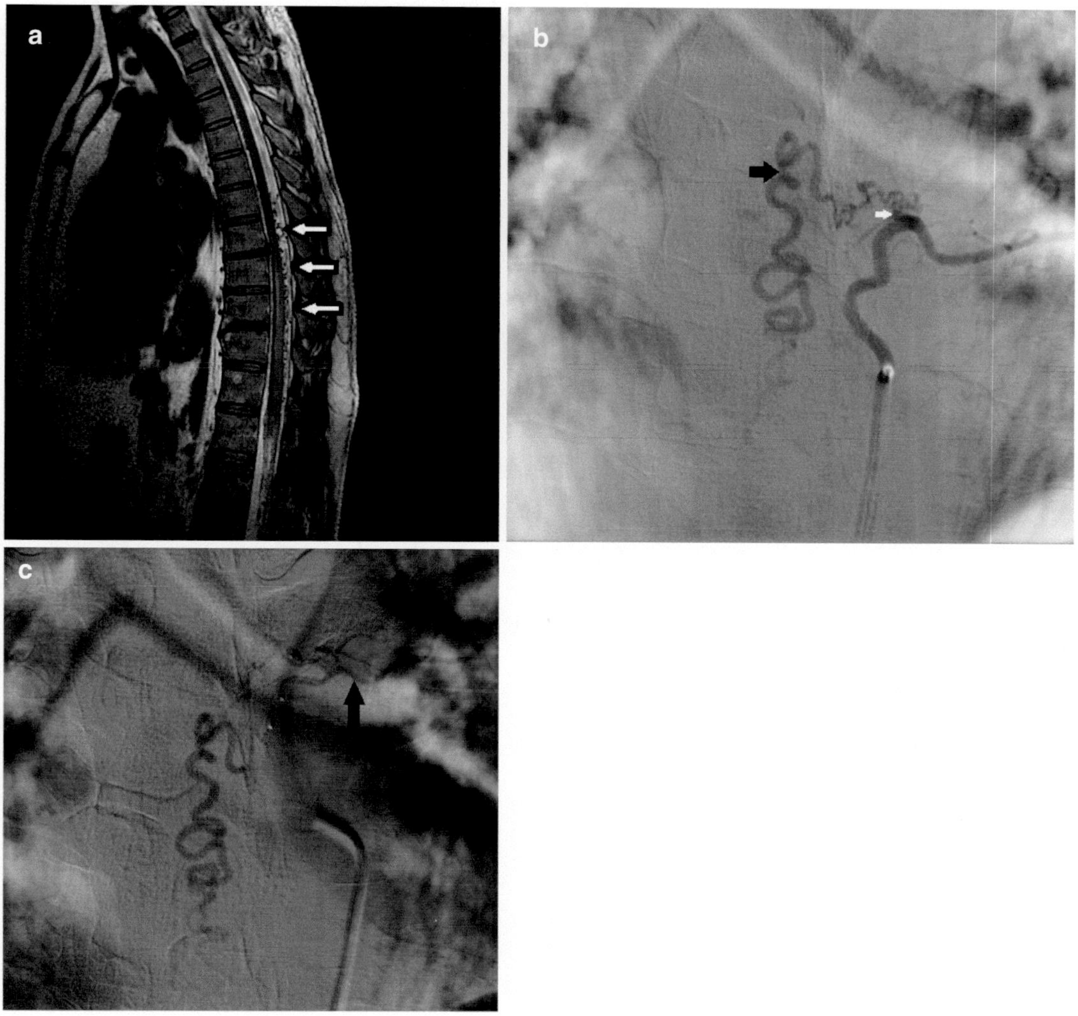

Fig. 3.1 (**a**) Sagittal plane of T2-weighted MRI with typical "flow voids" corresponding to dilated posterior median vein. (**b**) DSA with left thoracic segmental artery injection; radicular artery (white arrow) gives origin to the arteriovenous net inside the radicular sleeve; note the extended and tortuous due to excessive drainage posterior median vein (black arrow). (**c**) Superselective distal injection; reflux of the contrast material shows intercostal branch (black arrow) unseen on previous angiogram

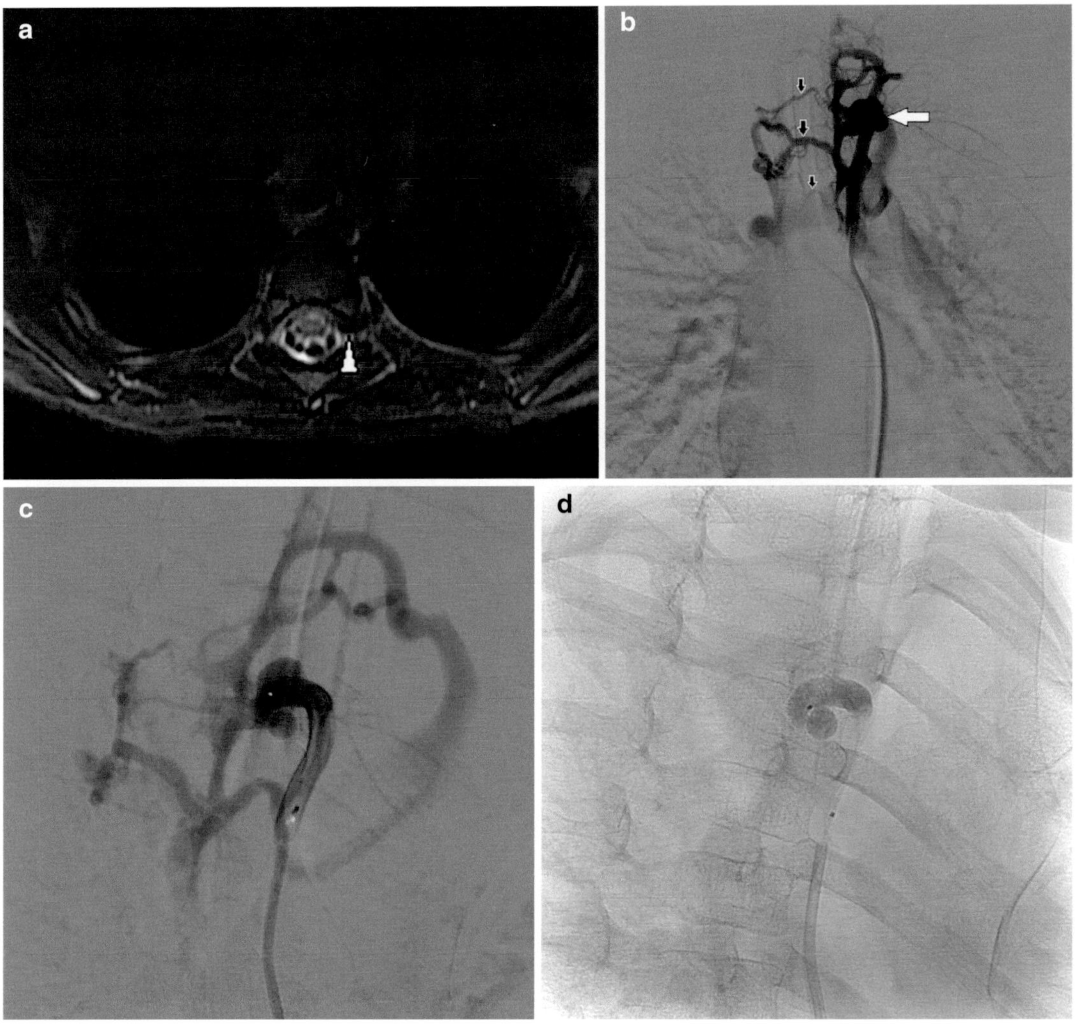

Fig. 3.2 (**a**) Thoracic slice of the T2W MRI of a 9-year-old child reveals significant "flow void" in the region of left radicular sleeve (white arrow). (**b**) DSA with left thoracic segmental injection showing prominent AV shunting between posterior radicular artery and posterior radicular vein with prominent varix (white arrow) at the fusion site. Note the retrograde filling of the coronal veins (black arrows). (**c**) Microcatheter tip is navigated into the fistula. (**d**) LEA cast with complete occlusion of the AV lesion

3.2 Type II

This cohort includes nidus arteriovenous malformations (also known as glomus malformations). The distinctive feature of type II lesions is the presence of intramedullary arteriovenous nidus. Pathophysiology and histological properties in the group are identical to cerebral AVMs (with adjustments for localization and distinct spatial anatomy). Glomus malformations are the second most common spinal AV lesions following radicular DAVFs and account for approximately 30% of cases [3]. Among them, 70% are located in the thoracolumbar region, and 30% are located in the cervical segments, with caudo-medullar AVMs being a different nosological group associated with tethered spinal cord syndrome [14]. In contrast with type I, where clinical presentation is usually related to congestive myelopathy, type II lesions (as well as their cerebral "siblings") often tend to manifest with hemorrhage (the annual rate is estimated to be 4% for previously unruptured AVMs and 10% for those with history of hemorrhages) [15]. However, venous congestion is still a factor in pathogenesis of spinal nidus malformations [16]. Surgical treatment proposedly gains the most radical results [15], while endovascular measures allow to achieve cure in approximately 30% of cases [16, 17]. Needless to say, that constant progress in endovascular materials and techniques should increase the endovascular curability of spinal AVMs, though in contrast with brain AVMs, even the large retrospective cohort studies seem to be impossible due to the relative rarity of the lesions. Radiosurgery, while hasn't been proven as a curative method, is still capable to obliterate some nodes and should be considered as an option for the cases where local anatomy rules out microsurgery or endovascular intervention [18].

Vascular anatomy is the major factor in the technical possibility of complete endovascular obliteration. For thoracolumbar lesions, it is important to recognize major spinal trunks warped by the high-flow anomaly. Decision to embolize should only be made when one can be sure that the anterior or posterior spinal arteries will not be compromised by either propagation of embolic agent or by critical reflux. Not to mention that in comparison with cerebral AVMs, thoracolumbar spine AVMs usually do not have multiple catheterizable feeders, owing to the segmental nature of spinal circulation. See Fig. 3.3 for an illustrative case of thoracolumbar type II AVM.

Cervical region differs from other segments by more "rostral" multiple source inflow, with the involvement of costocervical and thyrocervical trunks and vertebral arteries. Cervical AVMs have more variability in the inflow and outflow, but due to extremely high stakes of the cervical medullar edema, open surgery should probably routinely follow embolization at least in limited decompressive form. See Fig. 3.4 for an example of cervical glomus AVM.

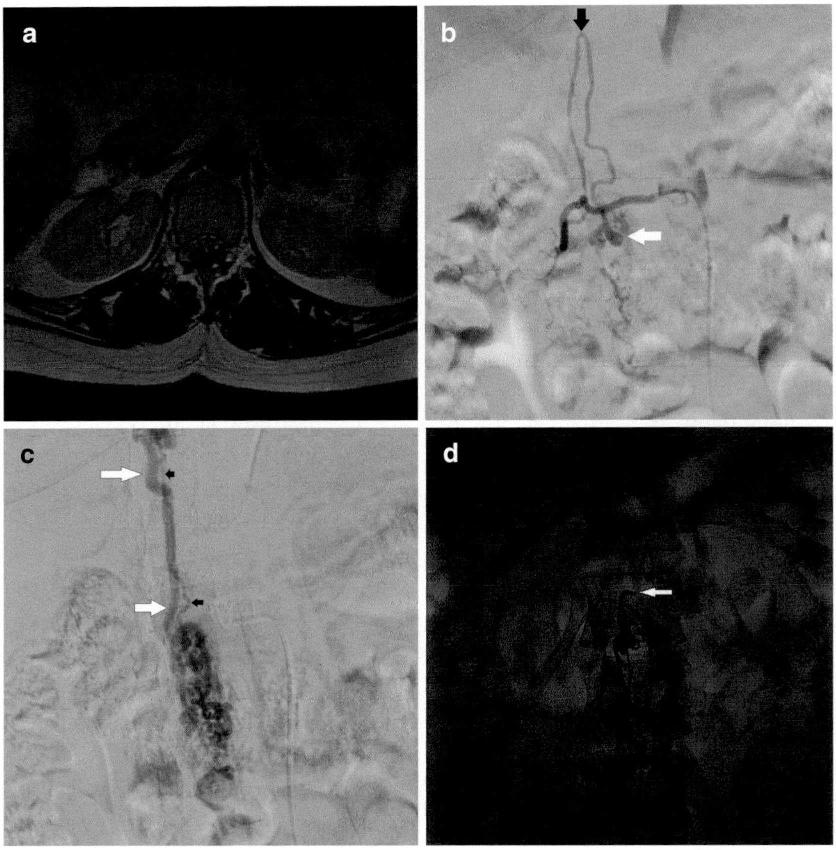

Fig. 3.3 (**a**) Axial plane of T2-weighted MRI with "flow voids" in a pattern of intramedullary lesion. (**b**) Right lumbar segmental artery injection (early phase) reveals intranidal aneurysms (white arrow), which are common in type II lesions. Note the characteristic "hairpin" turn of the radiculomedullary artery (black arrow). (**c**) Late phase shows the AVM nidus, along with the anterior spinal artery (black arrows) and early filling of dilated anterior spinal vein. (**d**) Single-shot fluoroscopy image with EVOH cast. Note that reflux did not propagate further than the point of "sharp turn" of the feeder, to avoid risks of ASA occlusion. The patient, in this case, did not develop additional neurological symptoms

Fig. 3.4 (**a–c**) AP (left) and lateral (right) DSA. Left thyrocervical trunk injection (**a**) showing intramedullary AV nidus at the level of C4 with numerous intranidal aneurysms (white arrows) and distinct venous varices (black arrows) Superselective series confirms the intranidal position of the catheter tip (**b**). LEA cast following complete occlusion (**c**). (**d**) Axial (left) and sagittal (right) planes of the flat-panel scan showing the LEA cast; due to the risk of medullary edema, the patient has been scheduled for decompression surgery immediately following the procedure

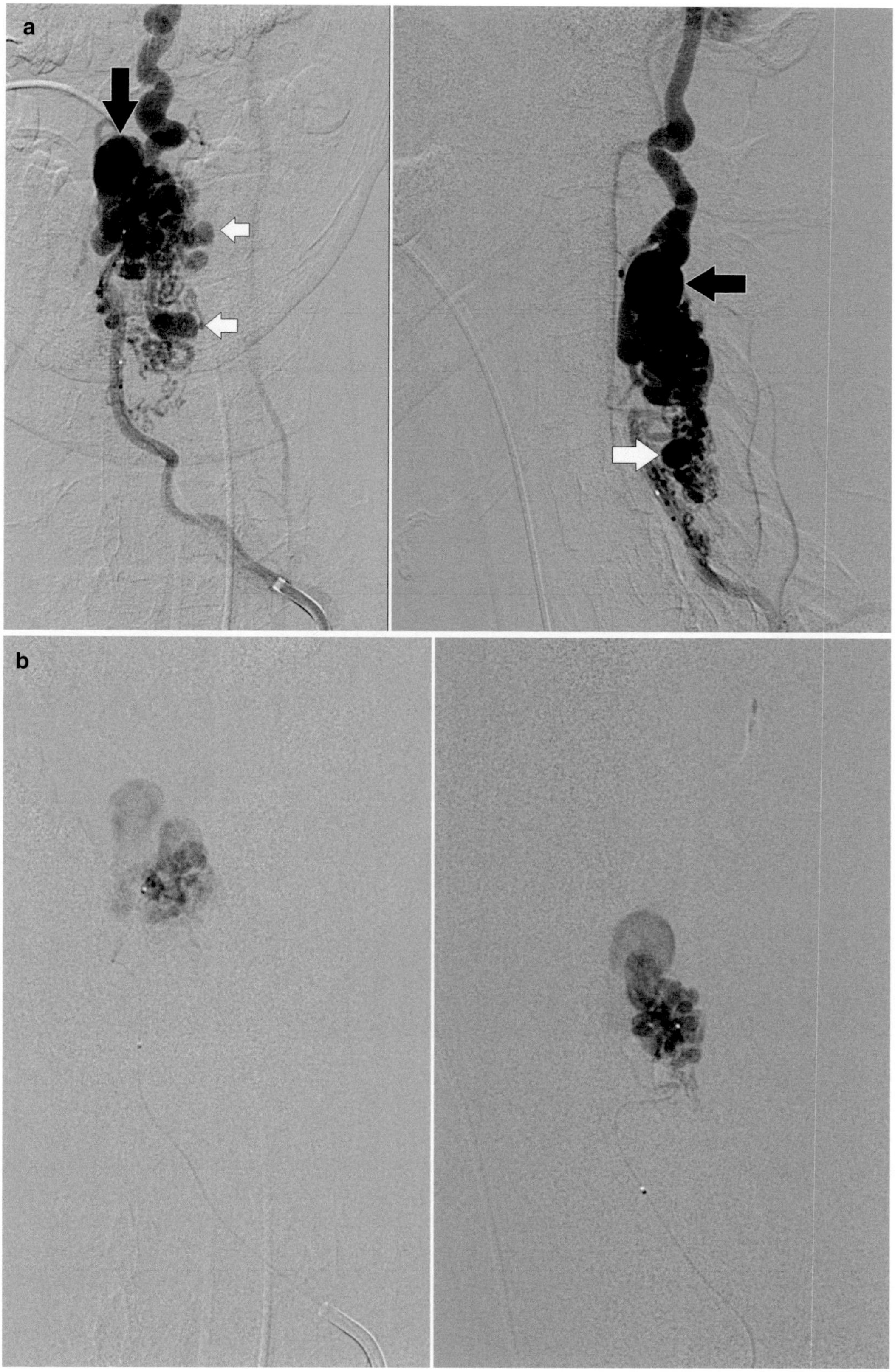
a
b

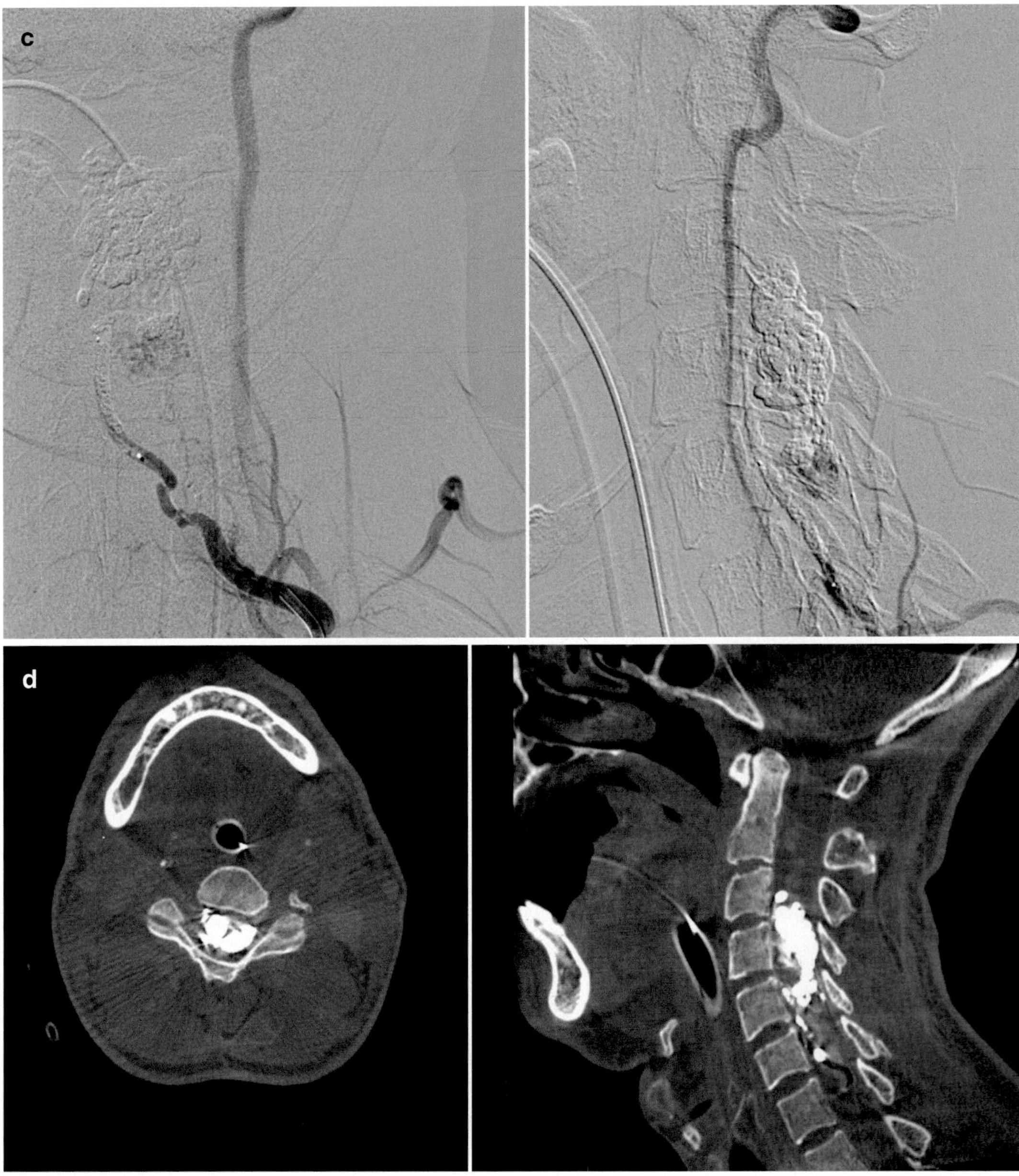

Fig. 3.4 (continued)

3.3 Type III

Juvenile spinal AVM is another distinct nosology that comprises of lesions that involve not only the spinal cord but also most of the tissues (i.e., vertebrae and muscles) in the involved metamere, thus the alternative name "metameric." These lesions are extremely rare and are thought to be of congenital origin [19]. By far the most complex among all spinal vascular lesions, metameric

AVMs require tedious multivessel catheter injections to assert the extent of the disease. While there are scant reports of successful treatment by either endovascular [20] or combined methods [21], the authors of this chapter prefer to use extremely individual approach to treatment with partial embolization of approachable parts that have the highest probability to affect the course of the disease. In Fig. 3.5, we have an illustration of partial embolization for extra-intradural lesion.

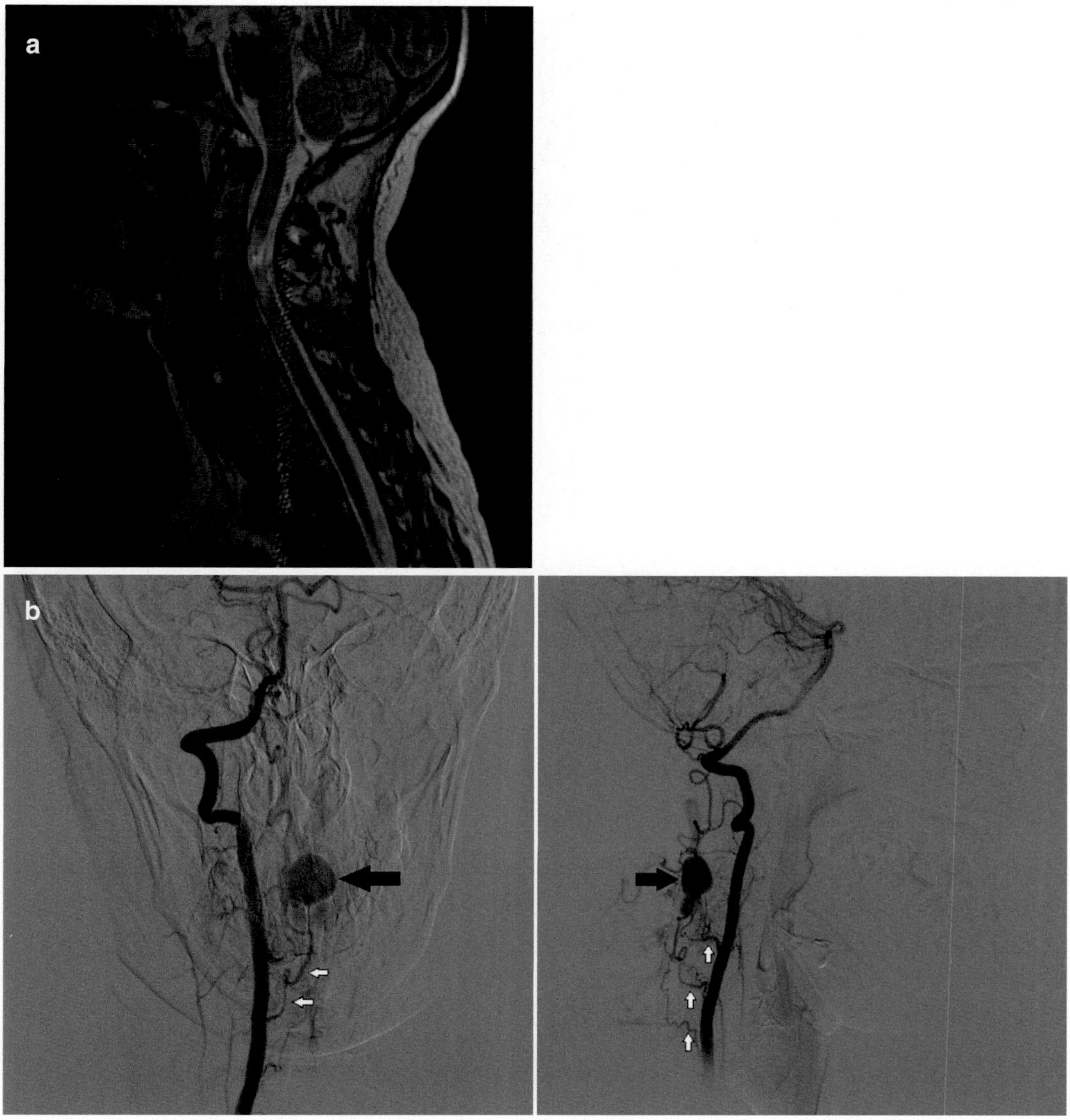

Fig. 3.5 (**a**) T2W MRI of a 13-year-old child with progressive myelopathy reveals type III lesion. (**b–e**) AP (left) and lateral (right) DSA projections. Right vertebral injection (**b**) reveals intramedullary AV shunt with prominent varix (black arrow) fed through muscular branches of vertebral artery (white arrows) with late-phase (**c**) cranial reflux. Left thyrocervical trunk injection (**d**) and right subclavian injection (**e**) reveal multiple soft tissue AV lesions of the posterior neck region. (**f**) Oblique projection shows superselective microcatheter placement for glue embolization, as a preoperative measure, following vertebral injection (**g**) that reveals no residual intramedullary shunt

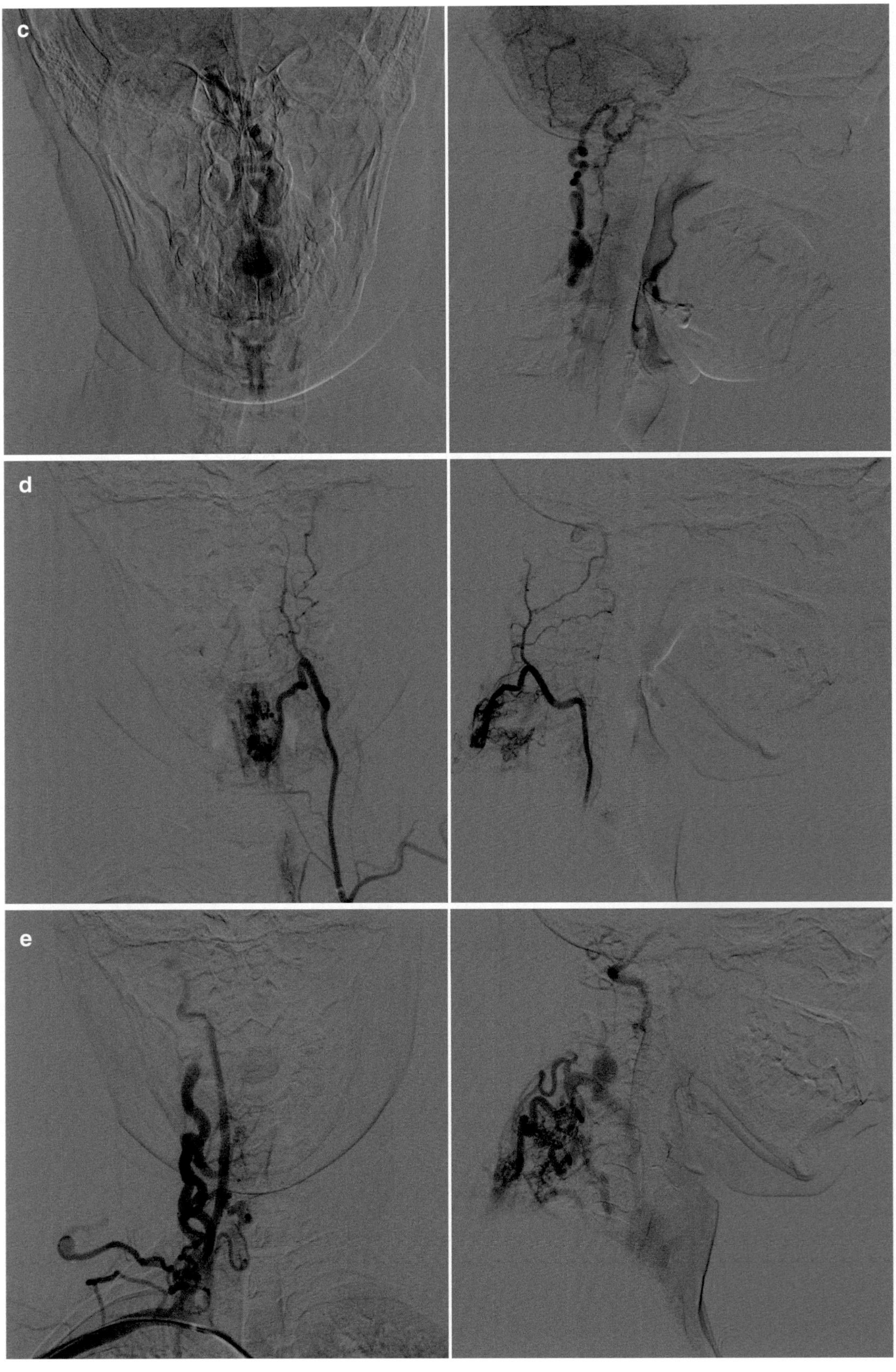

Fig. 3.5 (continued)

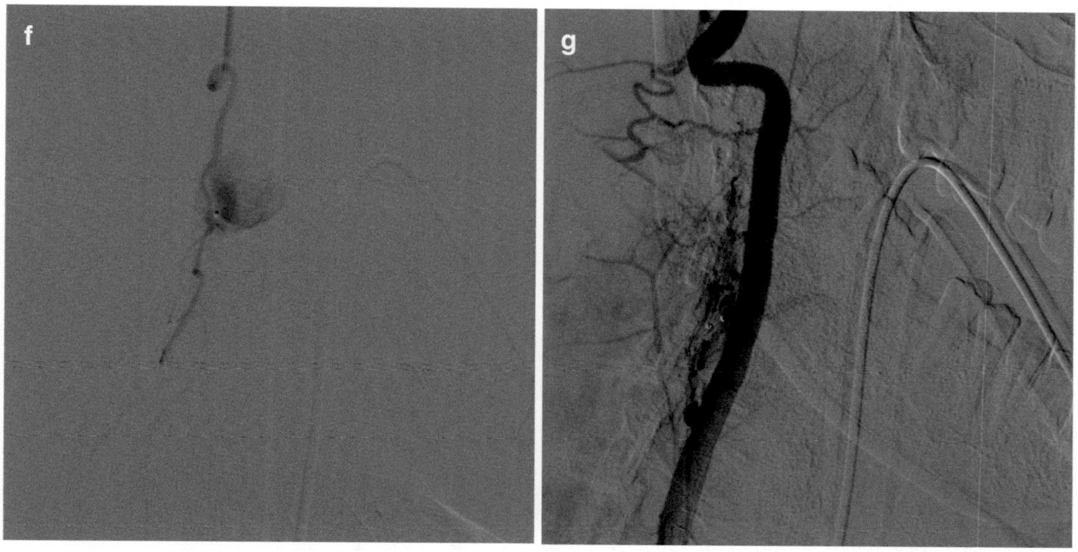

Fig. 3.5 (continued)

3.4 Type IV

The fourth group of spinal cord AV lesions is the perimedullary arteriovenous fistulas. In contrast to type II lesions, those fistulas are restricted to the pial surface and consist of the shunt between the spinal cord artery and coronal venous plexus. Some authors also subdivide the nosocomial group further into three subgroups [4] depending on the inflow and drainage. These lesions are rare and account for approximately 12% of spinal vascular malformations [22]. While most patients present with myeloradiculopathy, there are known cases of spinal subarachnoid hemorrhage related to type IV lesions [23].

Mentioned ABC classification subdivides the pathology as follows:

(a) Solitary ASA supply with ascending venous drainage. Patients from this subgroup are the most obvious candidates for open surgery, due to the difficult (and often impossible) catheterization.
(b) Anterior and posterolateral spinal artery feeders with ascending venous drainage. Embolization as either curative procedure or preoperative measure is the treatment of choice.
(c) Anterior and posterolateral spinal artery feeders with high-speed outflow into dilated segmental veins. Embolization is the most obvious modality and provides high cure rate [23] as a solitary method.

Figures 3.6, 3.7, and 3.8 provide illustrative cases for type IV lesions.

There is also a known group of rare spinal extradural lesions [24], but due to anatomical reasons, they lay beyond the scope of this chapter.

While, technically, embolization of spinal AV lesions does not differ significantly from embolization of cerebral malformations, regardless of the embolic agent, there are several pitfalls of spinal endovascular techniques:

1. Spinal DSA rarely allows visualizing vascular structures as clearly as cerebral DSA does, due to constant movement of the overlying structures as well as the abundance of small angiographic negative vessels.
2. Spinal DSA, in addition to the need of multilevel catheterization, is often tedious and requires not only a decent catheterization technique but also high level of surgical endurance.

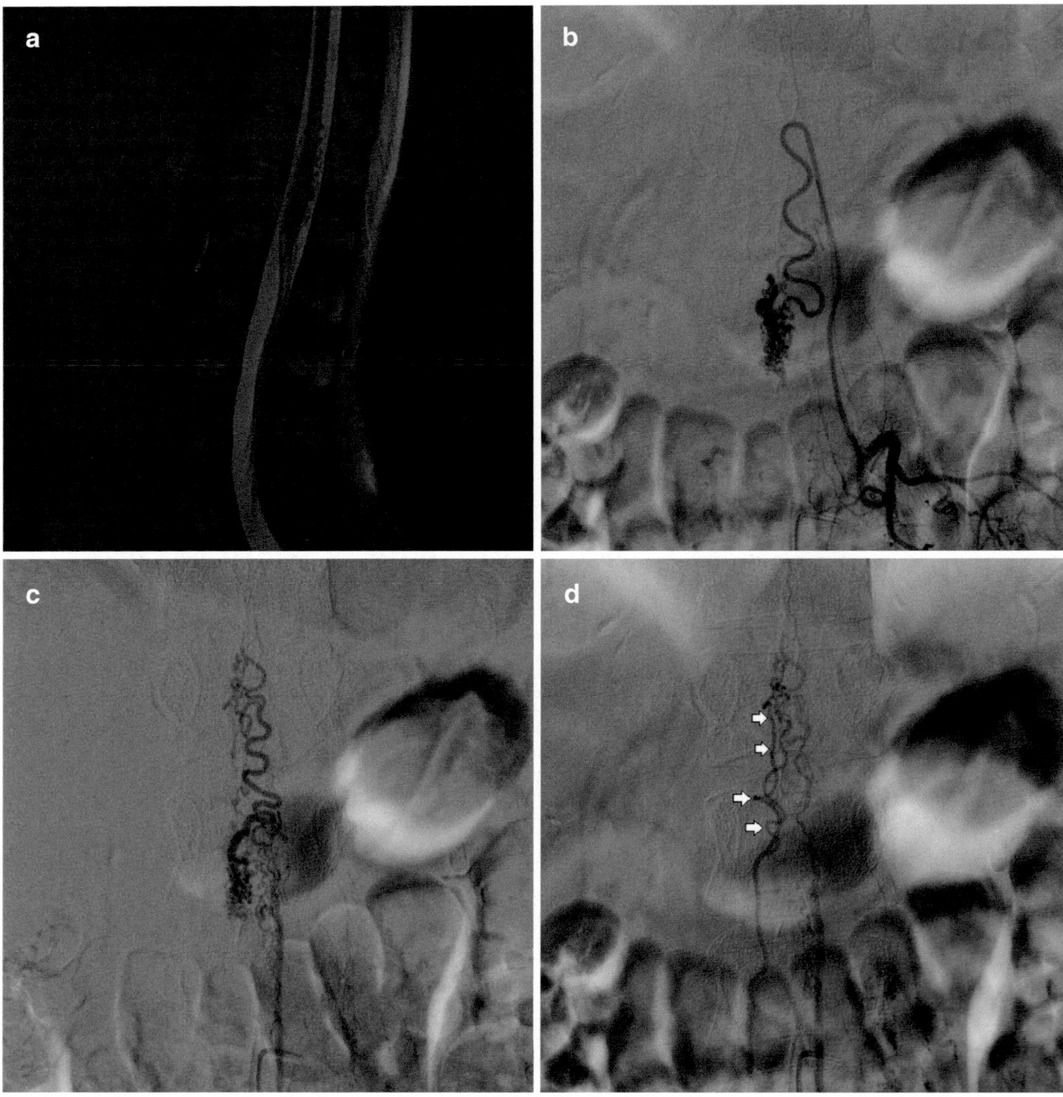

Fig. 3.6 (**a**) Sagittal plane T2W MRI with perimedullary "flow voids". (**b–d**) AP DSA. Left lumbar segmental injection reveals AV net fed through radiculomedullary artery (**b**), and mid-phase (**c**) shows complex venous efferents of perimedullary plexus, while late phase (**d**) shows vicinity of the ASA (arrows) with the nidus. No safe embolization is possible under those circumstances

3. The price of error is often ridiculously high, for example, failure to discriminate radicular artery from radiculomedullary artery will result in dramatic consequences for ambulatory capability of the patient.

Understanding of vascular concepts, spatial vascular anatomy, and, especially, angiographic anatomy of spinal vessels that are or may be involved is the crucial skill for both open vascular and endovascular specialists.

Thus, surgeon must develop good understanding of angiographic nuances of arteriovenous lesions in combination with clear knowledge of spatial vascular anatomy before the start of the career of spinal endovascular surgeon. Authors of this chapter, for example, had a broad experience with endovascular treatment of cerebral lesions

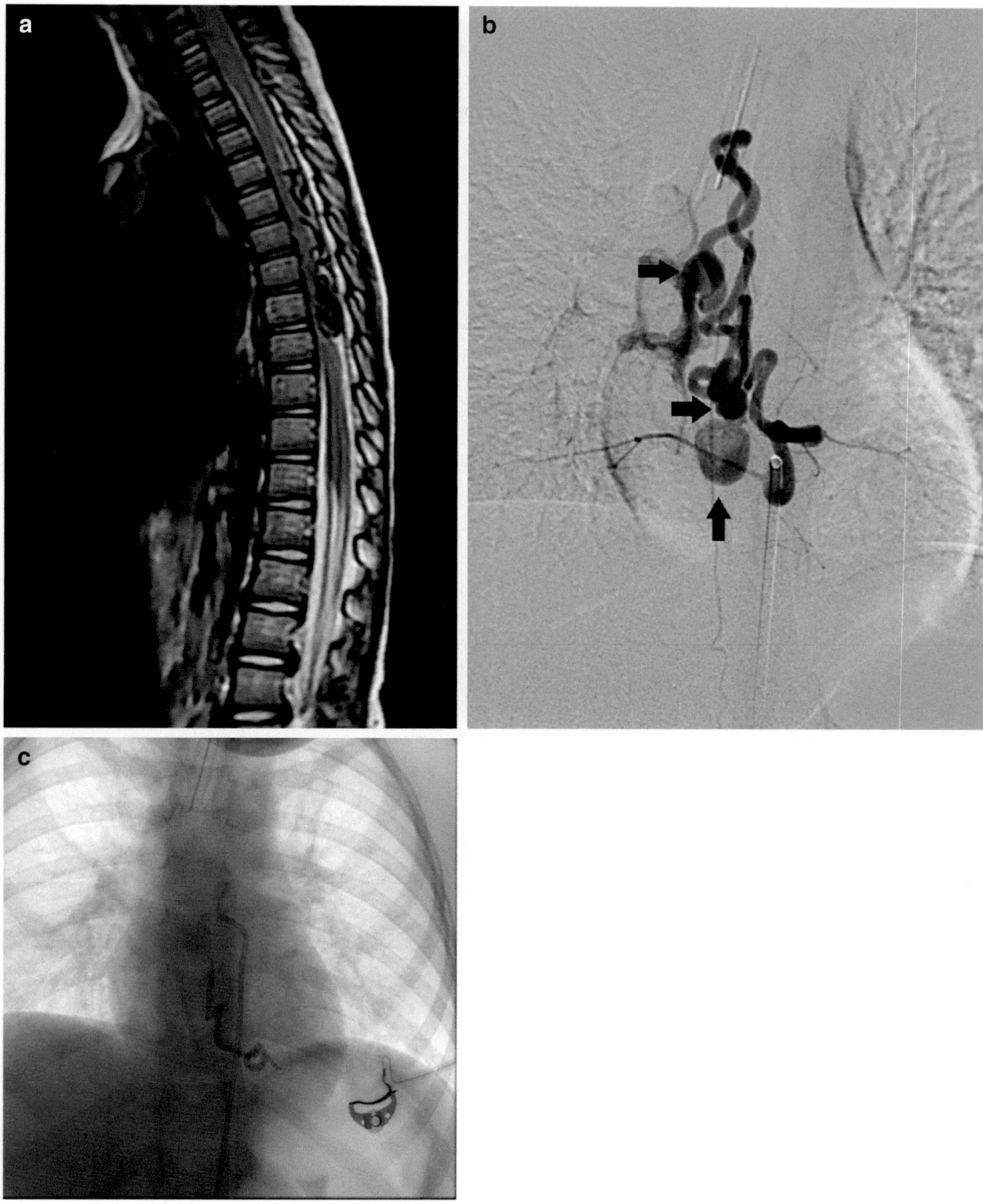

Fig. 3.7 (**a**)Sagittal plane T2W MRI of a 10-year-old child shows perimedullary vascular lesion. (**b**) Thoracic segmental artery injection reveals high-flow fistula with venous varices (black arrows). (**c**) Single-shot fluoroscopic image shows LEA casts propagated up to the venous site through two feeders

prior to their first spinal embolization. In addition, in our opinion, neurosurgeons with some experience in spinal surgery develop the knowledge of corresponding endovascular anatomy with more ease.

Extremely important to perform as many diagnostic spinal angiograms as possible, visual experience of multiple runs at multiple levels with normal and pathological vessels is the most valuable asset in decision-making. This is the

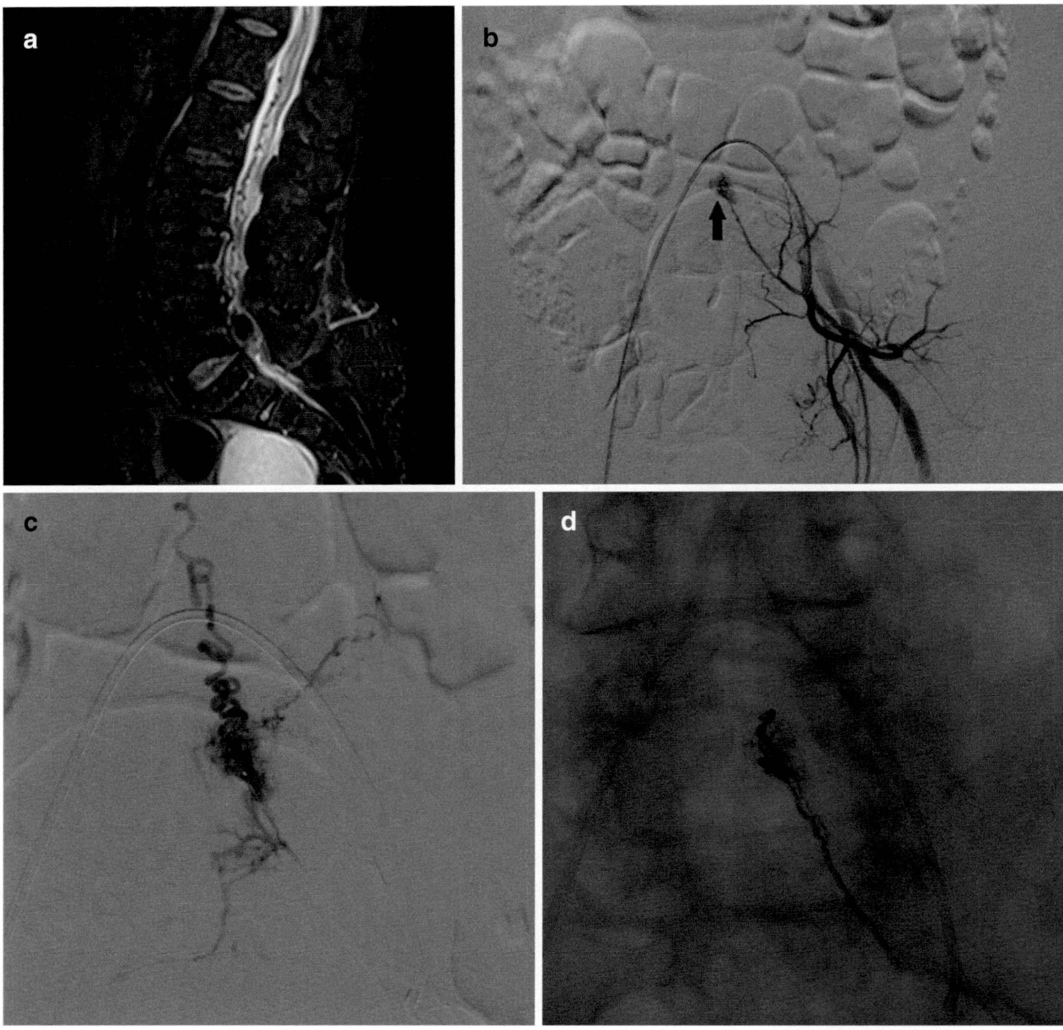

Fig. 3.8 (**a**) Sagittal plane T2W MRI with the "flow voids" at caudo-medullary region. (**b**) Left internal iliac injection reveals vascular net (arrow) supplied by segmental artery. (**c**) Superselective angiogram shows complex venous drainage through the anterior spinal vein and caudal venous plexus. (**d**) Single-shot image with LEA cast completely filling the vascular net

only way to cultivate strict understanding of vascular structures and the ability to discriminate AV lesion into one of the multiple groups, regardless of implied classification.

Overall, even the most common type I lesions are quite rare in clinical practice. Moreover, there are no possible circumstances where the patient with spinal AV lesion could not be transferred between clinics. Thus, the best possible way to build the center with high capabilities in treatment of spinal vascular pathology is to refer the patients from whole region into single center. This is the only possibility to increase the caseload to the volumes sufficient for acquisition of the broad experience.

References

1. Di Chiro G, Doppman J, Ommaya AK. Selective arteriography of arteriovenous aneurysms of spinal cord. Radiology. 1967;88:1065–77.

2. Borden JA, Wu JK, Shucart WA. A proposed classification for spinal and cranial dural arteriovenous fistulous malformations and implications for treatment. J Neurosurg. 1995;82:166–79.
3. Bao YH, Ling F. Classification and therapeutic modalities of spinal vascular malformations in 80 patients. Neurosurgery. 1997;40:75–81.
4. Spetzler RF, Detwiler PW, Riina HA, Porter RW. Modified classification of spinal cord vascular lesions. J Neurosurg. 2002;96:145–56.
5. Zozulya Y, Slin'ko E, Focus IA-Q-N. Undefined spinal arteriovenous malformations: new classification and surgical treatment. Neurosurg Focus. 2006;20(5):E7; thejns.org.
6. LasjauniasP,BerensteinA.SurgicalNeuroangiography: volume 5. Neurosurgery. 2006;34(3):555–6. https://doi.org/10.1227/0006123-199403000-00031.
7. Takai K. Spinal arteriovenous shunts: angioarchitecture and historical changes in classification. Neurol Med Chir (Tokyo). 2017;57:356.
8. Krings T, Geibprasert S. Spinal dural arteriovenous fistulas. AJNR Am J Neuroradiol. 2009;30:639.
9. Jellema K, Tijssen CC, Van GJ. Spinal dural arteriovenous fistulas: a congestive myelopathy that initially mimics a peripheral nerve disorder. Brain. 2006;129:3150–64.
10. Sim SY. Pathophysiology and classification of intracranial and spinal dural AVF. J Cerebrovasc Endovasc Neurosurg. 2022;24:203.
11. Ropper AE, Gross BA, Du R. Surgical treatment of type I spinal dural arteriovenous fistulas. Neurosurg Focus. 2012;32(5):E3. https://doi.org/10.3171/2012.1.FOCUS11344.
12. Koch MJ, Stapleton CJ, Agarwalla PK, Torok C, Shin JH, Coumans JV, Borges LF, Ogilvy CS, Rabinov JD, Patel AB. Open and endovascular treatment of spinal dural arteriovenous fistulas: a 10-year experience. J Neurosurg Spine. 2017;26:519–23.
13. Perez Perez VH, Hernesniemi J, Small JE. Anatomy of the great posterior radiculomedullary artery. AJNR Am J Neuroradiol. 2019;40:2010.
14. Niimi Y, Berenstein A. Endovascular treatment of spinal vascular malformations. Neurosurg Clin N Am. 1999;10:47–71.
15. Gross BA, Du R. Spinal glomus (type II) arteriovenous malformations: a pooled analysis of hemorrhage risk and results of intervention. Neurosurgery. 2013;72:25–32.
16. Kataoka H, Miyamoto S, Nagata I, Ueba T, Hashimoto N. Venous congestion is a major cause of neurological deterioration in spinal arteriovenous malformations. Neurosurgery. 2001;48:1224–30.
17. Corkill RA, Mitsos AP, Molyneux AJ. Embolization of spinal intramedullary arteriovenous malformations using the liquid embolic agent, onyx: a single-center experience in a series of 17 patients. J Neurosurg Spine. 2007;7:478–85.
18. Zhan PL, Jahromi BS, Kruser TJ, Potts MB. Stereotactic radiosurgery and fractionated radiotherapy for spinal arteriovenous malformations—a systematic review of the literature. J Clin Neurosci. 2019;62:83–7.
19. Gross BA, Du R. Spinal juvenile (type III) extradural-intradural arteriovenous malformations: clinical article. J Neurosurg Spine. 2014;20:452–8.
20. Drake B, Patro S, Quateen A, Cora EA, Finitsis S, Sinclair J, Lesiuk H, Iancu D. Metameric spinal AVM: long-term symptomatic relief achieved by embolization of the extradural component. Interv Neuroradiol. 2019;25:469–73.
21. Spetzler RF, Zabramski JM, Flom RA. Management of juvenile spinal AVM's by embolization and operative excision. Case report J Neurosurg. 1989;70:628–32.
22. Rosenblum B, Oldfield EH, Doppman JL, Di Chiro G. Spinal arteriovenous malformations: a comparison of dural arteriovenous fistulas and intradural AVM's in 81 patients. J Neurosurg. 1987;67:795–802.
23. Mourier KL, Gobin YP, George B, Lot G, Merland JJ. Intradural perimedullary arteriovenous fistulae: results of surgical and endovascular treatment in a series of 35 cases. Neurosurgery. 1993;32:885–91.
24. Clarke MJ, Patrick TA, White JB, Cloft HJ, Krauss WE, Lindell EP, Piegras DG. Spinal extradural arteriovenous malformations with parenchymal drainage: venous drainage variability and implications in clinical manifestations. Neurosurg Focus. 2009;26(1):E5. https://doi.org/10.3171/FOC.2009.26.1.E5.

4 Pathophysiology and Classification of Spinal Vascular Malformations

Osama Mahmoud Ramadan
and Mohamed Khallaf

Abstract

Spinal vascular malformations (sVMs), encompassing spinal arteriovenous malformations and fistulas, represent a rare and intricate neurosurgical challenge. Various mechanisms are proposed to elucidate neurological deterioration associated with arteriovenous shunting. These mechanisms include venous hypertension, venous congestion, hemorrhage, vascular steal, or mass effect, which may be exacerbated by the presence of venous varices or aneurysmal dilations. The classification of sVMs depends upon their anatomic location and features. The two widely used classifications are (1) the American/French/English connection and (2) the Spetzler system. Additionally, various classification systems have been delineated throughout the past century.

Keywords

Pathophysiology · Classification · Spinal · Vascular malformations

O. M. Ramadan (✉) · M. Khallaf
Department of Neurosurgery, Faculty of Medicine, Assiut University, Assiut, Egypt
e-mail: oramadan@aun.edu.eg

4.1 Introduction

Spinal arteriovenous malformations (sAVMs) and fistulas (sAVFs) represent about 4% of all intradural spinal cord lesions. Despite their rarity, they are challenging lesions [1]. The first observed spinal vascular lesion was in Germany by Berenbruch in 1890. This lesion was recognized later at autopsy as sVM [2]. About 20 years later, Fedor Krause was considered to be the first to realize a spinal lesion after laminectomy as a vascular lesion. He didn't do any attempt to excise the lesion [3]. Charles Albert Elsberg who was a pioneer in spinal surgery did the first trial to resect a spinal vascular lesion 2 years later. The patient didn't improve on follow-up [4]. In 1926, two French physicians named Foix and Alajouanine described a case of rapid neurological deterioration due to thrombosis of a sAVM, a syndrome termed subacute necrotic myelopathy. This syndrome is named after their name later on [5].

SVMs were considered challenging cases with high rate of morbidity and mortality. However with advent of microsurgical and endovascular techniques, new multimodality treatment protocols have been established that changed the vision to the management of these lesions. Conservative treatment, surgical excision, endovascular embolization and/ or radiosurgery are among the variety of techniques.

X. Lv (ed.), *Endovascular and Neurovascular Surgery for Spinal Vascular Malformations*,
https://doi.org/10.1007/978-981-97-4661-3_4

4.2 Anatomy

Blood vessels originate from the mesoderm during development. As nerve roots begin to form, they bring along a radicular artery on their path toward connecting with the spinal cord. Subsequently, certain radicular arteries undergo enlargement to supply areas beyond their corresponding spinal cord level. Conversely, some arteries undergo spontaneous regression, contributing to the absence of the theoretically expected 31 radicular arteries. This dynamic process of growth and regression shapes the vascular network associated with the developing spinal cord [6].

The frontal two-thirds of the spinal cord receive blood supply from the anterior spinal artery (ASA) (Fig. 4.1). The ASA has its origin in the two branches of the vertebral arteries and follows a course along the anterior medial fissure. Additionally, there are contributions from approximately six to eight segmental radiculomedullary arteries. It's noteworthy that during the embryonic period, there are initially 31 pairs of segmental arteries at each level, but most of them undergo regression over time. Some of the commonly observed segmental radiculomedullary arteries include the C3 artery (also known as the artery of cervical enlargement, originating from the vertebral artery), C6 artery (from the deep cervical artery), C8 artery (from the costocervical trunk), T4/T5, and the artery of Adamkiewicz. The latter typically arises on the left side between the T9 and L2 levels [7].

The posterior one-third of the spinal cord depends on a pair of posterior spinal arteries (PSA). These arteries have their origins in the intradural segment of the vertebral artery or the posterior inferior cerebellar artery. Additionally, they receive contributions from 10 to 23 radiculopial branches [7].

The posterior vascular system is also known as the dorsolateral pial supply or centripetal system. This network emits radial arteries that encircle the spinal cord, forming connections with the ventral system. Moreover, it releases axially oriented perforating branches into the white matter. At the lower part of the spinal cord, the anterior spinal artery (ASA) and posterior spinal artery (PSA) systems interconnect around the conus [8].

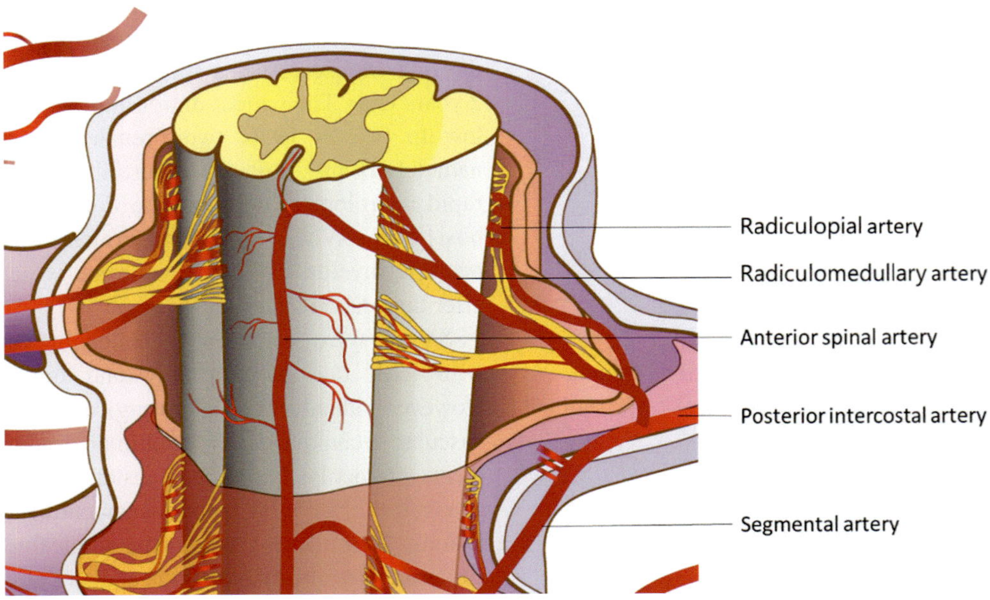

Fig. 4.1 Blood supply of the spinal cord (Courtesy of Dr. Hongyue Ma, M.D., at School of Medicine and School of Clinical Medicine, Tsinghua University, Beijing)

The venous system initiates with a series of radially oriented intrinsic spinal cord veins and small superficial pial veins, leading to the superficial longitudinal median spinal cord veins. Eventually, these veins drain into a network resembling the arterial system, including the anterior and posterior median spinal veins, creating an extensive interconnected network with transmedullary anastomoses [9].

4.3 Pathophysiology

Many theories have been postulated to explain the neurological deterioration associated with sVMs. As with the presence of abnormal arteriovenous shunting, there is a resulting venous hypertension. Many surgeons in the past have documented the presence of elevated venous pressure to reach as 70% as the systemic blood pressure [10].

Venous hypertension is considered as a primary leading cause of neurological deterioration in sVMs. In the latest researches, animal experiments have documented the relation between venous hypertension and myelopathy. There are pathological correlations including glial cell proliferation, neuronal degeneration, hyalinized small blood vessels, and perivascular/intraparenchymal lymphocytic infiltration [11].

Twenty-five percent of patients with sVMs present with rupture of their lesions evidenced by intraparenchymal hemorrhage and subarachnoid hemorrhage, which is considered as another leading cause of neurological deterioration.

Hemorrhage causes its damage through direct and indirect ways: direct way through disruption of fiber tract and indirect way via mass effect. Also, mass effect can be caused by venous varices and aneurysmal dilatation. Generally speaking, sAVM and sAVF produce changes to the normal blood flow and perfusion pressure to the spinal cord through pathological fistulous connections producing what is called vascular steal phenomenon [12].

4.4 Classification of Spinal Vascular Malformation

Many classifications have been suggested to sVM according to the anatomic locations and features. The two major systems or classifications are the American/French/English connection and the Spetzler system. In 1858, Virchow put the first classification system after observing a lesion at autopsy, and he referred to it as a vascular tumor. He divided the lesions into angioma cavernosum or angioma racemosum. Absence of parenchyma between the vascular network is considered angioma cavernosum [13]. Angioma racemosum is subdivided into telangiectasias and arteriale sive venosum or arteriovenous shunts. After that, in 1916, Elsberg has published a new system that included angiomas, aneurysms of the spinal vessels and dilated posterior spinal veins, or hemorrhoids of the spinal cord [4].

Twelve years later, in 1928, Cushing and Bailey proposed a new system excluding hemangioblastomas from sVMs, and a distinct category is assigned to venous angiomas or telangiectasias that progressed to develop an anomalous arteriovenous fistulous classification [14]. Another classification system was described by Bergstrand [15] in 1936 and Wyburn-Mason in 1943, but all these classifications were of little benefits as the vascular spinal anatomy had not been yet fully described [16]. In the 1960s, a series of breakthroughs led to significant strides in comprehending and managing sVMs. This included advancement in the operating microscope and the microsurgical instruments and evolution in interventional radiology with selective spinal angiography and embolization.

Three major centers—including the National Institutes of Health in Bethesda leaded by neuroradiologist John Doppman, the National Hospital for Neurology and Neurosurgery in London in which neurosurgeon Valentine Logue worked with neuroradiologist Brian Kendall, and the Hospital Lariboisière in Paris where the driving force was neuroradiologist René Djindjian—

were included in this system. While the three centers operated autonomously, there was substantial intellectual interchange, and their collaborative efforts significantly contributed to advancements in comprehending the angioarchitecture, pathophysiological mechanisms, and treatment of spinal vascular lesions. This system classified the sVMs into three major types and a fourth subtype. Type I consist of single radicular artery draining into a congested spinal vein on the posterior aspect of the dural sheath, i.e., dural AV fistula. The first description of this type was published by Kendall and Logue in 1977 [17].

In 1995, Borden published a classification system that combined the cranial and spinal dural-based lesions in a single entity oriented toward treatment paradigms. This is a subclassification for type I sVMs, and the researchers refer to it as the arteriovenous fistulous malformations (AVFMs) [18]. Type I lesions refer to lesions that have anterograde flow and drain into Batson's plexus of veins. Type II lesions refer to lesions that drain into retrograde way into spinal perimedullary veins. Type III lesions refer to lesions supplied by meningeal branches from radicular artery and drain into dorsal spinal coronal venous plexus through subarachnoid veins. Lesions having single arterial feeder are classified as subtype (a), while lesions having two arterial feeders or more are classified as subtype (b). In 15–20% of cases, other AVMs may be associated with these lesions, so full angiographic examination of the cranial and spinal levels is recommended.

It is worth to know that spinal dural AVF is slow-flow lesion, while spinal AVMs are considered high-flow lesion with high tendency to rupture and to be presented by hemorrhage and sudden onset of neurological deterioration. As the spinal dural AVFs are slow-flow lesions, they produce their effect through venous congestion and hypertension. On the other hand, spinal AVMs produce their effect via hemorrhage, mass effect, venous hypertension, and vascular steal phenomenon due to the high flow characteristic of these lesions.

A pooled analysis was done by Gross and revealed that the annual hemorrhage rate was 4% before treatment increasing to 10% for sAVMs with previous hemorrhage [19].

In 1997, Niimi and Berenstein classified vascular lesions of the spine into two main categories: spinal vascular lesions and spinal cord vascular lesions. Within spinal vascular lesions, they further divided them into dural and extradural fistulas. In the case of spinal cord vascular lesions, they used the term spinal cord vascular malformations, comprising two types: isolated, encompassing AVMs (arteriovenous malformations) and AVFs (arteriovenous fistulas), and multiple, including metameric and nonmetameric forms [19]. In the same year, Bao and Ling provided a classification for spinal cord vascular lesions, categorizing them into intramedullary AVMs (arteriovenous malformations), intradural AVFs (arteriovenous fistulas), dural AVFs, paravertebral AVMs, and Cobb's syndrome. Within the intramedullary lesions, they identified glomus and juvenile forms. In the case of intradural AVFs, they further subdivided them into types I, II, and III based on their size and degree of blood flow. Paravertebral AVMs involve the paravertebral muscles, as well as the paravertebral and epidural space. Cobb's syndrome encompasses multiple structures within the same metamere [20].

Rosenblum and colleagues delineated two primary types of spinal arteriovenous malformations (AVMs) after studying the arteriogram of 81 patients from the medical records, classifying them based on the location of the vascular nidus: dural versus intradural. Intradural AVMs were further categorized into intramedullary and dural AVFs (arteriovenous fistulas). Intramedullary lesions were then subtyped into glomus (compact) and juvenile (diffuse) AVMs. Dural AVFs were characterized by a supply from a dural artery, with fistulous drainage into spinal veins, at least partially within the cord or pia. In contrast, intramedullary lesions were supplied by medullary arteries, and the arteriovenous shunt was situated partially in the spinal cord or pia mater. Dural AVFs received their supply from a radicular branch along the dural nerve root sleeve, draining through an AVF into the coronal venous plexus. This classification system did not encompass descriptions of extradural-intradural or conus AVMs [21].

4.5 The Spetzler et al. Classification System

From the enriched experience of the pioneer Robert F. Spetzler in treating over 130 spinal cord vascular lesions and after conducting a comprehensive review of the pertinent literature, the author and his colleagues present a refined classification system for spinal cord vascular [22].

Spinal vascular lesions can be divided into three categories: tumors, aneurysms, and arteriovenous lesions. Neovascular lesions include hemangioblastoma and cavernous malformations, both of which are sporadic and familial. The second type is a rare spinal aneurysm. The third type, spinal arteriovenous disease, is divided into arteriovenous fistula (AVF) and arteriovenous malformation (AVM). Arteriovenous fistula is divided into epidural fistula and intradural fistula, and intradural lesions are classified as dorsal or ventral. Arteriovenous malformations can be further divided into extradural-intradural, intradural, and intramedullary malformations and conus medullaris, which is a new category of AVMs. This classification is simplified in Fig. 4.2.

The revised classification system for spinal cord vascular lesions, based on pathophysiology, neuroimaging features, intraoperative observations, and neuroanatomy, renders forth several advantages. Firstly, it encompasses all surgical vascular lesions impacting the spinal cord. Secondly, it aids in treatment decisions by categorizing lesions according to their location and pathophysiology. Lastly, it eliminates the confusion stemming from the multitude of unrelated nomenclatural terms prevalent in the literature.

4.5.1 Extradural sAVFs

Before the Spetzler classification, these lesions are considered to be dural-based lesions (type I). The difference is that these lesions arise from a connection from epidural segment of the radicular artery and an epidural venous plexus. The fistula is located extradural not on the nerve root sleeve as compared with type I lesion. The excess of venous channels in the epidural space makes this lesion tend to present with venous engorgement and mass effect, and so venous hypertension and steal phenomenon are also observed.

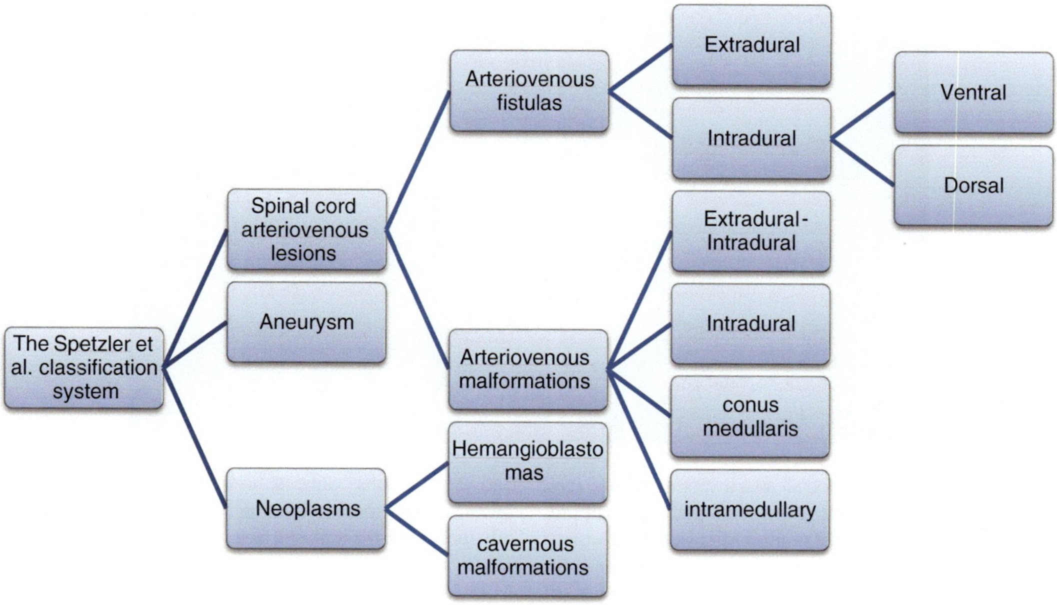

Fig. 4.2 Diagram showing Spetzler classification system of spinal vascular lesion

Further classification of this type was described by Leonardo Rangel-Castilla who published it in 2011. In type A spinal extradural AVFs, the arteriovenous shunting takes place in the epidural space. These types exhibit an intradural draining vein, leading to venous hypertension, spinal cord edema, and the development of myelopathy or cauda equina syndrome. On the other hand, type B1 malformations are limited to the epidural space without any intradural draining vein. This results in compression of the spinal cord and/or nerve roots, leading to myelopathy and/or radiculopathy. Type B2 malformations are also confined to the epidural space, lacking an intradural draining vein and presenting no mass effect, making them asymptomatic [23].

4.5.2 Intradural Dorsal sAVFs

This lesion looks like classic type I to a large extent. This consists of a midline fistula between a radicular artery as it pierces the dural sleeve of a nerve root and a medullary vein (Fig. 4.3).

Trauma or spontaneous thrombosis may cause venous outflow obstruction and subsequent arterialization of the venous plexus, which cause formation of this lesion [24].

4.5.3 Intradural Ventral sAVFs

This type of lesion consists of a fistula between ASA and radicular vein, which directly drain into coronal venous plexus, so with venous hyperten-

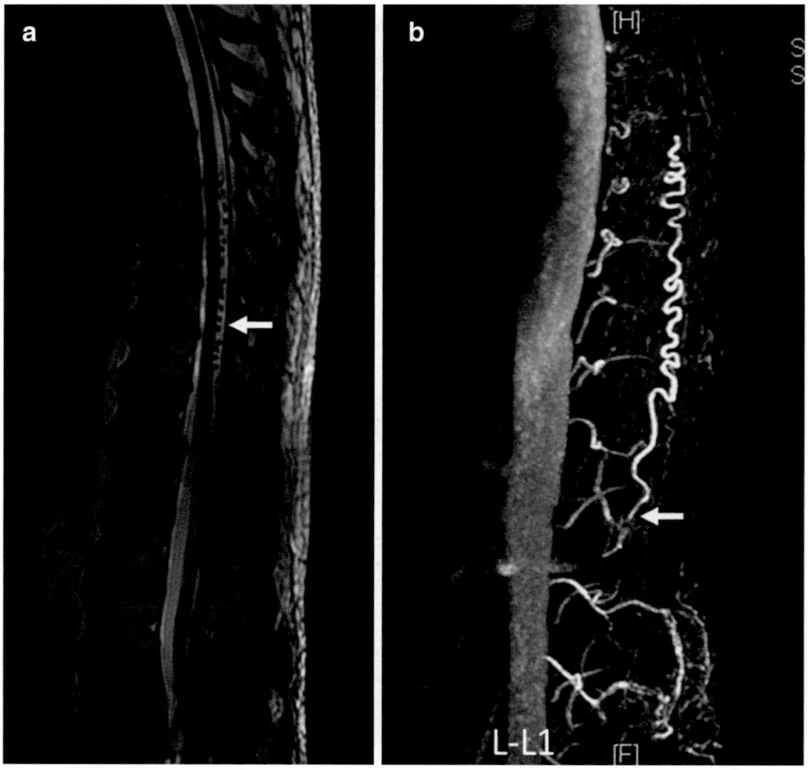

Fig. 4.3 An intradural dorsal arteriovenous fistula (i.e., type I AVM or spinal dural AVF). A 68-year-old man presented with lumbago. (**a**) T2 sagittal MRI showing tortuous vasculature on the dorsal aspect of the spinal cord and signal change within the cord representing edema (arrow). (**b**) On MR angiography, pay attention to the fistula connection between the dural branch of the posterior radicular artery and the radicular vein, as well as the resulting venous plexus congestion and dilation (arrow). The fistula is usually located on the inner surface of the dura mater and laterally at the nerve root sleeve (Courtesy of Dr. Xianli Lv, M.D., Associate Professor, Department of Neurosurgery, Beijing Tsinghua Changgung Hospital, School of Clinical Medicine, Tsinghua University, Beijing, China)

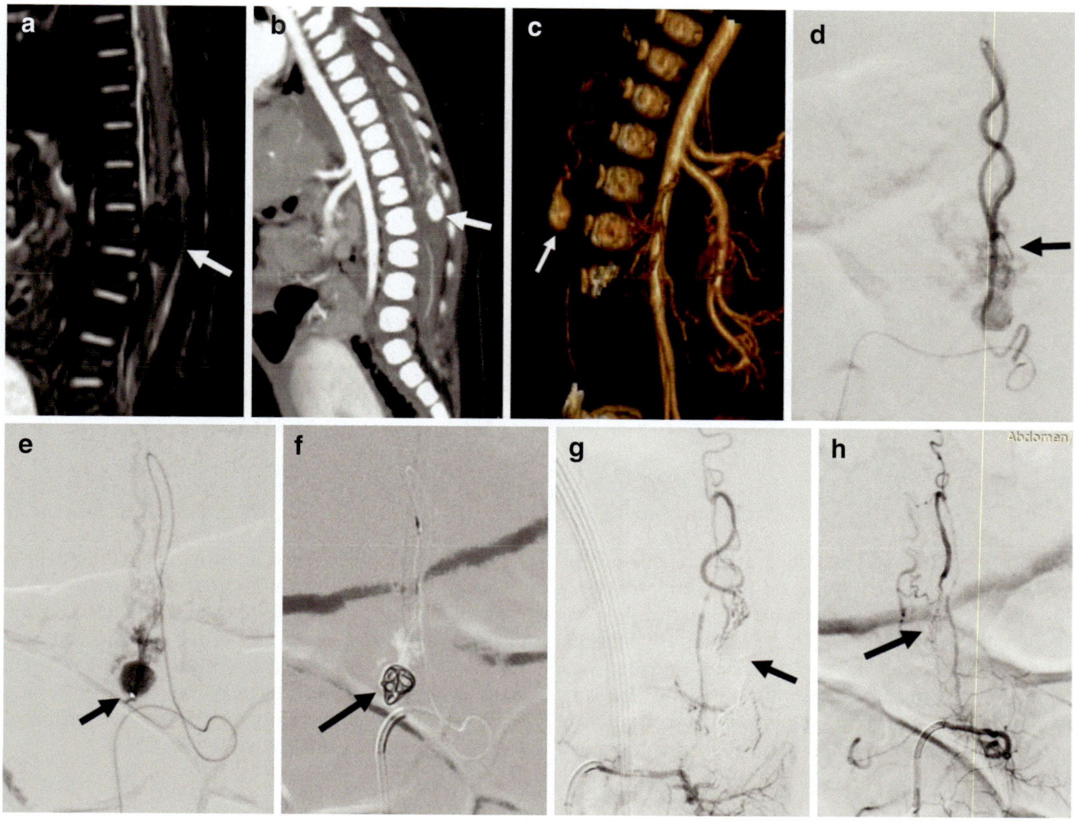

Fig. 4.4 An intradural ventral arteriovenous fistula (i.e., type IV AVM or perimedullary AVF). A 2-month-old male infant presented with constant crying. (**a**) Spinal cord MRI examination, T2-weighted, revealed spinal vascular malformation with bleeding at L2 level (arrow). (**b**) Enhanced CT examination, sagittal view, revealed enhanced vascular lesions around the spinal cord (arrow). (**c**) Enhanced CT reconstruction showed dilated blood vessels (arrow). (**d**) Microcatheter superselective angiography of radial artery at L2 showed a perimedullary arteriovenous fistula (arrow). (**e**) Microcatheter superselective angiography showed the microcatheter reached the aneurysmal dilated draining vein through the posterior radiculomedullary artery (arrow). (**f**) Roadmapping image showed coil embolization of the aneurysmal dilated draining vein and fistula via the microcatheter (arrow). After embolization, the radial artery angiography, lateral (**g**) and anterior (**h**) images, showed complete occlusion of the fistula and disappearance of abnormal venous drainage (arrows). (Courtesy of Dr. Xianli Lv, M.D., Associate Professor, Department of Neurosurgery, Beijing Tsinghua Changgung Hospital, School of Clinical Medicine, Tsinghua University, Beijing, China)

sion, this makes it liable to rupture because of the high-flow fistula (Fig. 4.4).

Thus, venous hypertension, mass effect, and hemorrhage are modes of pathophysiology. Steal phenomenon is observed due to the high flow [25].

4.5.4 Extradural-Intradural sAVMs

They correspond to type III AVMs. Extensive engagement of adjacent structures, such as the skin, muscle, bone, spinal cord, and nerve roots, characterizes these vascular lesions (Fig. 4.5).

In cases where the somite is entirely affected, it is termed Cobb's syndrome. These types of AVMs typically manifest with venous engorgement, mass effect, and arterial steal phenomenon [26].

4.5.5 Intramedullary sAVMs

These correspond to type II AVM, and this type is considered the true spinal AVM. It consists of

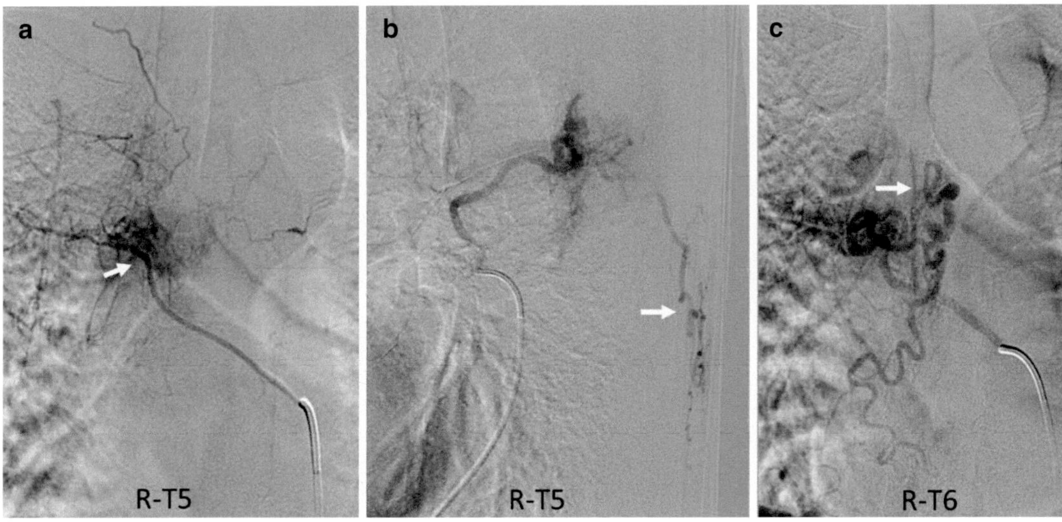

Fig. 4.5 An extradural-intradural arteriovenous malformations (i.e., type III AVM or metameric AVM). A 30-year-old woman presented with pain and weakness in the right lower limb and frequent urination. Pay attention to two different components of the lesion—intradural and epidural—involving the vertebral body and the ventral epidural space. The AP (**a**) and lateral (**b**) projections of selective catheterized of the right T5 segmental artery revealed a large metameric arteriovenous malformation (arrows). The right AP (**c**) projection of the selective catheterized of the right T6 segmental artery showed the enlarged radicular artery associated flow-related and intranidal aneurysms. (Courtesy of Dr. Xianli Lv, M.D., Associate Professor, Department of Neurosurgery, Beijing Tsinghua Changgung Hospital, School of Clinical Medicine, Tsinghua University, Beijing, China)

single or multiple arterial feeders from ASA or PSA with compact nidus and draining into coronal plexus of veins (Fig. 4.6) [24].

4.5.6 Conus Medullaris sAVMs

They are new entity in the classification and were first described by Spetzler in 2002 as a separate type. These spinal arteriovenous malformations (sAVMs) receive contributions from numerous feeders originating from both the anterior spinal artery (ASA) and posterior spinal artery (PSA). The nidus is typically centered around the conus medullaris, resulting in noticeable venous dilatation due to the substantial open space in that region. The pathophysiology of these lesions involves venous hypertension, ischemia, and mass effect, often leading to the occurrence of cauda equine syndrome (Fig. 4.7) [22].

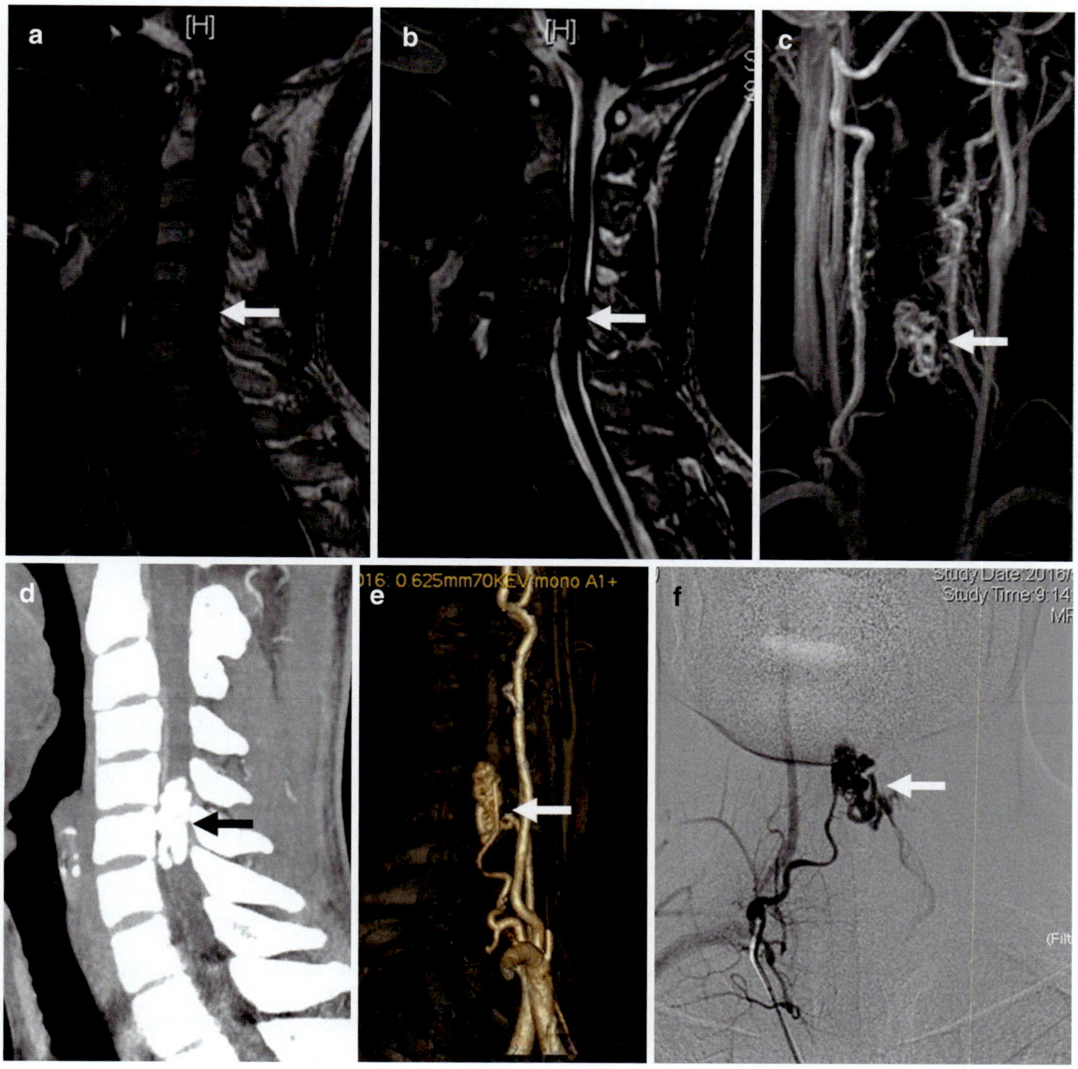

Fig. 4.6 An intramedullary arteriovenous malformation (i.e., type II AVM or glomus AVM). A 37-year-old man presented with neck and shoulder pain. (**a**) T1 sagittal MRI. (**b**) T2 sagittal MRI. (**c**) MR angiography. (**d**) Enhanced CT scanning. (**e**) CT angiography. (**f**) AP projection of the right thyrocervical trunk angiography. The intramedullary tortuous vasculature of the spinal cord and signal change within the cord representing edema (arrows). (Courtesy of Dr. Xianli Lv, M.D., Associate Professor, Department of Neurosurgery, Beijing Tsinghua Changgung Hospital, School of Clinical Medicine, Tsinghua University, Beijing, China)

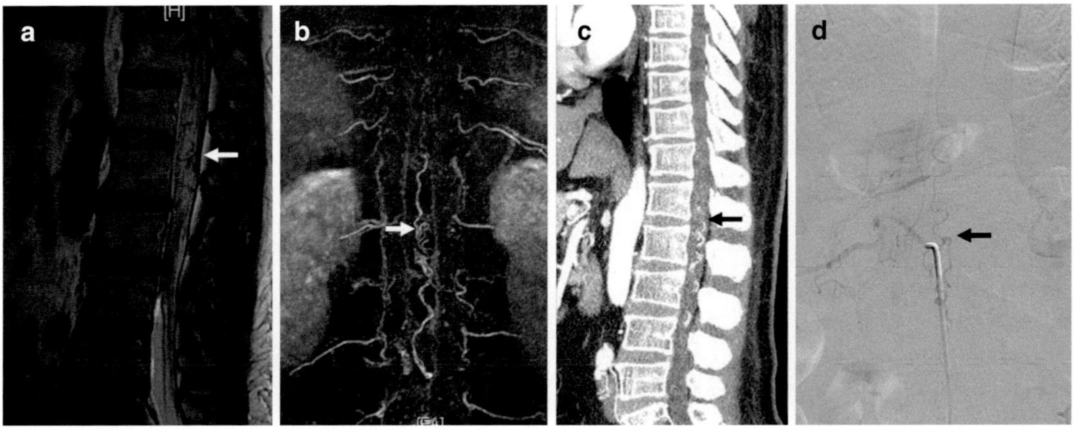

Fig. 4.7 A conus medullaris sAVM (i.e., type IV AVM or perimedullary AVF). A 49-year-old male patient presented with weakness of both lower limbs, difficulty of defecating, and urinary incontinence. (**a**) Spinal cord MRI examination, T2-weighted. (**b**) MR angiography. (**c**) Enhanced CT scanning. (**d**) The right L1 segmental artery angiography, AP projection. Revealed spinal vascular malformation at L1–2 levels (arrows). (Courtesy of Dr. Xianli Lv, M.D., Associate Professor, Department of Neurosurgery, Beijing Tsinghua Changgung Hospital, School of Clinical Medicine, Tsinghua University, Beijing, China)

References

1. Krings T, Mull M, Gilsbach JM, Thron A. Spinal vascular malformations. Eur Radiol. 2005;15:267–78.
2. Berenbruch K. Ein Fall von multiplen Angiolipomen kombiniert mit einem Angiom des Ruckenmark. Medical Faculty Universitat Tubingen; 1890.
3. Krause F. Surgery of the brain and spinal cord: based on personal experiences. Rebman; 1912.
4. Elsberg CA. Diagnosis and treatment of surgical diseases of the spinal cord and its membranes. WB Saunders; 1916.
5. Foix C, Alajounanine T. La my_elite central angiohypertrophique _evolution progressive: Parapl_egie amyotrophique lentement ascendan d'abord spasmodique, puis flasque. Rev Neuro. 1926;2:1–42.
6. Grunwald I, Thron A, Reith W. Spinal angiography: vascular anatomy, technique and indications. Radiologe. 2001;41:961–7.
7. Thron A. Vascular anatomy of the spinal cord: neuroradiological investigations and clinical syndromes. Berlin: Springer; 1988.
8. Romanes GJ. The arterial blood supply of the human spinal cord. Spinal Cord. 1965;2(4):199–207.
9. Ishizaka K, Kudo K, Fujima N, Zaitsu Y, Yazu R, Tha KK, Terae S, Haacke EM, Sasaki M, Shirato H. Detection of normal spinal veins by using susceptibility-weighted imaging. J Magn Reson Imaging. 2010;31(1):32–8.
10. Niimi Y, Berenstein A. Endovascular treatment of spinal vascular malformations. Neurosurg Clin N Am. 1999;10:47–71.
11. Lenck S, Nicholson P, Tymianski R, Hilditch C, Nouet A, Patel K, Krings T, Tymianski M, Radovanovic I, Mendes PV. Spinal and paraspinal arteriovenous lesions: uncovering vascular pathology of the spine. Stroke. 2019;50(8):2259–69.
12. Patchana T, Savla P, Taka TM, Ghanchi H, Wiginton J 4th, Schiraldi M, Cortez V. Spinal arteriovenous malformation: case report and review of the literature. Cureus. 2020;12(11):e11614. https://doi.org/10.7759/cureus.11614.
13. Virchow R. Die Krankhaften Geschwulste. Berlin: Hirschwald; 1864.
14. Cushing H, Bailey P. Tumors arising from the blood vessels of the brain: angiomatous malformations and hemangioblastomas. CC Thomas; 1928.
15. Bergstrand H, Olivecrona H, Tönnis W. Gefässmissbildungen und gefässgeschwülste des gehirns. In: Gefässmissbildungen und gefässgeschwülste des gehirns; 1936. p. 181.
16. Wyburn-Mason R. The vascular abnormalities and tumours of the spinal cord and its membranes. H. Kimpton; 1943.
17. Kendall BE, Logue V. Spinal epidural angiomatous malformations draining into intrathecal veins. Neuroradiology. 1977;13:181–9.
18. Borden JA, Wu JK, Shucart WA. A proposed classification for spinal and cranial dural arteriovenous fistulous malformations and implications for treatment. J Neurosurg. 1995;82(2):166–79.
19. Gross BA, Du R. Spinal glomus (type II) arteriovenous malformations: a pooled analysis of hemorrhage risk and results of intervention. Neurosurgery. 2013;72(1):25–32.

20. Bao YH, Ling F. Classification and therapeutic modalities of spinal vascular malformations in 80 patients. Neurosurgery. 1997;40(1):75–81. https://doi.org/10.1097/00006123-199701000-00017.
21. Rosenblum B, Oldfield EH, Doppman JL, Di Chiro G. Spinal arteriovenous malformations: a comparison of dural arteriovenous fistulas and intradural AVM's in 81 patients. J Neurosurg. 1987;67(6):795–802.
22. Spetzler RF, Detwiler PW, Riina HA, Porter RW. Modified classification of spinal cord vascular lesions. J Neurosurg. 2002;96(2 Suppl):145–56. https://doi.org/10.3171/spi.2002.96.2.0145.
23. Rangel-Castilla L, Holman PJ, Krishna C, Trask TW, Klucznik RP, Diaz OM. Spinal extradural arteriovenous fistulas: a clinical and radiological description of different types and their novel treatment with Onyx. J Neurosurg Spine. 2011;15(5):541–9.
24. Kim LJ, Spetzler RF. Classification and surgical management of spinal arteriovenous lesions: arteriovenous fistulae and arteriovenous malformations. Neurosurgery. 2006;59(5):S3–195.
25. Rangel-Castilla L, Russin JJ, Zaidi HA, Martinez-del-Campo E, Park MS, Albuquerque FC, McDougall CG, Nakaji P, Spetzler RF. Contemporary management of spinal AVFs and AVMs: lessons learned from 110 cases. Neurosurg Focus. 2014;37(3):E14.
26. Xu DS, Sun H, Spetzler RF. Spinal arteriovenous malformations: surgical management. Handb Clin Neurol. 2017;143:153–60.

Pathophysiology of Spinal Vascular Malformations

5

Kevin Abel Sene and Xianli Lv

Abstract

Spinal vascular malformations (SVMs) are diverse anomalies characterized by abnormal blood vessel formations in the spinal cord. Understanding the pathophysiology of these malformations is essential for accurate diagnosis, targeted treatment, and improved patient outcomes. SVMs are a rare, but potentially devastating, group of abnormalities affecting the delicate network of blood vessels around the spinal cord. These tangled knots of arteries and veins disrupt the normal flow of blood, posing a significant threat to neurological function. SVMs encompass a spectrum of types, each with its unique characteristics and clinical implications. They are classified into arteriovenous malformations (AVMs), cavernous malformations (CMs), and dural arteriovenous fistulas (DAVFs), each with distinct pathophysiological features. AVMs are characterized by direct connections between arterial and venous vessels, bypassing the normal capillary network. This abnormal vascular connection leads to high-flow arterialized venous drainage, resulting in venous hypertension, vessel rupture, and subsequent hemorrhage. The pathogenesis of AVMs involves genetic factors, aberrant angiogenesis, and impaired vascular development. DAVFs are abnormal connections between arteries and veins within the dural covering of the brain or spinal cord. DAVFs are characterized by the presence of an abnormal direct connection between dural arteries and venous structures, bypassing the normal capillary network. This arteriovenous shunt leads to increased blood flow and pressure within the venous system, causing venous congestion and subsequent hemodynamic changes. While the exact mechanisms underlying SVMs remain incompletely understood, recent advances in molecular genetics and imaging techniques have shed light on the underlying pathophysiological processes. Studies have identified several oncogenic signaling pathways, angiogenic factors, and gene mutations implicated in SVM development and progression.

Understanding the pathophysiology of SVMs enables clinicians to make accurate diagnoses and select appropriate therapeutic strategies. Imaging modalities such as magnetic resonance imaging (MRI), computed tomography angiography (CTA), and digital subtraction angiography (DSA) aid in visualizing the vascular abnormalities and guide

K. A. Sene
International Department, Chifeng University Affiliated Hospital, Chifeng University, Chifeng, Inner Mongolia, China

X. Lv (✉)
Department of Neurosurgery, Beijing Tsinghua Changgung Hospital, School of Clinical Medicine, Tsinghua University, Beijing, China

X. Lv (ed.), *Endovascular and Neurovascular Surgery for Spinal Vascular Malformations*,
https://doi.org/10.1007/978-981-97-4661-3_5

treatment planning. SVMs encompass a spectrum of vascular malformation pathologies within the spinal cord. Advancements in understanding the underlying pathophysiology have improved the diagnosis, management, and treatment of these conditions. Further research is needed to elucidate the genetic and molecular mechanisms driving SVM development, with the ultimate goal of developing targeted therapies and improving patient outcomes.

Keywords

Spinal vascular malformation · Arteriovenous malformation · Dural arteriovenous fistula · Perimedullary arteriovenous fistula · Juvenile arteriovenous malformation

5.1 Introduction

Spinal vascular malformations (SVMs) are a diverse group of abnormalities involving the blood vessels within or around the spinal cord. These anomalies can disrupt the normal blood flow and often lead to a range of neurological symptoms and complications. SVMs can be categorized into three main types: arteriovenous malformations (AVMs), cavernous malformations (CMs), and dural arteriovenous fistulas (DAVFs). The exact causes of SVMs are often unclear, and they may occur sporadically or be associated with genetic or hereditary conditions. Certain risk factors, such as trauma, radiation exposure, or prior spinal surgeries, have been implicated in the development or progression of SVMs. Additionally, some SVMs may be present at birth (congenital) or develop over time (acquired). Clinical presentation of SVMs can vary widely depending on the location, size, and type of the malformation. Common symptoms include back or neck pain, weakness, sensory disturbances, difficulty walking, and bowel or bladder dysfunction. Severe cases may lead to paralysis or even life-threatening complications, such as intramedullary hemorrhage or spinal cord infarction.

5.2 Spinal Vascular Malformation Classification

Spinal vascular malformations can be classified into several types based on their anatomical and hemodynamic characteristics. Here is a detailed breakdown of the different types:

Type I: Dural arteriovenous fistula (DAVF).

Type II: Glomerular spinal AVMs (nidal AVMs).

Type III: Juvenile AVM.

Type IV: Intradural perimedullary AVF.

Each type of spinal vascular malformation has distinct characteristics and requires specific diagnostic and treatment approaches. It is important to accurately classify the malformation to guide appropriate management decisions. It is worth noting that the classification system provided here is a general framework and may be subject to updates and refinements as new research and clinical evidence emerge.

5.3 Type I: Dural Arteriovenous Fistula (DAVF)

Spinal dural arteriovenous fistulas (DAVFs) are abnormal connections between arteries and veins within the dura mater of the spinal cord. The spinal DAVF is located on the dural sheath of the spinal nerve root, where the radicular meningeal artery lies in close proximity to the radicular vein (Fig. 5.1). The pathophysiology of DAVFs involves various key mechanisms that contribute to the clinical manifestations and complications associated with this condition. The exact cause of spinal DAVFs is not yet fully understood. DAVFs may originate from congenital factors such as an abnormal embryonic development of the blood vessels in the spinal cord's protective covering, known as the dura mater. This abnormal development could result in the formation of

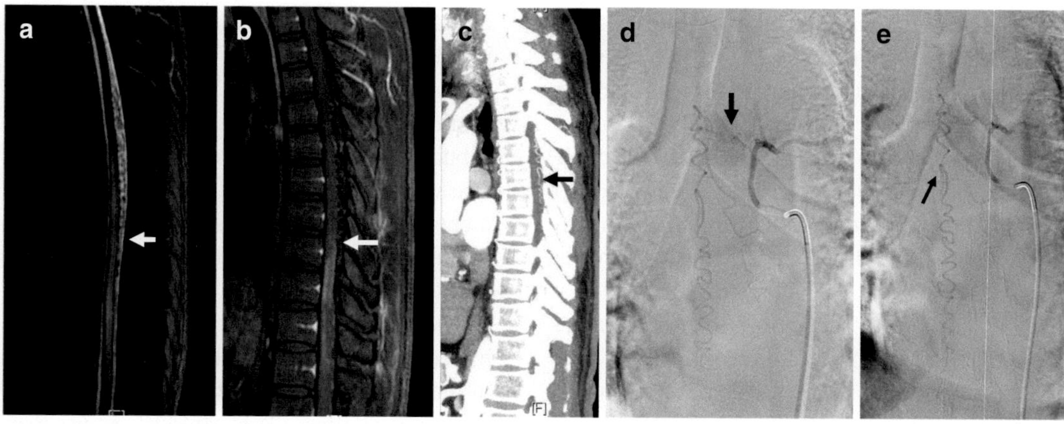

Fig. 5.1 A 57-year-old male patient presented with weakness, numbness in both lower limbs, and weakness of urination. (**a**) Spinal MRI examination revealed a flow void signal on the dorsal side of the thoracic spinal cord accompanied by parenchymal edema of the spinal cord (arrow). (**b**) Enhanced spinal MRI examination showed enhanced dorsal blood vessels in the thoracic spinal cord and thoracic spinal cord edema (arrow). (**c**) Enhanced CT scanning showed enhanced blood vessels on the dorsal side of the spinal cord (arrow). (**d**) Left T5 segmental artery angiography, early arterial phase, showed the left T4 level dural arteriovenous fistula, with the arteriovenous shunt located in the left T4 intervertebral foramen and supplied by the radiomeningeal artery (arrow). (**e**) Left T5 segmental artery angiography, late arterial phase, showed venous drainage from the left T4 level dural arteriovenous fistula to the surface of the spinal cord, with significantly dilated drainage veins (arrow)

abnormal connections between arteries and veins. DAVFs are more commonly observed in older individuals, suggesting that age-related changes in blood vessels may contribute to their development. Over time, the walls of blood vessels can weaken, potentially leading to the formation of abnormal connections. Trauma to the spinal cord or surrounding structures may contribute to the formation of DAVFs. In some cases, the trauma may damage blood vessels and disrupt their normal structure, leading to the development of abnormal connections. Inflammatory conditions affecting the spinal cord or the dura mater may promote the development of DAVFs. Inflammation can cause changes to blood vessel walls, making them more prone to abnormal connections. Degenerative changes in the spinal cord or the dura mater, such as degenerative disc disease or spinal stenosis, may facilitate the development of DAVFs. These changes can alter the blood flow dynamics and increase the risk of abnormal connections forming. It is important to note that while these factors are believed to be associated with the development of DAVFs, they do not explain every case. DAVFs can occur sporadically without a clear cause or predisposing factors. Further research is needed to fully understand the underlying mechanisms and causes of DAVFs. This specific spinal vascular malformation results in the development of several conditions.

5.3.1 Pathophysiology

The abnormal connection bypasses the capillary network, causing high-pressure flow in the dural veins and downstream cortical veins. This can lead to:

- *Venous congestion* [1, 2]: Distention of veins compresses neighboring structures like the brain and nerves, causing headaches, seizures, and neurological deficits.
- *Steal phenomenon*: High-pressure veins compete with smaller arterioles for blood flow, potentially depriving the brain of sufficient oxygen and nutrients, leading to ischemia (reduced blood supply) and neurological symptoms.

- *Edema and cerebral dysfunction*: Venous congestion and ischemia can cause fluid accumulation in the brain (edema) and impaired brain function.
- *Hemorrhage* [2]: The fragile nature of dural veins and fistulous connections can lead to spontaneous bleeding within the brain or into the subarachnoid space [2], causing strokes and other serious complications.
- *Thrombosis and ischemia*: In some cases, blood clots can form within the fistulous connections, leading to downstream ischemia and further neurological damage.

The abnormal shunting in SDAVFs leads to venous stasis and hypertension within the affected area. The increased venous pressure can cause dilation and engorgement of the veins. This venous congestion can further impair normal venous drainage from the spinal cord, leading to increased pressure within the spinal cord veins.

- *Arteriovenous shunting* [1, 2]: The abnormal connections, known as fistulas, allow high-pressure arterial blood to flow directly into the low-pressure venous system, bypassing the normal capillary network. This leads to the direct entry of arterial blood into the veins, causing an increase in venous pressure.
- *Venous congestion* [1, 2]: The direct flow of high-pressure arterial blood into the veins results in venous congestion within the affected spinal cord segments. The increased blood volume and pressure in the veins cause them to become engorged and dilated.
- *Compromised venous drainage* [1]: The venous congestion in SDAVFs impairs the normal venous drainage from the spinal cord. The abnormal connections within the dura mater disrupt the usual venous pathways, leading to a reduced ability for blood to flow out of the spinal cord adequately.
- *Pressure gradient imbalance*: The abnormal shunting of arterial blood into the venous system upsets the pressure gradient within the venous circulation of the spinal cord. The increased inflow of arterial blood and reduced outflow result in an imbalance, leading to elevated venous pressure.
- *Venous hypertension* [1, 2]: The venous congestion [1] and compromised drainage contribute to venous hypertension in SDAVFs. The veins within the affected spinal cord segments experience increased pressure due to the abnormal shunting and impaired venous outflow.
- *Vascular remodeling*: Prolonged venous hypertension [2] can lead to structural changes in the blood vessels, a process known as vascular remodeling. The affected veins may undergo dilation, tortuosity, and thickening as a response to the increased pressure.

The venous congestion and increased pressure within the spinal cord veins can compromise the blood supply to the spinal cord tissue. This can result in ischemia and hypoxia, leading to neuronal dysfunction and damage.

5.4 Type II: Glomerular Spinal AVMs (Nidal AVMs)

Glomerular spinal AVMs are typically congenital in nature, meaning they are present at birth, although symptoms may not manifest until later in life (Fig. 5.2). These malformations involve abnormal tangles of blood vessels within the spinal cord, disrupting the normal blood flow and causing a range of neurological problems [3]. The cause of glomerular spinal AVMs is believed to be related to abnormal development of blood vessels during fetal development. Genetic factors may also play a role in some cases. The severity of symptoms can range from mild to severe, and early diagnosis is crucial for optimal management.

5.4.1 Pathophysiology

Glomerular spinal AVMs (nidal AVMs) are a specific type of spinal cord vascular malformation characterized by their intricate, tangled network of abnormal blood vessels within the spinal cord.

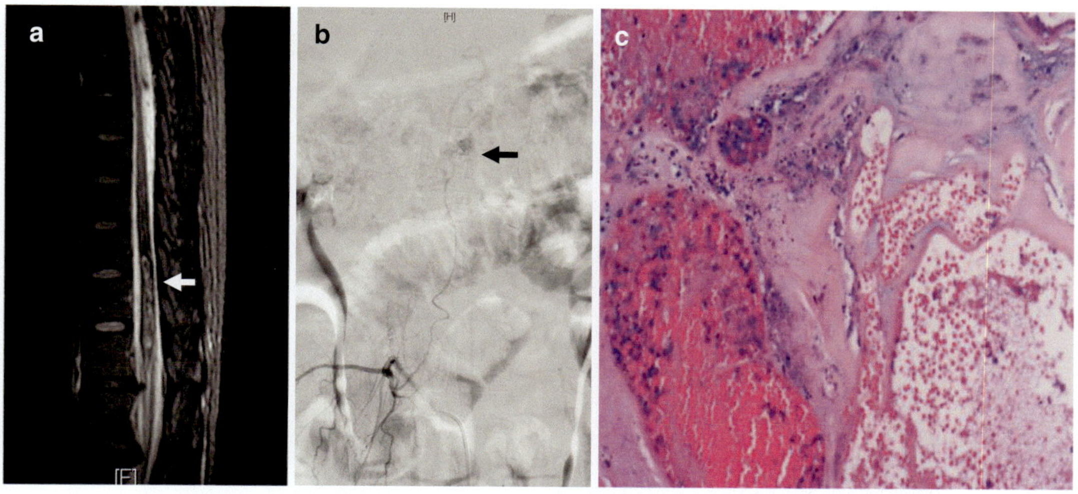

Fig. 5.2 A 30-year-old female patient presented with paralysis and numbness in both lower limbs, as well as difficulty in defecation. (**a**) Spinal MRI examination, T2-weighted, revealed intraparenchymal hemorrhage of the spinal cord (arrow). (**b**) Right L2 segmental artery angiography, early arterial phase, showed a glomerular spinal AVM at the T12 level supplied by the radiomedullary artery (arrow). (**c**) Histopathological examination (H&E staining) showed dilated thin-walled blood vessels of varying sizes were seen in the tissue with wall degeneration and a small amount of muscular blood vessels, accompanied by fresh and old bleeding

Their pathophysiology, the mechanisms underlying their dysfunction, involves several key factors.

Glomerular AVMs have numerous feeding arteries supplying the malformation, often bypassing the normal capillary network of the spinal cord. This direct connection between arteries and veins creates a high-pressure, low-resistance pathway for blood flow. This "arteriovenous shunting" diverts blood away from healthy spinal cord tissue, leading to ischemia causing neurologic deficits. Increased pressure in the spinal cord veins can lead to edema, further compromising neuronal function. The fragile, abnormal vessels within the nidus are prone to rupture, causing intramedullary hemorrhage leading to immediate and often severe neurological damage and subarachnoid hemorrhage potentially causing irritation and inflammation. The high-pressure flow within the AV malformation can "steal" blood from surrounding normal tissue, further exacerbating ischemia. The growing nidus can directly compress surrounding spinal cord tissue, contributing to neurological symptoms. Glomerular AVMs are thought to result from errors in early embryonic vascular development, leading to the formation of the tangled nidus. Overall, the complex interplay of these factors contributes to the diverse clinical presentation of glomerular spinal AVMs, with symptoms ranging from sensory and motor deficits to pain, weakness, and paralysis.

5.5 Type III: Juvenile AVM

Juvenile arteriovenous malformation typically involves a larger, tangled network of abnormal blood vessels compared with other types of spinal AVMs. They are multiple feeders meaning they are supplied by multiple arteries, making them more challenging to treat (Fig. 5.3). Both intramedullary and extracellular involvements: the abnormal vessels can be located both within the spinal cord itself (intramedullary) and surrounding it (extramedullary) [3, 4]. They often have high blood flow rates, increasing the risk of complications. Type III spinal AVMs most commonly affect children and young adults [4]. Perimedullary AVF and intramedullary AVM are dissimilar with dural AVF in clinical characteristics [5].

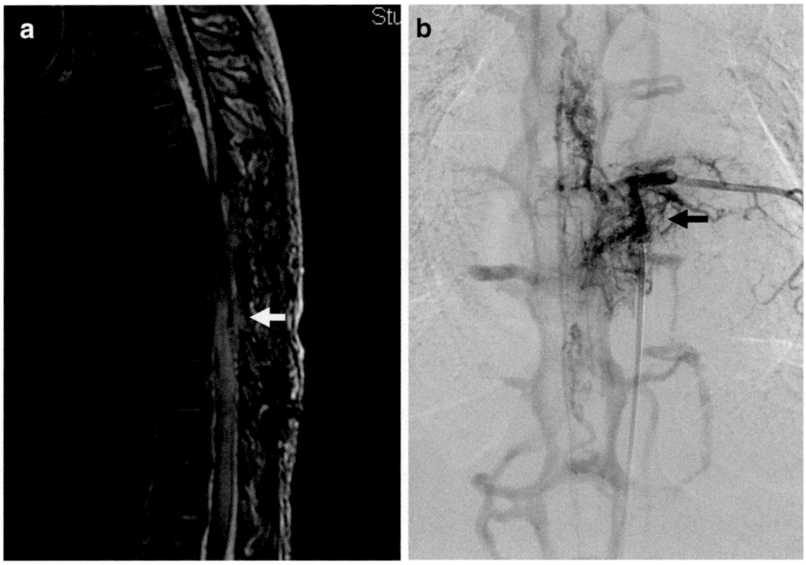

Fig. 5.3 An 18-year-old male patient presented with weakness in both lower limbs and urinary dysfunction. (**a**) Spinal MRI examination, T2-weighted, revealed parenchymal edema of the spinal cord and vascular malformations in the muscles and subcutaneous tissues surrounding the spine (arrow). (**b**) Left T8 segmental artery angiography, early arterial phase, showed juvenile type of the spinal AVM involving the spinal cord, vertebral body, muscle, and subcutaneous tissue of the same segment supplied by the radial artery (arrow)

5.5.1 Pathophysiology

These are rare vascular malformations involving abnormal connections between arteries and veins within the spinal cord. Their pathophysiology involves several key aspects. They are believed to be primarily caused by malformations during embryonic development, leading to the abnormal formation of these arteriovenous connections. They typically occur in the cervical or thoracic region of the spinal cord and are characterized by a complex nidus of vessels with both direct and indirect arteriovenous shunts. These shunts disrupt the normal flow of blood through the capillary network, causing high-pressure venous flow. The shunts bypass the capillary network, leading to increased pressure in the veins. This can reduce arterial perfusion. The high-pressure veins compete with smaller arterioles for blood flow, potentially leading to ischemia and damage to the spinal cord. Venous congestion and compromised perfusion can lead to fluid accumulation (edema) and damage to the spinal cord tissue (myelopathy). The fragile nature of these vessels can lead to spontaneous bleeding within the spinal cord, further exacerbating neurological deficits.

5.6 Type IV: Intradural Perimedullary AVF

Intradural perimedullary arteriovenous fistula (AVF) is a rare vascular abnormality that occurs within the dura mater (Fig. 5.4). This condition involves an abnormal connection between arteries and veins in the spinal cord, leading to altered blood flow patterns. Intradural perimedullary AVFs are typically acquired conditions, meaning they develop later in life rather than being present at birth [5]. They are often associated with underlying vascular malformations or previous trauma to the spinal cord. They are believed to result from the weakening or rupture of small blood vessels within the spinal cord.

5.6.1 Formation

Congenital vs. acquired: The exact cause remains unclear, though most believe they are primarily congenital. Malformations during embryonic development likely lead to abnormal formation

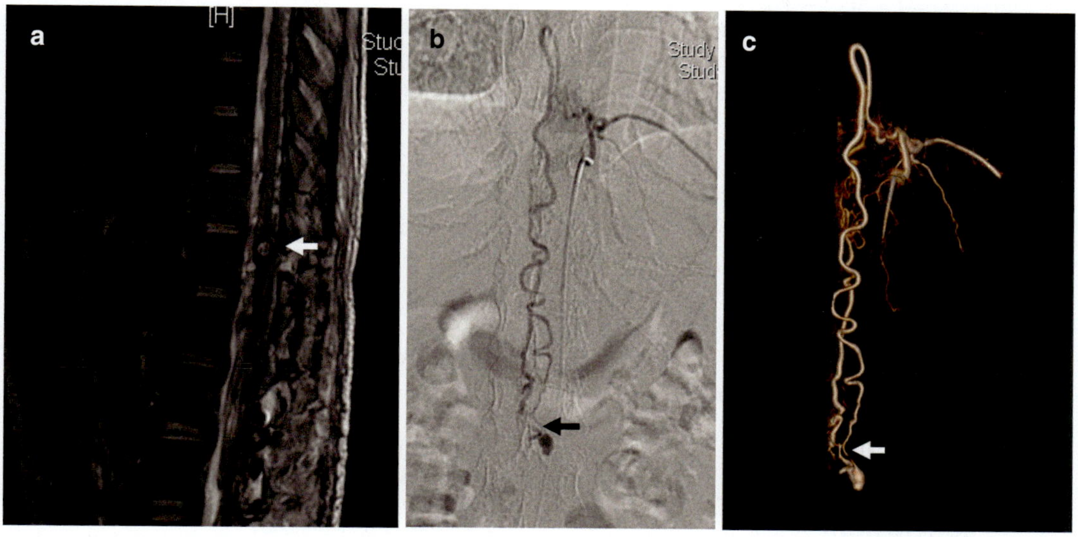

Fig. 5.4 A 38-year-old female patient presented with weakness in both lower limbs, unconsciousness during urination, and difficulty during urination. (**a**) Spinal MRI examination, T2-weighted, revealed intraparenchymal vascular lesion of the spinal cord accompanied by flow void signal around the spinal cord (arrow). (**b**) Left T8 segmental artery angiography, early arterial phase, showed an intradural perimedullary AVF at the T12 level supplied by the radiomedullary artery (arrow). (**c**) 3D reconstruction of the left T8 segmental artery angiography showing the arteriovenous shunt (arrow)

of these arteriovenous connections. Some cases might be acquired due to trauma or inflammation disrupting the vasculature.

Location: Perimedullary AVFs typically occur in the cervical or thoracic region and less frequently in the lumbar or sacral areas.

Types: They are further classified based on the number of fistulous connections:

Type I: Single fistula with direct arteriovenous communication.

Type II: Multiple fistulas with a single venous drainage point.

Type III: Multiple fistulas with multiple venous drainage points.

5.6.2 Pathophysiology

Intradural perimedullary arteriovenous fistulas (AVFs) are rare vascular malformations within the spinal cord, characterized by abnormal connections between arteries and veins directly within the pia mater surrounding the spinal cord. Understanding their pathophysiology involves exploring the factors leading to their formation and the consequences they have on the surrounding nervous tissue.

The abnormal direct connection bypasses the normal capillary network, leading to high-pressure venous flow.

This can:

- *Increase venous congestion*: Increased pressure distends the veins, potentially compressing the surrounding spinal cord and nerve roots.
- *Reduce arterial perfusion*: Steal phenomenon occurs where high-pressure veins compete with smaller arterioles for blood flow, potentially compromising spinal cord perfusion.
- *Edema and myelopathy*: Venous congestion and compromised perfusion can lead to edema and damage to the spinal cord tissue (myelopathy). This manifests as neurological symptoms like weakness, numbness, pain, and bowel/bladder dysfunction.

- *Hemorrhage*: The fragile nature of these fistulas can lead to spontaneous bleeding within the spinal cord, further exacerbating neurological deficits.

The pathophysiology of intradural perimedullary AVF can result in a range of symptoms, including progressive neurological deficits, sensory disturbances, motor weakness, pain, and bowel or bladder dysfunction. Prompt diagnosis and appropriate management are crucial to prevent further neurological deterioration and optimize outcomes.

5.7 Conclusion

In conclusion, spinal vascular malformations (SVMs) disrupt normal blood flow in the spinal cord and surrounding structures, leading to a cascade of complex pathophysiological mechanisms that can severely impact neurological function. Understanding these mechanisms, including venous hypertension, steal phenomenon, and potential hemorrhages, is crucial for accurate diagnosis, effective treatment selection, and predicting patient outcomes. While different types of SVMs present unique challenges, a comprehensive understanding of their underlying pathophysiology empowers healthcare professionals to provide optimal care and improve the lives of individuals affected by these complex conditions. Ultimately, ongoing research into SVM pathophysiology holds the promise of developing even more effective treatment strategies and enhancing long-term prognoses for these individuals.

References

1. Abecassis IJ, Osbun JW, Kim L. Chapter 13—classification and pathophysiology of spinal vascular malformations. In: Handbook of clinical neurology; 2017. p. 135–43. https://doi.org/10.1016/B978-0-444-63640-9.00013-8.
2. Lv X, editor. Intracranial and spinal dural arteriovenous fistulas. Singapore: Springer Nature; 2022. https://doi.org/10.1007/978-981-19-5767-3.
3. Tjoumakaris S, editor. Arteriovenous fistulas—diagnosis and management. InTech; 2013. https://doi.org/10.5772/50823.
4. Lv X. "A nightmare of complex infantile type spinal dural arteriovenous malformation." Paper presented at the meeting for the Neurointerventional Nightmares Summit, December 2–3; 2021. https://assets.nightmares-summit.com/www.nightmares-summit.com/index.htm
5. Lv X, Li Y, Yang X, Jiang C, Wu Z. Endovascular embolization for symptomatic perimedullary AVF and intramedullary AVM: a series and literature review. Neuroradiology. 2012;54:349–59.

6 Spinal Dural Arteriovenous Fistulas

Manoj Kumar Mahata

Abstract

Spinal dural arteriovenous fistula (SDAVF) is a rare and often poorly diagnosed spinal pathology. They mainly occur in males in the fifth or sixth decade of life, with the most common involving the thoracolumbar region, although SDAVF can occur anywhere along the spinal cord. The clinical symptoms presented often have insidious and nonspecific onset, such as weakness of the lower limbs and pain. The symptoms may slowly develop into severe myelopathy with paraplegia within a few years. These symptoms and accompanying imaging findings are often attributed to more common and occasionally coexisting pathological processes, such as degenerative spinal stenosis or demyelinating/inflammatory myelitis. Early diagnosis of SDAVFs is important. Defects may be reversible, but delayed treatment may lead to irreversible neurological dysfunction. Imaging diagnosis mainly relies on magnetic resonance imaging (MRI) and traditional spinal angiography. Once SDAVF is detected, the treatment method is intravascular embolization or surgical obliteration of the fistula.

Keywords

Spinal · Dural arteriovenous fistula · Embolization · Glue · Onyx · Paraplegia

6.1 Introduction

Although it is the most common spinal vascular malformation, spinal dural arteriovenous fistulas (SDAVFs) are rare and still underdiagnosed. If not properly treated, they may lead to a considerable incidence rate and progressive spinal cord symptoms. Due to the nonspecific clinical symptoms, neuroradiologists are usually the first clinical doctors to propose this diagnostic possibility, and this diagnosis initially depends mainly on MR imaging. However, in order to thoroughly understand this disease and develop treatment strategies, selective spinal digital subtraction angiography (DSA) is still necessary. Spinal dural arteriovenous fistula (SDAVF) is a rare but serious vascular malformation of the spinal cord that can cause significant neurological deficits if left untreated. SDAVFs are caused by abnormal connections between arteries and

M. K. Mahata (✉)
Department of Interventional Neuroradiology, Fortis Hospital, Kolkata, India

X. Lv (ed.), *Endovascular and Neurovascular Surgery for Spinal Vascular Malformations*,
https://doi.org/10.1007/978-981-97-4661-3_6

veins within the dura mater, the outermost layer of the spinal cord [1]. These abnormal connections lead to increased blood flow and pressure within the spinal cord, which can cause progressive myelopathy and neurological dysfunction. In this chapter, we will review the clinical presentation, diagnosis, and management of SDAVFs [2].

6.2 Embryology

The embryological basis of SDAVFs can be understood by exploring the development of the spinal cord and its vasculature.

During embryonic development, the spinal cord and its associated structures form from the neural tube. At around 4 weeks of gestation, the neural tube folds to form the brain and the spinal cord. As the spinal cord develops, it becomes surrounded by a series of membranes known as the meninges, which provide protection and support [1, 3].

The vasculature of the spinal cord also develops during this time. The spinal arteries arise from the dorsal aorta and supply blood to the developing spinal cord. These arteries give rise to smaller vessels known as the radicular arteries, which provide blood supply to the nerve roots.

The venous drainage of the spinal cord develops in a more complex manner. During development, there are several primitive veins that drain the spinal cord and its associated structures. These veins eventually coalesce to form the anterior and posterior spinal veins, which then drain into the segmental veins of the vertebral column.

As the spinal cord develops, it becomes surrounded by a network of small blood vessels known as the perimedullary plexus. This plexus is supplied by the radicular arteries and drains into the anterior and posterior spinal veins.

In some cases, an abnormal connection can develop between a radicular artery and a vein in the perimedullary plexus, resulting in an SDAVF. The exact cause of this abnormality is not well understood, but it is thought to be related to incomplete regression of primitive embryonic vessels [4].

6.3 Clinical Presentation

The clinical presentation of SDAVFs can vary depending on the location and severity of the fistula. The most common presenting symptoms include progressive myelopathy, sensory deficits, motor deficits, and sphincter disturbances. The onset of symptoms is usually gradual and may not be noticed until the condition has progressed significantly. In some cases, SDAVFs can cause acute neurological deterioration, which requires urgent intervention [5].

The neurological deficits associated with SDAVFs are caused by a combination of direct spinal cord compression and venous congestion. The progressive myelopathy typically affects the lower extremities first and can progress to involve the upper extremities. Sensory deficits usually present as a loss of vibration and proprioception, with intact pain and temperature sensation. Motor deficits can range from mild weakness to complete paralysis, depending on the severity of the fistula. Sphincter disturbances can present as urinary or fecal incontinence or retention.

Classification of spinal vascular malformations: Multiple classification schemes for spinal vascular malformations have been proposed. The Bicetre Hospital divided spinal cord arteriovenous malformations into three main groups:

1. Genetic hereditary lesions that are caused by a genetic disorder affecting the vascular germinal cells. Spinal cord arteriovenous malformations associated with hereditary hemorrhagic telangiectasia (HHT) belong to this category.

2. Genetic nonhereditary lesions that share metameric links, such as the Cobb syndrome (or metameric spinal arteriovenous malformation) that affects the entire myelomere. These patients typically exhibit multiple spinal arteriovenous shunts involving the nerve root, bone, and paraspinal, subcutaneous, and skin tissue. Klippel-Trenaunay and Parkes Weber syndromes belong to this group.
3. Single lesions that may reflect incomplete expression of one of the above conditions, including spinal cord, nerve root, and filum terminale lesions. Spinal cord arteriovenous malformations (like brain arteriovenous malformations) are shunts fed by the normal supply of neural tissue arteries (i.e., the intrinsic arteries of the spinal cord), while SDAVFs (like intracranial DAVFs) are supplied by radiculomeningeal arteries, which are similar to intracranial meningeal arteries, and are drained by radicular veins, which are similar to intracranial pial veins.

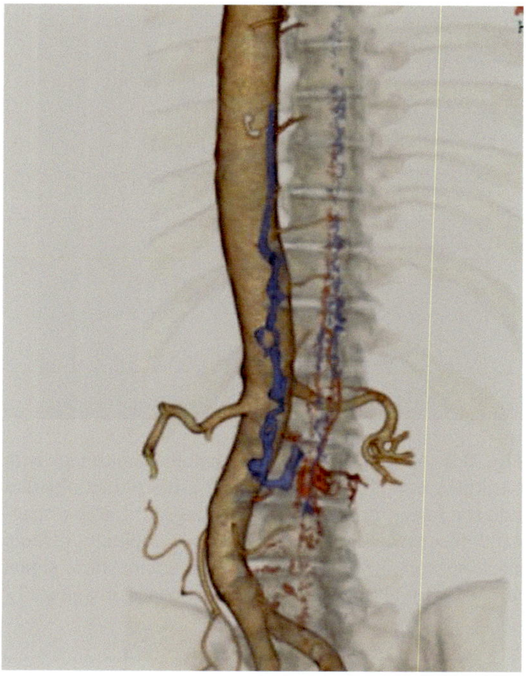

Fig. 6.1 CT angiography images showing a spinal DAVF arising from L3 segmental artery with intradural venous reflux

6.4 Diagnosis

The diagnosis of SDAVFs is based on a combination of clinical examination, imaging studies, and angiography. Magnetic resonance imaging (MRI) of the spine is the most sensitive noninvasive test for detecting SDAVFs. The MRI findings can suggest the diagnosis. MR or CT angiography can confirm the presence of the fistula (Figs. 6.1 and 6.2) [6].

Digital subtraction angiography (DSA) is the gold standard for diagnosing SDAVFs. It involves the injection of contrast dye into the spinal artery to visualize the abnormal connection between the arteries and veins. The angiographic findings can help to determine the location, size, and severity of the fistula, which can guide treatment decisions [7, 8]. DSA with maximum intensity projection can precisely locate point of fistulous connection along with venous ectasia (Fig. 6.3) [6].

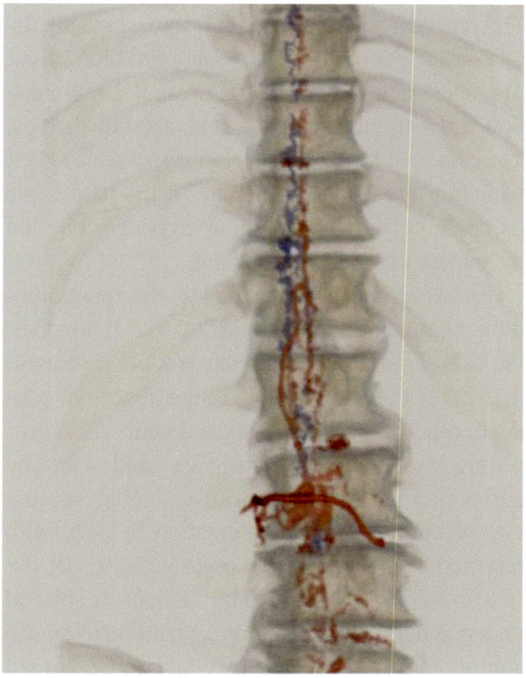

Fig. 6.2 CT angiography images showing a spinal DAVF arising from L3 segmental artery with intradural venous reflux

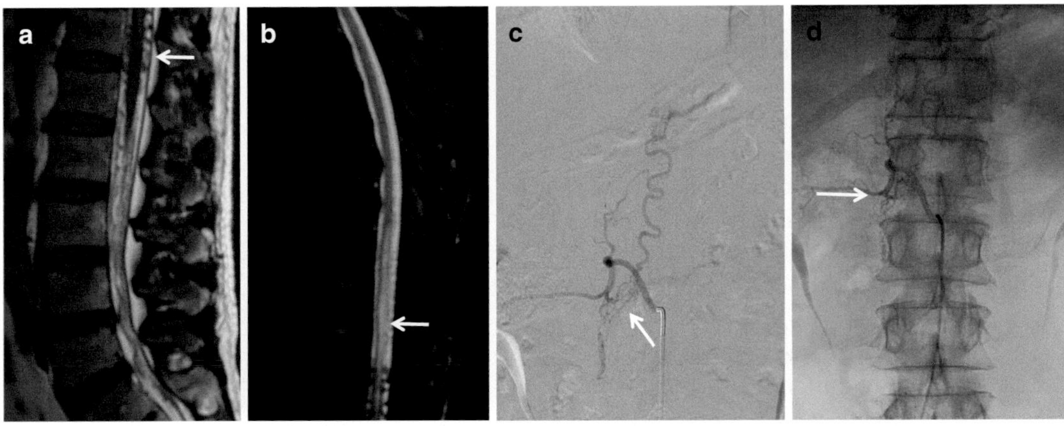

Fig. 6.3 A 53-year-old male patient presented with weakness in both lower limbs and urinary tract obstruction for 1 year, progressive worsening. (**a**) Lumbar magnetic resonance imaging, T2 phase, sagittal position, showing spinal cord and pericauda equina flow signal (arrow). (**b**) Thoracic magnetic resonance imaging, T2 phase, sagittal position, showing perispinal flow signal and spinal cord edema (arrow). (**c**) The right lumbar artery angiography shows a dural arteriovenous fistula (arrow). (**d**) Non-subtractive images showed that the fistula was located in the right first lumbar intervertebral foramen

6.5 Management

The management of SDAVFs requires a multidisciplinary approach that includes neurosurgeons, interventional neuroradiologists, and neurologists. The primary goal of treatment is to occlude the fistula and to restore normal spinal cord blood flow. Treatment options include endovascular embolization, microsurgical resection, and radiation therapy. The choice of treatment depends on several factors, including the location and size of the fistula, the presence of associated venous hypertension, and the patient's overall health status.

Endovascular embolization is the most common treatment option for SDAVFs. It involves the use of catheters to deliver embolic agents to the site of the fistula to block the abnormal connection between the arteries and veins. This procedure is minimally invasive and can be performed under local anesthesia. The success rate of endovascular embolization is high, with reported occlusion rates of up to 90% [9, 10].

Patient preparation: The patient is placed under general anesthesia and positioned on the angiography table. The procedure is performed under strict sterile conditions. Vital signs, including blood pressure and heart rate, are closely monitored throughout the procedure.

Arterial access: An arterial access is obtained through the femoral artery using a standard Seldinger technique. A sheath is placed, and a diagnostic angiogram is performed to identify the feeding arteries of the SDAVF (Fig. 6.3).

Superselective catheterization: A microcatheter is advanced over a guidewire into the feeding artery of the SDAVF under fluoroscopic guidance. Superselective catheterization is essential to ensure accurate placement of the embolic agent and to minimize the risk of damage to the normal spinal cord vasculature.

Dye injection and angiography: Contrast dye is injected through the microcatheter, and angiography is performed to identify the exact location of the SDAVF and to determine the extent of the fistula.

Embolization: Once the SDAVF is identified, an embolic agent is injected into the microcatheter to occlude the abnormal connection between the radicular artery and the perimedullary plexus. Several types of embolic agents can be used, including coils, glue, and liquid embolic agents. The choice of embolic agent depends on the size and location of the SDAVF (Figs. 6.4 and 6.5).

Post-embolization angiography: After the embolic agent is injected, a final angiogram is performed to confirm the occlusion of the SDAVF and to ensure that there is no residual flow.

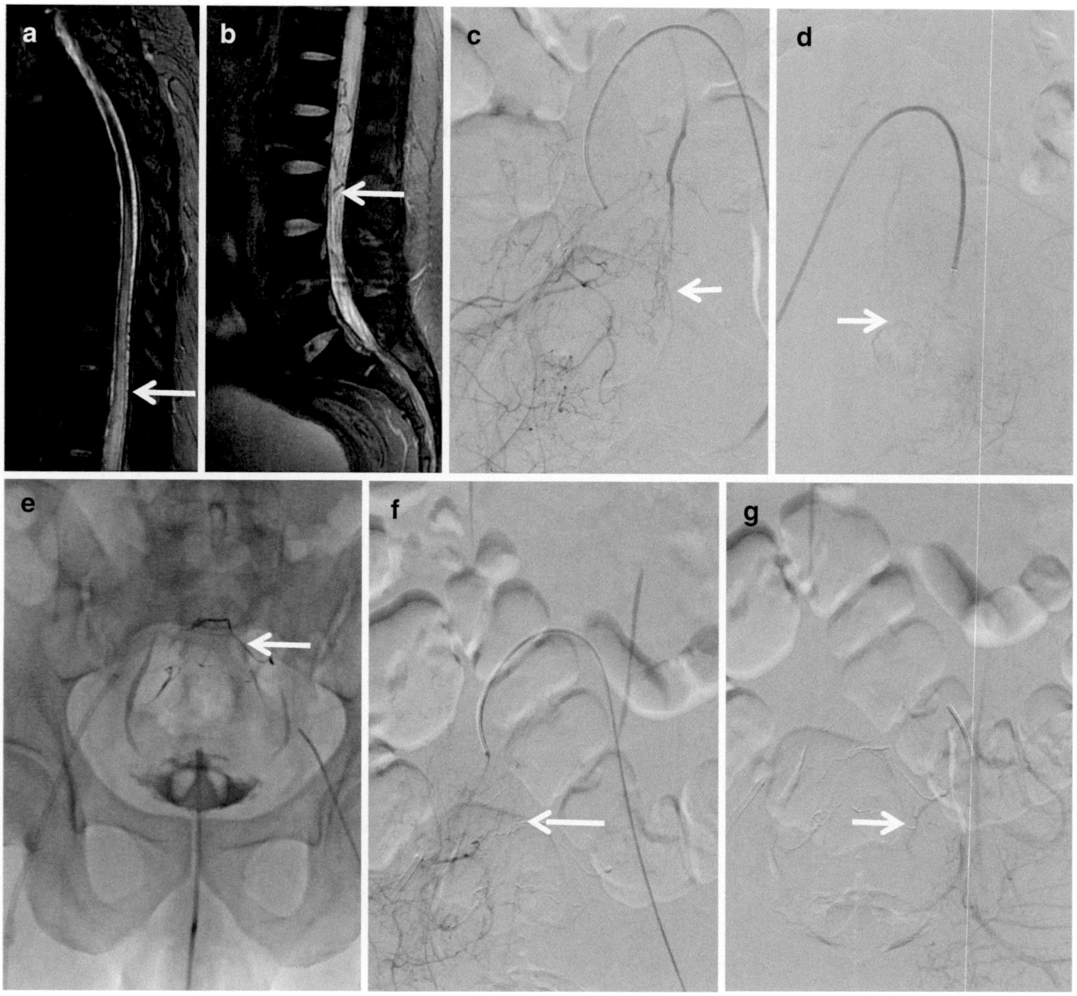

Fig. 6.4 A 44-year-old male presented with progressive worsening of bilateral lower limb weakness for 6 weeks. (**a**) Thoracic magnetic resonance imaging, T2 phase, sagittal position, showing perispinal flow signal and spinal cord edema (arrow). (**b**) Lumbar magnetic resonance imaging, T2 phase, sagittal position, showing spinal cord and pericauda equina flow signal (arrow). (**c**) The right internal iliac artery angiography shows the right sacral 2 dural arteriovenous fistula (arrow). (**d**) Left internal iliac artery angiography shows left sacral 2 dural arteriovenous fistula (arrow). (**e**) The non-subtracted image shows the Onyx cast after bilateral anterior sacral artery embolization. (**f**) The right internal iliac artery angiography shows complete disappearance of the lesion fistula. (**g**) Left internal iliac artery angiography shows complete disappearance of the lesion fistula

Closure: Once the procedure is complete, the microcatheter is removed, and hemostasis is achieved at the femoral access site.

Post-procedural monitoring: The patient is closely monitored for several hours after the procedure for any signs of complications, including bleeding, hematoma, and neurological deficits.

In conclusion, endovascular embolization is a minimally invasive procedure that can be used to treat spinal dural arteriovenous fistulas. The procedure involves accessing the arterial system, identifying the feeding artery of the SDAVF, superselective catheterization, angiography, embolization, and post-procedural monitoring. This technique can be highly effective in treating SDAVFs and can result in significant improvements in neurological function.

Microsurgical resection is another treatment option for SDAVFs. It involves the surgical

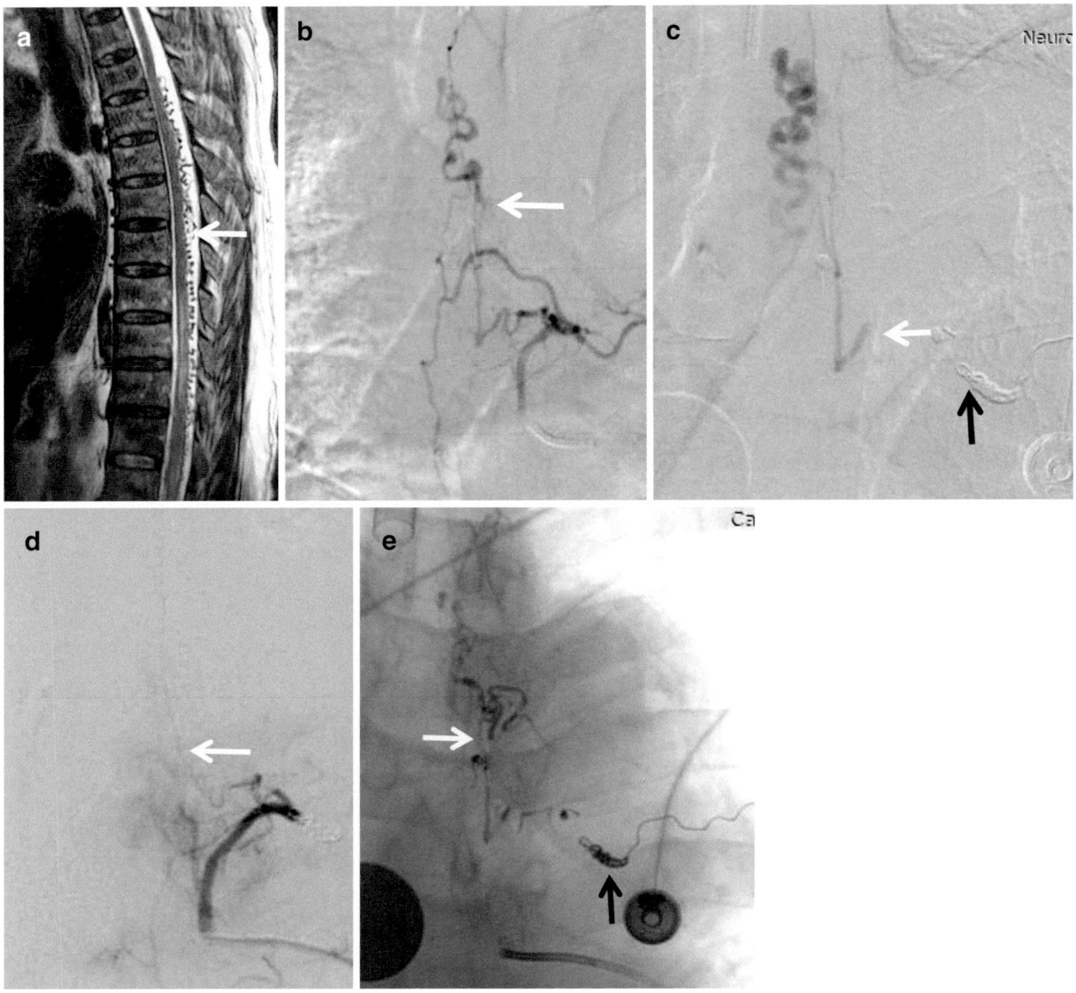

Fig. 6.5 An 85-year-old male patient presented with progressive worsening of lower limb weakness for 3 days. (**a**) Thoracic magnetic resonance imaging, T2 phase, sagittal position, showing perispinal flow signal and spinal cord edema (arrow). (**b**) Left thoracic 6 intercostal artery angiography shows left thoracic 6 dural arteriovenous fistula (arrow). (**c**) Micrograph of the left radiodural artery shows the fistula (white arrow). Embolize the left intercostal artery with coils (black arrow) to ensure that the tip of the microcatheter reaches the distal of the radiomedullary artery. (**d**) After Onyx embolization, the left intercostal artery angiography showed complete disappearance of the lesion fistula and preservation of the radiomedullary artery (arrow). (**e**) The non-subtracted image shows Onyx casting (white arrow) and the coil mass (black arrow)

removal of the abnormal connection between the arteries and veins within the dura mater. This procedure is more invasive than endovascular embolization and requires general anesthesia. The success rate of microsurgical resection is high, with reported cure rates of up to 80%.

Radiation therapy is a less common treatment option for SDAVFs. It involves the use of high-energy radiation to damage the abnormal blood vessels within the dura mater. This procedure is noninvasive and can be performed on an outpatient basis.

References

1. Krings T, Geibprasert S. Spinal dural arteriovenous fistulas. AJNR Am J Neuroradiol. 2009;30(4):639–48.
2. Jellema K, Tijssen CC, van Gijn J. Spinal dural arteriovenous fistulas: a clinical review. Lancet Neurol. 2006;5(10):961–70.

3. Luetmer PH, Lane JI, Gilbertson JR, et al. Preangiographic evaluation of spinal dural arteriovenous fistulas with elliptic centric contrast-enhanced MR angiography and spin-echo MR imaging. AJNR Am J Neuroradiol. 2002;23(5):858–67.
4. Spetzler RF, Detwiler PW, Riina HA, et al. Modified classification of spinal cord vascular lesions. J Neurosurg Spine. 2002;96(2 suppl):145–56.
5. Krings T, Geibprasert S. Spinal dural arteriovenous fistulas. Neuroimaging Clin N Am. 2012;22(4):725–38.
6. Tanaka M. Spinal dural AVFs: classifications and advanced imaging. In: Esposito G, Regli L, Cenzato M, et al., editors. Trends in cerebrovascular surgery and interventions [internet]. Cham (CH): Springer. https://www.ncbi.nlm.nih.gov/books/NBK573754/; 2021. https://doi.org/10.1007/978-3-030-63453-7_19.
7. Rangel-Castilla L, Spetzler RF. Management of spinal dural arteriovenous fistulas: a review. Neurosurg Focus. 2012;32(5):E13.
8. Borden JA, Wu JK, Shucart WA. A proposed classification for spinal and cranial dural arteriovenous fistulous malformations and implications for treatment. J Neurosurg. 1995;82(2):166–79.
9. Kiyosue H, Hori Y, Okahara M, et al. Treatment of spinal dural arteriovenous fistulae: a multidisciplinary approach. Neurol Res. 2012;34(4):356–66.
10. Chen CJ, Chen ST, Hsieh YK, et al. Endovascular treatment of spinal dural arteriovenous fistulas. Neurosurgery. 2009;64(2 suppl): E301–8.

7 Endovascular Therapeutic Considerations for Cervical Epidural Arteriovenous Fistula

Jinlu Yu

Abstract

A cervical epidural arteriovenous fistula (CEAVF) is an uncommon arteriovenous shunt in the epidural space. CEAVFs can be classified into type A and type B. Type B can be further divided into two subtypes: B1 and B2. Endovascular treatment (EVT) has shown clinical utility. However, deep understanding of the role of EVT is necessary due to the rarity and intricate pathomechanics of CEAVFs. Therefore, a systematic review was performed by searching the PubMed database. The clinical data were extracted. A total of 20 articles reporting 22 patients with a single CEAVF were identified. The patients were 42.3 ± 17.6 years old, and 42.9% were female. Type B1 accounted for 81.8% of CEAVFs, and 73.7% of CEAVFs with exact location data were at the C4–7 levels. Multiple feeding arteries per arteriovenous fistula were present in 72.8% of CEAVFs. The vertebral artery was the most common feeding artery, accounting for 67% of CEAVFs. The draining vein had a venous pouch in 86.4% of CEAVFs. When EVT was performed, complete obliteration was obtained in 68.2% of CEAVFs. During follow-up, 78.9% of patients made a complete or significant recovery, and 21.1% showed moderate improvement. Therefore, EVT is effective for CEAVFs. Complete obliteration of nearly 70% of CEAVFs can be achieved via EVT. In this study, nearly 80% of patients made a complete or significant recovery during follow-up.

J. Yu (✉)
Department of Neurosurgery, First Hospital of Jilin University, Changchun, China
e-mail: jlyu@jlu.edu.cn

Keywords

Cervical · Epidural arteriovenous fistula · Endovascular treatment · Prognosis · Review

7.1 Introduction

A spinal epidural arteriovenous fistula (AVF) is uncommon and located in the epidural space; it is an arteriovenous shunt between the branches of the feeding arteries and the epidural venous plexus without the nidus-like structure [1]. Normally, the spinal epidural venous plexus is a communicating system; it has multiple outflows at nearly every segmental level, and spinal epidural AVFs can be silent due to multiple draining paths [2]. However, when spinal epidural AVF has a mass effect or blockade of the outflow that results in reflux into the medullary vein, it becomes symptomatic, presenting with progressive radiculopathy and myelopathy [3]. At this time, treatment is mandatory at the earliest opportunity.

X. Lv (ed.), *Endovascular and Neurovascular Surgery for Spinal Vascular Malformations*,
https://doi.org/10.1007/978-981-97-4661-3_7

In Huang et al. report, the most common location of spinal epidural AVF is the cervical region (53%), followed by lumbosacral (30%) and thoracic (17%) regions [4]. Cervical epidural AVF (CEAVF) is complex due to its high location and difficult treatment [5]. The ideal treatment for a CEAVF is the obliteration of shunts leading to the successive disappearance of the AVF as well as extra- and intradural drainers [6]. Currently, therapeutic approaches include microsurgical shunt detachment, endovascular treatment (EVT), or a combination of both [7]. Of these methods, EVT is gaining popularity, including transarterial embolization (TAE) or transvenous embolization (TVE) and combinations of both [6, 8–10].

Deep understanding of the role of EVT for CEAVFs is necessary due to the rarity and intricate pathomechanics. Therefore, we performed a systematic review of the English-language literature to address this complex issue.

7.2 Materials and Methods

7.2.1 Search Strategy

This systematic review was conducted in accordance with the Preferred Reporting Items for Systematic Reviews and Meta-Analyses (PRISMA) guidelines [11]. The search terms were as follows: "spinal epidural arteriovenous fistula" or "spinal extradural arteriovenous fistula" or "cervical epidural arteriovenous fistula" or "cervical extradural arteriovenous fistula." Eligible English-language articles were identified by searching the PubMed database (the last search date was 1 October 2022). The reference lists of the identified articles were also searched manually for additional relevant studies.

7.2.2 Inclusion and Exclusion Criteria

The inclusion criteria were as follows: (a) the full text of the article was available; (b) complete clinical data were available; (c) the fistula was located in the epidural space of the cervical spine and accepted EVT; and (d) for CEAVFs in the high cervical spine (C1 and C2), the fistula was drained by the vertebral venous plexus (Fig. 7.1a).

The exclusion criteria were as follows: (a) patients with congenital diseases, such as neurofibromatosis, congenital vascular syndrome, Cowden syndrome, congenital Klippel-Trenaunay syndrome, or fibromuscular dysplasia; (b) CEAVFs with direct vertebral venous fistula; and (c) CEAVFs in the high cervical spine (C1 and C2) in which the fistula only drained into the intracranial venous system without the vertebral venous plexus (Fig. 7.1b). A flowchart of the selection process is shown in Fig. 7.2.

7.2.3 Classification of CEAVFs

CEAVFs were categorized according to the classification scheme proposed by Rangel-Castilla et al. [12]. They were divided into types A and B according to their drainage components (Fig. 7.3). Type A has both epidural venous drainage and a vein that pierces the dura, travels intradurally, and drains into the perimedullary venous plexus. Type B, which has no intradural draining vein, can be further divided into two subtypes: B1 and B2. Type B1 is accompanied by compression myelopathy from epidural venous drainage; type B2 has no radiographic or clinical mass effect and is asymptomatic.

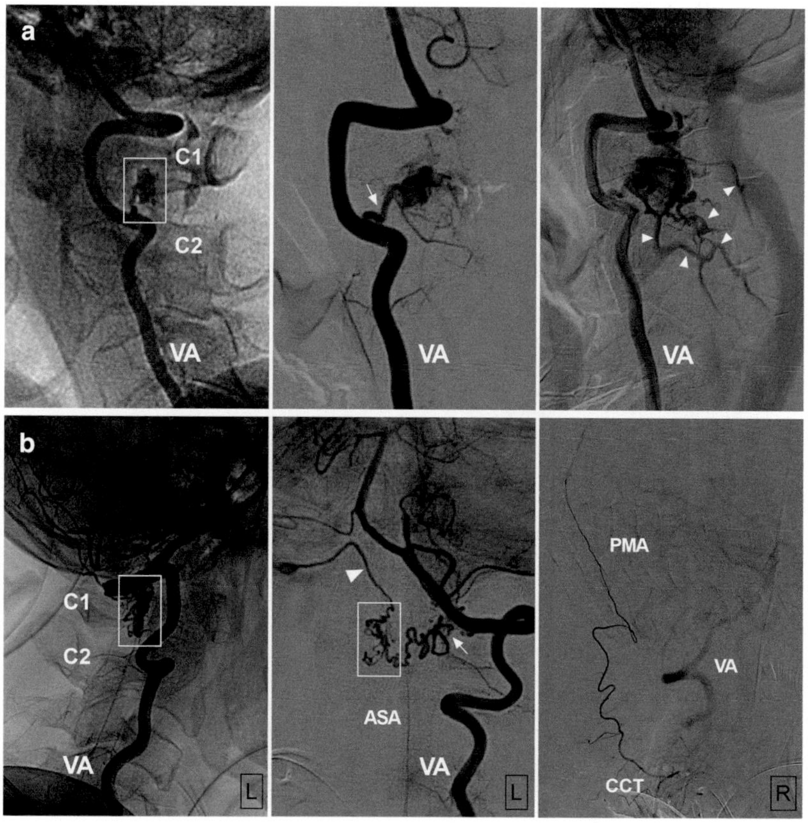

Fig. 7.1 Inclusion and exclusion criteria for high CEAVF. The images are of the cases from our institute. (**a**) Example of an included CEAVF. The left image shows that the CEAVF (frame) is located between C1 and C2; the middle image shows that the CEAVF is fed by a branch of the VA (arrow); the right image shows that the CEAVF drains into the vertebral venous plexus (triangles). (**b**) Example of an excluded CEAVF. The left image shows that the CEAVF (frame) is located between C1 and C2; the middle image shows that the CEAVF (frame) is fed by a tangled branch of the left VA (arrow) and drains into the sigmoid sinus via a vein (triangle); the right image shows that the posterior meningeal artery originates from the costocervical trunk. Abbreviations: *ASA* anterior spinal artery, *CEAVF* cervical epidural arteriovenous fistula, *C1 and C2* the first and second cervical vertebrae, *CCT* costocervical trunk, *L* left, *PMA* posterior meningeal artery, *R* right, *VA* vertebral artery

7.2.4 Collected Data

The collected data included age, sex, CEAVF type, medical history and clinical presentation, preoperative Aminoff-Logue scale score (Table 7.1) [13], fistula location, feeding artery, draining vein (with/without a venous pouch), EVT path and outcome, complications, follow-up, and prognosis.

7.2.5 Data Description

Continuous variables are expressed as the mean ± standard deviation.

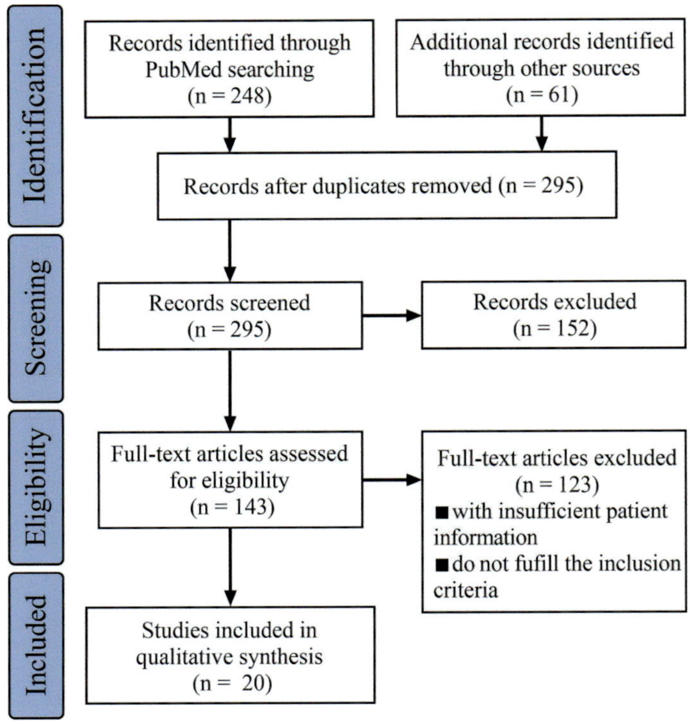

Fig. 7.2 Flowchart of the search strategy

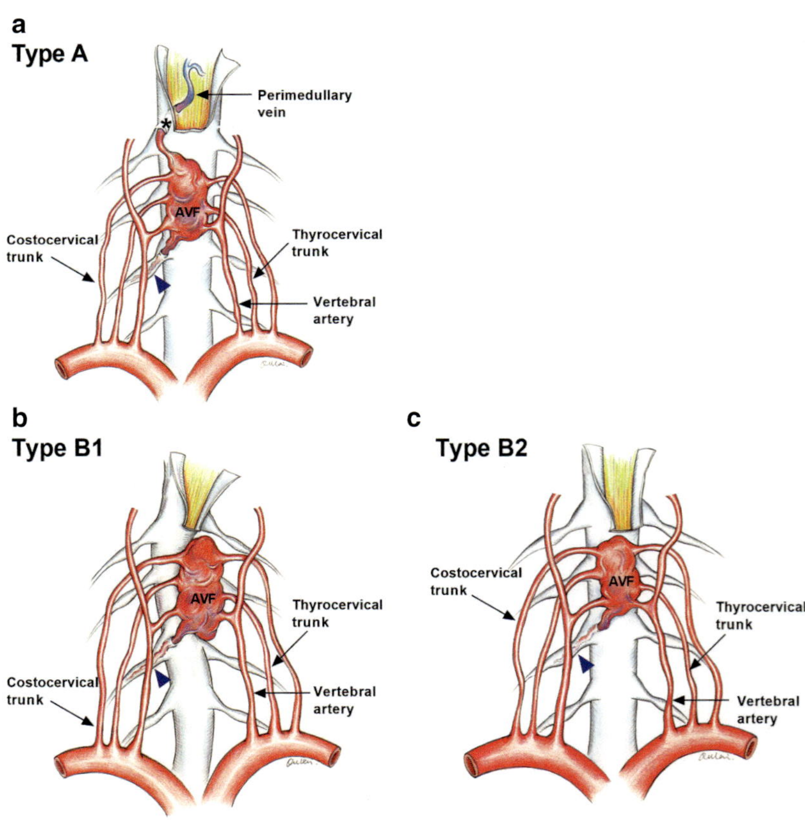

Fig. 7.3 Classification of CEAVFs. (**a**) A CEAVF of type A has both epidural venous drainage (blue triangle) and a vein that pierces the dura and drains into the perimedullary vein (asterisk). (**b**) A CEAVF of type B1 has only epidural venous drainage (blue triangle) and causes compression myelopathy. (**c**) A CEAVF of type B2 has only epidural venous drainage (blue triangle) and has no mass effect that compresses the cervical cord. The feeding arteries of CEAVFs can include the vertebral artery, thyrocervical artery, and costocervical artery. Abbreviations: *AVF* arteriovenous fistula, *CEAVF* cervical epidural arteriovenous fistula. *Note*: The figure has been created by Dr. Lai Qu for the book, she agrees to transfer the right to publish the figure in a commercial book.

Table 7.1 Aminoff-Logue scale [13]

Grade	Motor	Urinary
0	Normal	Normal
1	Leg weakness, abnormal stance or gait, unrestricted activity	Hesitancy, urgency but no incontinence
2	Restricted activity	Occasional incontinence or retention
3	A crutch or other support is needed to walk	Total incontinence or retention
4	Crutches are needed to walk	
5	Cannot stand; bedridden or confined to wheelchair	

7.3 Results

A total of 20 articles reporting 22 patients (22 CEAVFs) were identified (Table 7.2) [1, 12, 14–31]. In addition to the 22 patients identified in the literature, we also present 1 typical case for illustration (Figs. 7.4 and 7.5); this case was excluded from the final analysis due to the lack of follow-up images.

7.3.1 General Information

The patients ranged from 4 to 68 years old (mean 42.3 ± 17.6 years). The sexes of 21 patients were recorded; 42.9% (9/21) of these patients were female, while 57.1% (12/21) were male. Type A AVF accounted for 18.2% (4/22) of cases, and type B1 accounted for the remaining 81.8% (18/22). Information on individual medical history and onset was available in 15 patients; sudden onset occurred in 26.7% (4/15) of cases, comprising 3 cases of hemorrhage and 1 case of tetraparesis, while 73.3% (11/15) had progressive onset with a duration of 1 month to 4 years. Preoperative scores on the Aminoff-Logue scale were available for 13 patients; their scores ranged from 0 to 8 (mean 2.3 ± 2.9).

7.3.2 Imaging Characteristics

Nineteen CEAVFs had their exact locations recorded; 26.3% (5/19) of these AVFs were at C1–3, and 73.7% (14/19) were at C4–7. Regarding the feeding arteries, 27.2% (6/22) of CEAVFs had a single feeding artery, while 72.8% (16/22) had more than one; the vertebral artery (VA) was involved in 68.2% (15/22) of CEAVFs, the costocervical trunk (CCT) in 59.1% (13/22), and the thyrocervical trunk (TCT) in 54.5% (12/22). All CEAVFs were drained by the vertebral venous plexus; 18.2% (4/22) involved an intramedullary vein, and 86.4% (19/22) had a venous pouch.

7.3.3 Therapeutic Outcomes

Complete obliteration via TAE was achieved in 50% (11/22) of CEAVFs, and complete obliteration via TVE was achieved in 18.2% (4/22) of CEAVFs. Incomplete obliteration occurred in 31.8% (7/22) of CEAVFs, including 5 that were treated by TAE, 1 that was treated by TVE, and 1 that was treated with a combined TAE/TVE procedure; surgical disconnection was performed for 2 CEAVFs that showed incomplete obliteration via EVT. The presence or absence of complications was recorded in 21 patients; the rate was 9.5% (2/21), including 1 case of mass effect treated by hematoma evacuation as well as 1 case of increased symptoms addressed by conservative treatment.

Accurate follow-up time was recorded in 18 patients; the duration ranged from 10 days to 8 years. During follow-up, two CEAVFs that were incompletely embolized underwent complete occlusion. EVT outcomes were recorded in v42.1% (8/19) of patients, significant improvement in 36.8% (7/19), and moderate improvement in 21.1% (4/19) of patients. The results are summarized in Table 7.3.

Table 7.2 Patients' primary clinical data

No.	Author (year)	Age/ sex	Type	Length of history; symptoms	Motor/ urinary	Location	Feeding artery	Draining vein	Venous pouch	Treatment	Complications	Follow-up period	Prognosis
1	Cahan et al. (1987) [14]	51/F	B1	NM; unilateral radiculopathy	0/0	C4 and C5	Unilateral VA, TCT, and CCT	VVP	Y	Complete TAE with NBCA	N	NM	Complete recovery
2	Cahan et al. (1987) [14]	19/M	A	SAH	NA	C5	Unilateral VA	VVP + IMV	Y	Complete TAE with detachable balloon	N	NM	NM
3	Willinsky et al. (1990) [15]	36/M	A	7 months; quadriparesis	5/3	C7	Unilateral VA and CCT	VVP + IMV	Y	Complete TAE with NBCA	N	7 months	Moderate improvement
4	Willinsky et al. (1993) [16]	57/M	B1	4 years; unilateral limb weakness, urinary hesitancy	2/1	C4 and C5	Bilateral VA, TCT, and CCT	VVP	Y	VA occlusion; incomplete TAE with particles and TVE with balloon and coil	N	12 months	Moderate improvement
5	Kohno et al. (1996) [17]	51/M	B1	2 months; unilateral arm weakness	1/0	C2 and C3	Unilateral VA, TCT, and CCT	VVP	Y	Incomplete TAE with coil and NBCA; surgery	N	12 months	Significant improvement
6	Goyal et al. (1999) [18]	68/M	B1	NM; cervical myelopathy	NM	C	Bilateral VA, ECA, TCT, and CCT	VVP	Y	Complete TVE with coil and NBCA	N	NM	Significant improvement
7	Asai et al. (2001) [19]	24/M	B1	4 months; quadriparesis	NM	C5–T2	Bilateral TCT and CCT	VVP	N	Incomplete TAE with coil and NBCA; surgery	N	2 months	Significant improvement

8	Chuang et al. (2003) [20]	4/F	B1	Several hours; epidural hematoma	NA	C6 and C7	Unilateral CCT	VVP	Y	Complete TAE with NBCA	Space-occupying effect, treated by hematoma evacuation	16 months	Moderate improvement
9	Chul Suh et al. (2004) [21]	50/F	B1	3 months; neck pain	0/0	C5	Unilateral VA and CCT	VVP	Y	Incomplete TVE with coil	N	8 years	Complete recovery
10	Kawabori et al. (2009) [22]	65/F	A	2 months; monoplegia of the arm	2/0	C5 and C6	Unilateral TCT	VVP + IMV	Y	Incomplete TAE with coil and NBCA	N	DSA at 10 days showed complete embolization	Significant improvement
11	Rangel-Castilla et al. (2011) [12]	57/M	B1	6 months; bilateral leg weakness	1/0	C6 and C7	Unilateral TCT	VVP	Y	Complete TVE with coil and onyx	N	12 months	Complete recovery
12	Dabus et al. (2011) [23]	60/F	B1	NM; unilateral arm numbness	1/0	C5	Bilateral VA and CCT	VVP	Y	Complete TVE with coil and onyx	N	1 month	Complete recovery
13	Miyamoto et al. (2013) [24]	24/M	B1	Sudden tetraparesis	5/3	C1–C3	Unilateral VA	VVP	N	Incomplete TAE with NBCA	N	4 months	Moderate improvement
14	Ramanathan et al. (2014) [25]	46/NM	A	4 months; bilateral leg weakness	1/0	C7	Unilateral TCT	VVP + IMV	Y	Complete TAE with onyx	N	4 months	Complete recovery
15	Nakagawa et al. (2014) [26]	54/M	B1	SAH	NA	C2	Bilateral VA and ASA (with aneurysm)	VVP	Y	Incomplete TAE with NBCA	N	DSA at 12 months showed complete embolization	Complete recovery
16	Kasliwal et al. (2015) [27]	17/F	B1	4 months; quadriparesis	NM	C2	Unilateral VA and occipital artery	VVP	Y	VA trapping; complete TAE with coil and onyx	N	6 months	Significant improvement
17	Romano et al. (2016) [28]	42/F	B1	NM; unilateral arm radiculopathy	0/0	C2 and C3	Unilateral VA and TCT	VVP	N	VA trapping	N	1 month	NM

(continued)

Table 7.2 (continued)

No.	Author (year)	Age/ sex	Type	Length of history; symptoms	Motor/ urinary	Location	Feeding artery	Draining vein	Venous pouch	Treatment	Complications	Follow-up period	Prognosis
18	Song et al. (2019) [29]	57/M	B1	NM	NM	C6	Bilateral CCT	VVP	Y	Complete TVE with coil	NM	NM	NM
19	Goyal et al. (2020) [30]	55/M	B1	1 year; quadriparesis	NM	C4	Bilateral TCT; unilateral VA and CCT	VVP	Y	Complete TAE with NBCA	N	1 month	Complete recovery
20	Shetty et al. (2021) [1]	37/M	B1	NM; paraparesis and urinary retention	3/2	C	Unilateral TCT and upper intercostal artery	VVP	Y	Complete TAE with NBCA and onyx	N	3 months	Significant improvement
21	Shetty et al. (2021) [1]	24/F	B1	NM; paraparesis and pain	NM	C	Unilateral VA, TCT, and CCT	VVP	Y	Complete TAE with coiling and onyx	Increased symptoms	3 months	Significant improvement
22	Park et al. (2022) [31]	33/F	B1	1 month; trapezius pain	0/0	C5–C7	Unilateral VA, TCT	VVP	Y	VA trapping; complete TAE with NBCA	N	12 months	Complete recovery

Abbreviations: *CCT* costocervical trunk, *ECA* external carotid artery, *F* female, *IMV* intramedullary vein, *M* male, *N* no, *NA* not applicable, *NBCA* N-butyl cyanoacrylate, *NM* not mentioned, *SAH* subarachnoid hemorrhage, *TAE* transarterial embolization, *TCT* thyrocervical trunk, *TVE* transvenous embolization, *VA* vertebral artery, *VVP* vertebral venous plexus, *Y* yes

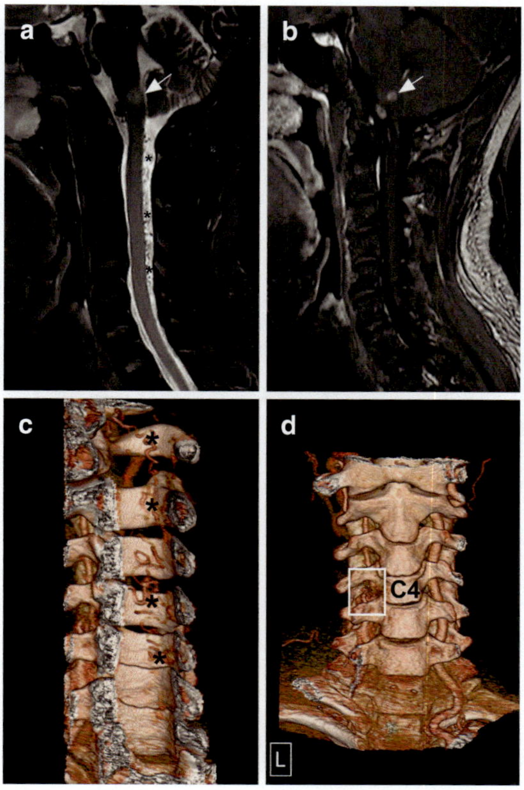

Fig. 7.4 Preoperative images of an illustrative case. The patient was a 42-year-old man who presented with progressive weakness of the limbs. (**a**) T2-weighted MRI shows dilated, serpentine veins behind the cervical spinal cord (asterisks) and high-signal edema (arrow) in the medulla oblongata. (**b**) Post-contrast MRI shows enhancement of the edema (arrow). (**c**) CTA shows the dilated veins (asterisks) in the cervical spinal canal. (**d**) CTA shows the location of the lesion (frame) by the left side of the C4 vertebra. Abbreviations: *CTA* computed tomography angiography, *L* left, *MRI* magnetic resonance imaging

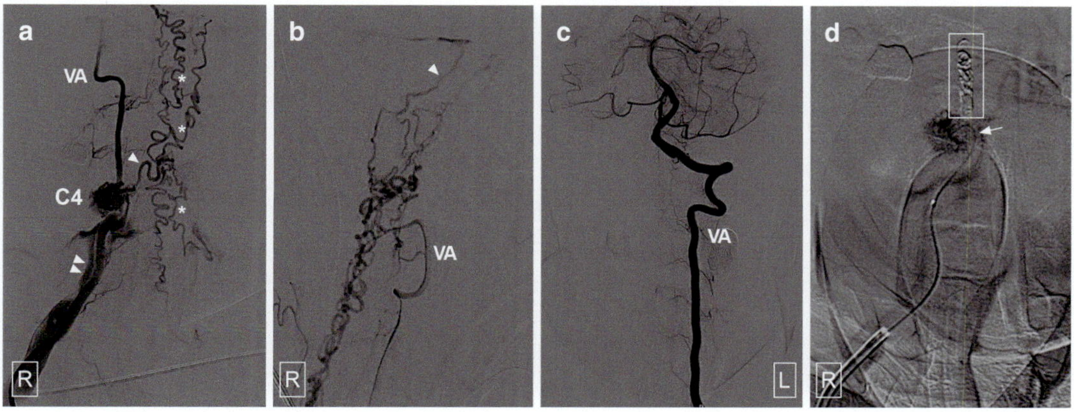

Fig. 7.5 Images showing the therapeutic process in an illustrative case. (**a**) Arterial-phase DSA of the right VA shows that the CEAVF is located epidurally at the C4 level beside the VA; the single triangle indicates the entrance of the drainage vein into the intradural space; the double triangles indicate the drainage of the vertebral venous plexus; the asterisks indicate the intramedullary vein drainage. (**b**) Late arterial-phase DSA shows intramedullary vein drainage into the brainstem venous system (triangle). (**c**) DSA showed that the left VA was normal. (**d**) After the right VA beyond the AVF was occluded with coiling (frame), the microcatheter went into the CEAVF via the feeding artery from the VA (arrow), and a superselective angiogram was performed. Then, Onyx was cast. (**e**) An unsubtracted image taken for DSA shows coils in the VA and Onyx in the CEAVF. (**f**) A superselective angiogram of the TCT (arrow) shows the incompletely embolized CEAVF, and the triangle indicates the intradural drainage. Then, Onyx was cast via the TCT. (**g** and **h**) DSA of the right subclavian artery shows the completely embolized CEAVF. (**h**) An unsubtracted image taken for DSA, which shows coils and Onyx. Abbreviations: *CEAVF* cervical epidural arteriovenous fistula, *DSA* digital subtraction angiography, *L* left, *R* right, *TCT* thyrocervical trunk, *VA* vertebral artery

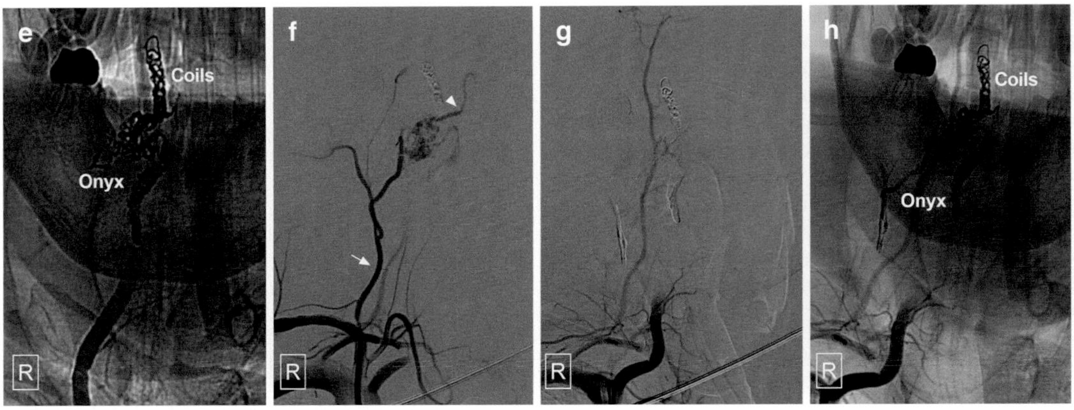

Fig. 7.5 (continued)

Table 7.3 Summarized patient data

Characteristic	Data
Age (years)	
Mean ± SD	42.3 ± 17.6
Range	4–68
Sex	
Female	42.9% (9/21)
Male	57.1% (12/21)
Classification	
Type A	18.2% (4/22)
Type B1	81.8% (18/22)
Presentation	
Sudden onset	26.7% (4/15)
Progressive onset	73.3% (11/15)
Aminoff-Logue scale score	
Mean ± SD	2.3 ± 2.9
Range	0–8
Location	
C1–C3	26.3% (5/19)
C4–C7	73.7% (14/19)
Feeding artery/arteries	
Single	27.2% (6/22)
Multiple	72.8% (16/22)
Vertebral artery	68.2% (15/22)
Costocervical trunk	59.1% (13/22)
Thyrocervical trunk	54.5% (12/22)
Draining vein	
Vertebral venous plexus	100% (22/22)
Intramedullary vein	18.2% (4/22)
Venous pouch	86.4% (19/22)
Treatment	
Complete transarterial embolization	50% (11/22)
Complete transvenous embolization	18.2% (4/22)
Incomplete endovascular embolization	31.8% (7/22)
Complications	9.5% (2/21)
Prognosis	
Complete recovery	42.1% (8/19)
Significant improvement	36.8% (7/19)
Moderate improvement	21.1% (4/19)

7.4 Discussion

A spinal epidural AVF is relatively uncommon and can produce neurological deterioration because a large fistula can lead to mass effects with subsequent radiculopathy/myelopathy or reflux into the intradural perimedullary veins, leading to congestion myelopathy [32]. They are often located in the ventral/ventrolateral wide epidural space outside the dura mater, with rich venous anastomoses (9). Lesions tend to occur in middle-aged people. In Huang et al.'s review of spinal epidural AVFs at all levels of the spine in 101 patients, the mean age was 46 years, and there was no significant difference in prevalence according to sex; in this review, CEAVFs accounted for more than 50% [4]. Therefore, for CEAVFs, the age and sex distributions may be similar. In the present review, the mean age was 42.3 ± 17.6 years, and 42.9% of patients were female; the results were similar.

The precise mechanism of CEAVF is still unclear, and most CEAVFs are considered acquired [33–36]. We present a male patient whose case supports this hypothesis; he had both CEAVF and dural AVF (DAVF), and thrombosis continuously progressed near the DAVF over a 3-month period (Fig. 7.6). As with DAVF,

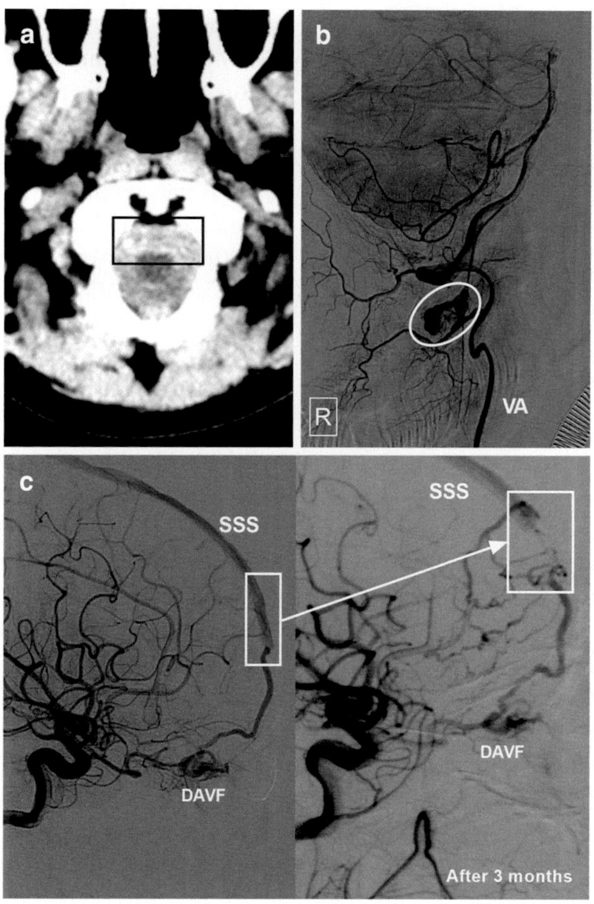

Fig. 7.6 A patient with multiple AVFs, including CEAVF and anterior fossa DAVF. The images are of the cases from our institute. (**a**) CT shows subarachnoid hemorrhage before the medulla oblongata (frame). (**b**) DSA of the right VA shows the location of the CEAVF (circle) at the high cervical level. (**c**) The left and right images show the DAVF of the anterior fossa. The frame in the left image shows that the SSS was not initially blocked, the frame in the right image shows that the SSS was blocked after 3 months of follow-up, and the long arrow emphasizes the change. Abbreviations: *CEAVF* cervical epidural arteriovenous fistula, *CT* computed tomography, *DAVF* dural arteriovenous fistula, *DSA* digital subtraction angiography, *R* right, *SSS* superior sagittal sinus, *VA* vertebral artery

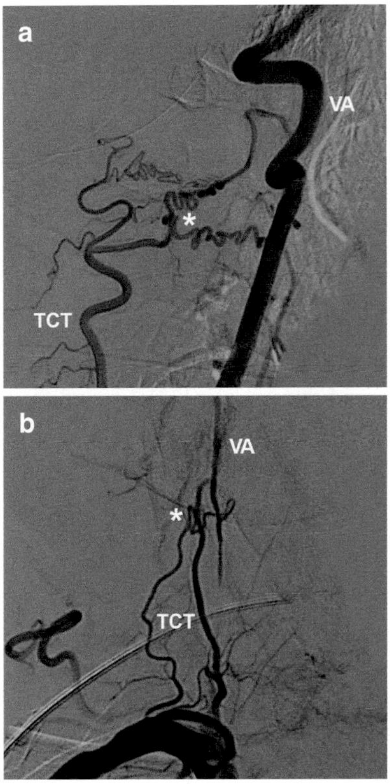

Fig. 7.7 Anastomosis between VA and TCT. The images are of the cases from our institute, and the anastomosis between VA and TCT became apparent after VA occlusion. (**a**) DSA shows anastomosis between the VA and TCA at the high cervical level (asterisk). (**b**) DSA shows the anastomosis between the VA and TCA at the middle cervical level (asterisk). Abbreviations: *DSA* digital subtraction angiography, *TCT* thyrocervical trunk, *VA* vertebral artery

CEAVFs may be initiated by thrombosis in the epidural space; after epidural thrombosis, intravenous stasis and/or acute hydrostatic disturbances within epidural compartments might reinforce the development of venous thrombosis [37]. Then, the epidural arteries around the thrombus were recruited, including the numerous osseous and epidural branches of the VA, the TCT, and the CCT, and they were often anastomosed (Fig. 7.7) [21, 38]. Because of the relatively rich supply of feeding arteries and abundant epidural space, CEAVF tends to occur at the C4–7 spinal canal, and even the bone can be involved [29]. In our review, C4–7 levels accounted for 73.7% of CEAVFs.

CEAVFs with a single feeding artery were relatively rare; multiple feeding arteries were more common, and the VA was also the most common feeding artery [4, 12, 18, 19, 26]. In our review, the model of multiple feeding arteries accounted for 72.8% of patients, and the VA was also the most common feeding artery in 68.2% of cases. Anatomically, the cervical vertebral venous plexus is composed of vertical, valveless channels that extend along the entire course of the spinal canal; thus, the drainage of a CEAVF may be extensive [7, 39].

Normally, an antireflux-impeding mechanism between both the epidural and perimedullary venous systems works well, resulting from narrowing and zigzagging of the vein walls while crossing the dura [9]. Therefore, the drainage of CEAVF can be limited to the epidural venous plexus. In previous reports, type A is less common than type B, accounting for 3% of spinal epidural AVFs in all locations, which illustrates that it is uncommon for an epidural AVF to shunt arterialized blood into the spinal venous system [4, 40]. In this review, type A accounted for 18.2% of CEAVFs. CEAVFs are classified as type B (B1 or B2). Type B2 CEAVFs are rarely reported because they are asymptomatic (Fig. 7.1a) [4].

The natural history of type B2 CEAVFs is unknown: they may remain silent or develop a mass effect due to thrombosis and transform into type B1. Type B1 CEAVF appears difficult to stabilize, although, rarely, CEAVF can have spontaneous regression [41]. In this review, most defects of type B1 had a progressive history. During progression, if type B CEAVFs induce the acute disruption of dural antireflux mechanisms, the radicular vein can become involved, and type B CEAVFs evolve into type A [1, 42].

Here, it should be noted that type A CEAVF may be disguised as type B1 on digital subtraction angiography (DSA) by the occlusion of intradural reflux due to compression or thrombosis. For instance, in a report by Miyamoto et al., the patient suffered sudden tetraparesis; magnetic resonance imaging showed cervical cord edema, but DSA failed to show that the CEAVF had intradural reflux. A reasonable explanation was that a type A CEAVF took on the appearance of type B after occlusion of the intramedullary drainage [24]. Additionally, the patient in Fig. 7.6 suffered subarachnoid hemorrhage, and DSA showed CEAVF without intramedullary vein drainage, which further supports the hypothesis [43].

Type B1 and A CEAVFs can lead to severe spinal cord dysfunction through compression, venous hypertension, or hemorrhage, presenting with radiculopathy and myelopathy [2]. Therefore, these patients should undergo surgery or EVT. Type A CEAVFs have a significantly higher deterioration rate than type B CEAVFs, which makes early intervention more urgent [13, 40, 44, 45]. The goal of CEAVF treatment is to disconnect the arteriovenous shunt; in particular, intradural intramedullary drainage must be completely interrupted [46]. Precise localization of the fistula point is essential, and the fistulous zone is often the arterialized epidural pouch [9]. Fortunately, venous pouches were observed in 86.4% of CEAVFs in this review. Treatment should be aimed at the venous pouch.

Currently, EVT, including TAE, TVE, and combinations of the two, is becoming a popular method to treat CEAVFs [8, 46, 47]. EVT is effective alone or in combination. The rates of complete or near-complete occlusion of the spinal epidural AVF with EVT ranged from 73.3% to 94.4%, and the rates of symptom improvement ranged from 62.5% to 91% [29]. In this review, complete obliteration via TAE or TVE was achieved in 68.2% of CEAVFs, while embolization was incomplete in 31.8%, and most of the incompletely embolized CEAVFs were cured after follow-up or subsequent surgery. In a review by Huang et al., the initial rate of complete AVF obliteration by EVT was 55%, and the rate increased to 92% during the follow-up [4]. To improve the rate of complete occlusion, the new technique was helpful, such as the pressure cooker technique using the Scepter Mini dual-lumen balloon (MicroVention, Aliso Viejo, California, USA) or coiling to prevent collateral inflow [47, 48].

In general, EVT is safe; in this review, only 9.5% of CEAVFs developed complications due to the increased mass effect, and these complications were resolved by surgery and conservative treatment with observation. However, the resolution of all pathological signs on imaging did not guarantee complete recovery from clinical symptoms because the spinal cord was irreversibly injured in some cases. In this review, complete or significant recovery was observed in 78.9% of CEAVFs, and moderate improvement was observed in 21.1%.

Materials that can be used for embolization include N-butyl-2-cyanoacrylate glue, Onyx (Medtronic, Irvine, California, USA), and coils [36, 46, 47]. If the lesion has extremely high flow and expanded drainage channels, coils may be used to reduce blood flow, which can cause the liquid embolic agent to form a plug [49]. Intramedullary vein drainage must be obliterated, but care must be taken to prevent embolic agents from occluding the intramedullary arteries [50].

7.5 Conclusions

CEAVFs create a complex connection between feeding and drainage vessels in the epidural space. They can be classified into type A and type B. EVT is an effective treatment for CEAVFs. Complete obliteration of nearly 70% of CEAVFs can be achieved via EVT. In this study, nearly 80% of patients made a complete or significant recovery during follow-up.

Acknowledgments We thank Dr. Lai Qu (Intensive Care Unit, The First Hospital of Jilin University) for drawing Fig. 7.3.

References

1. Shetty GS, Singh V, Prasad SN, Phadke RV, Neyaz Z, Udiya A, et al. Spinal epidural fistulas–a separate entity to dural fistulas with different angioarchitecture and treatment approach. World Neurosurg. 2021;149:e600–e11.
2. Yu JX, Hong T, Ma YJ, Ling F, Zhang HQ. A new type of spinal epidural arteriovenous fistulas causes spinal epidural hemorrhage: an analysis of five cases and natural history consideration. World Neurosurg. 2017;103:371–9.

3. Reul J, Braun V. Spinal arteriovenous epidural fistula with acute paraplegia. Diagnosis and neurointerventional emergency treatment. A case report. Interv Neuroradiol. 2007;13(1):75–8.
4. Huang W, Gross BA, Du R. Spinal extradural arteriovenous fistulas: clinical article. J Neurosurg Spine. 2013;19(5):582–90.
5. Clarke MJ, Patrick TA, White JB, Cloft HJ, Krauss WE, Lindell EP, et al. Spinal extradural arteriovenous malformations with parenchymal drainage: venous drainage variability and implications in clinical manifestations. Neurosurg Focus. 2009;26(1):E5.
6. Niizuma K, Endo T, Sato K, Takada S, Sugawara T, Mikawa S, et al. Surgical treatment of spinal extradural arteriovenous fistula with parenchymal drainage: report on 5 cases. Neurosurgery. 2013;73(2 Suppl Operative):onsE287–94; discussion onsE93-4.
7. Takai K, Shojima M, Imai H, Saito N, Taniguchi M. Microsurgical and endovascular treatments of spinal extradural arteriovenous fistulas with or without intradural venous drainage. World Neurosurg. 2018;111:e819–e29.
8. Nasr DM, Brinjikji W, Clarke MJ, Lanzino G. Clinical presentation and treatment outcomes of spinal epidural arteriovenous fistulas. J Neurosurg Spine. 2017;26(5):613–20.
9. Mull M, Othman A, Dafotakis M, Hans FJ, Schubert GA, Jablawi F. Spinal epidural arteriovenous fistula with perimedullary venous reflux: clinical and neuroradiologic features of an underestimated vascular disorder. AJNR Am J Neuroradiol. 2018;39(11):2095–102.
10. Abecassis ZA, Emerson S, Zhang F, Ghodke B, Sekhar LN. Embolization and resection of epidural spinal arteriovenous malformations: case report. Oper Neurosurg (Hagerstown). 2022;24(1):e50–4.
11. Stewart LA, Clarke M, Rovers M, Riley RD, Simmonds M, Stewart G, et al. Preferred reporting items for systematic review and meta-analyses of individual participant data: the PRISMA-IPD statement. JAMA. 2015;313(16):1657–65.
12. Rangel-Castilla L, Holman PJ, Krishna C, Trask TW, Klucznik RP, Diaz OM. Spinal extradural arteriovenous fistulas: a clinical and radiological description of different types and their novel treatment with onyx. J Neurosurg Spine. 2011;15(5):541–9.
13. Aminoff MJ, Logue V. The prognosis of patients with spinal vascular malformations. Brain. 1974;97(1):211–8.
14. Cahan LD, Higashida RT, Halbach VV, Hieshima GB. Variants of radiculomeningeal vascular malformations of the spine. J Neurosurg. 1987;66(3):333–7.
15. Willinsky R, TerBrugge K, Lasjaunias P, Montanera W. The variable presentations of craniocervical and cervical dural arteriovenous malformations. Surg Neurol. 1990;34(2):118–23.
16. Willinsky R, terBrugge K, Montanera W, Wallace MC, Gentili F. Spinal epidural arteriovenous fistulas: arterial and venous approaches to embolization. AJNR Am J Neuroradiol. 1993;14(4):812–7.
17. Kohno M, Takahashi H, Ide K, Ishijima B, Yamada K, Nemoto S. A cervical dural arteriovenous fistula in a patient presenting with radiculopathy. Case report J Neurosurg. 1996;84(1):119–23.
18. Goyal M, Willinsky R, Montanera W, terBrugge K. Paravertebral arteriovenous malformations with epidural drainage: clinical spectrum, imaging features, and results of treatment. AJNR Am J Neuroradiol. 1999;20(5):749–55.
19. Asai J, Hayashi T, Fujimoto T, Suzuki R. Exclusively epidural arteriovenous fistula in the cervical spine with spinal cord symptoms: case report. Neurosurgery. 2001;48(6):1372–5; discussion 5–6.
20. Chuang NA, Shroff MM, Willinsky RA, Drake JM, Dirks PB, Armstrong DC. Slow-flow spinal epidural AVF with venous ectasias: two pediatric case reports. AJNR Am J Neuroradiol. 2003;24(9):1901–5.
21. Chul Suh D, Gon Choi C, Bo Sung K, Kim KK, Chul RS. Spinal osseous epidural arteriovenous fistula with multiple small arterial feeders converging to a round fistular nidus as a target of venous approach. AJNR Am J Neuroradiol. 2004;25(1):69–73.
22. Kawabori M, Hida K, Yano S, Asano T, Iwasaki Y. Cervical epidural arteriovenous fistula with radiculopathy mimicking cervical spondylosis. Neurol Med Chir (Tokyo). 2009;49(3):108–13.
23. Dabus G, Nimmagadda A, Russell EJ. Cervical epidural arteriovenous fistula presenting with radiculopathy: transvenous embolization using onyx. Interv Neuroradiol. 2011;17(3):380–5.
24. Miyamoto N, Naito I, Takatama S, Iwai T, Tomizawa S, Inoue HK. Spinal epidural arteriovenous fistulas with unusual manifestation of sudden onset of severe neurological deficits: case report. Neurol Med Chir (Tokyo). 2013;53(12):896–901.
25. Ramanathan D, Levitt MR, Sekhar LN, Kim LJ, Hallam DK, Ghodke BV. Management of spinal epidural arteriovenous fistulas: interventional techniques and results. J Neurointerv Surg. 2014;6(2):144–9.
26. Nakagawa I, Park HS, Hironaka Y, Wada T, Kichikawa K, Nakase H. Cervical spinal epidural arteriovenous fistula with coexisting spinal anterior spinal artery aneurysm presenting as subarachnoid hemorrhage–case report. J Stroke Cerebrovasc Dis. 2014;23(10):e461–e5.
27. Kasliwal MK, Dua SG, Mangubat EZ, Lopes DK. Compressive cervical myelopathy secondary to totally extradural spinal arteriovenous fistula. Neurol India. 2015;63(5):790–2.
28. Romano A, Consoli A, Tari Capone F, Biraschi F, Suma G, Mangiafico S, et al. An epidural arteriovenous fistula studied with time-resolved imaging of contrast kinetics (TRICKS) sequence. Neuroradiol J. 2016;29(6):455–7.
29. Song Y, Cho SH, Lee DW, Sheen JJ, Shin JH, Suh DC. Osseous versus nonosseous spinal epidural arteriovenous fistulas: experiences of 13 patients. AJNR Am J Neuroradiol. 2019;40(1):129–34.

30. Goyal S, Sinha AK, Agarwal HN. Completely extradural spinal arteriovenous fistula (abnormal direct connection between arteries and extradural venous plexus) with totally extradural venous drainage causing compressive cervical myelopathy. Asian J Neurosurg. 2020;15(4):1081–4.
31. Park D, Kim D, Kang DH, Lee S, Cho DC. Cervical radiculopathy caused by spinal epidural arteriovenous fistula (SEDAVF) without intradural drainage: a case report and literature review. Korean J Neurotrauma. 2022;18(1):145–9.
32. Najjar A, Zairi F, Sunna T, Weil A, Estrade L, Weill A, et al. Minimally invasive approach for the treatment of lumbar epidural arteriovenous fistulas with intradural venous reflux. Neurochirurgie. 2016;62(5):258–62.
33. Hui F, Trosselo MP, Meisel HJ, Alvarez H, Sequeira E, Lasjaunias P. Paraspinal arteriovenous shunts in children. Neuroradiology. 1994;36(1):69–73.
34. Paolini S, Colonnese C, Galasso V, Morace R, Tola S, Esposito V, et al. Extradural arteriovenous fistulas involving the vertebral artery in neurofibromatosis type 1. J Neurosurg Spine. 2008;8(2):181–5.
35. Hauck EF, Nauta HJ. Spontaneous spinal epidural arteriovenous fistulae in neurofibromatosis type-1. Surg Neurol. 2006;66(2):215–21.
36. Brinjikji W, Yin R, Nasr DM, Lanzino G. Spinal epidural arteriovenous fistulas. J Neurointerv Surg. 2016;8(12):1305–10.
37. Hiramatsu M, Ishibashi R, Suzuki E, Miyazaki Y, Murai S, Takai H, et al. Incidence and clinical characteristics of spinal arteriovenous shunts: hospital-based surveillance in Okayama, Japan. J Neurosurg Spine. 2021;36(4):670–7.
38. Louis RG Jr, Yen CP, Mohila CA, Mandell JW, Sheehan J. A rare intraosseous arteriovenous malformation of the spine. J Neurosurg Spine. 2011;15(3):336–9.
39. Griessenauer CJ, Raborn J, Foreman P, Shoja MM, Loukas M, Tubbs RS. Venous drainage of the spine and spinal cord: a comprehensive review of its history, embryology, anatomy, physiology, and pathology. Clin Anat. 2015;28(1):75–87.
40. Feng Y, Yu J, Xu J, He C, Bian L, Li G, et al. Natural history and clinical outcomes of paravertebral arteriovenous shunts. Stroke. 2021;52(12):3873–82.
41. Kinoshita M, Asai A, Komeda S, Yoshimura K, Takeda J, Uesaka T, et al. Spontaneous regression of a spinal extradural arteriovenous fistula after delivery by cesarean section. Neurol Med Chir (Tokyo). 2009;49(7):313–5.
42. Mathur S, Symons SP, Huynh TJ, Muthusami P, Montanera W, Bharatha A. First-pass contrast-enhanced MRA for pretherapeutic diagnosis of spinal epidural arteriovenous fistulas with intradural venous reflux. AJNR Am J Neuroradiol. 2017;38(1):195–9.
43. Puri AS, Telischak NA, Vissapragada R, Thomas AJ. Analysis of venous drainage in three patients with extradural spinal arteriovenous fistulae at the craniovertebral junction with potentially benign implication. J Neurointerv Surg. 2014;6(2):150–5.
44. Takai K, Taniguchi M. Comparative analysis of spinal extradural arteriovenous fistulas with or without intradural venous drainage: a systematic literature review. Neurosurg Focus. 2012;32(5):E8.
45. Nasr DM, Brinjikji W, Rabinstein AA, Lanzino G. Clinical outcomes following corticosteroid administration in patients with delayed diagnosis of spinal arteriovenous fistulas. J Neurointerv Surg. 2017;9(6):607–10.
46. Takai K, Endo T, Yasuhara T, Seki T, Watanabe K, Tanaka Y, et al. Microsurgical versus endovascular treatment of spinal epidural arteriovenous fistulas with intradural venous drainage: a multicenter study of 81 patients. J Neurosurg Spine. 2020;33(3):381–91.
47. Al-Abdulwahhab AH, Song Y, Kwon B, Suh DC. Embolization tactics of spinal epidural arteriovenous fistulas. Neurointervention. 2021;16(3):252–9.
48. Clarençon F, Shotar E, Pouvelle A, Premat K, Lenck S, Drir M, et al. Spinal epidural arteriovenous fistula embolization with ethylene vinyl alcohol (EVOH) copolymer using the scepter mini dual-lumen balloon. J Neurointerv Surg. 2021;13(5):492.
49. Lanzino G, D'Urso PI, Kallmes DF, Cloft HJ. Onyx embolization of extradural spinal arteriovenous malformations with intradural venous drainage. Neurosurgery. 2012;70(2):329–33.
50. Brinjikji W, Colombo E, Cloft HJ, Lanzino G. Clinical and imaging characteristics of spinal dural arteriovenous fistulas and spinal epidural arteriovenous fistulas. Neurosurgery. 2021;88(3):666–73.

8 Current Status of the Treatment for Spinal Dural Arteriovenous Fistulas

Jinlu Yu

Abstract

Spinal dural arteriovenous fistula (SDAVF) is a rare disease. Currently, the understanding of SDAVFs is not complete. Therefore, we performed a review of this condition. The following characteristics of SDAVF were discussed: natural history and current diagnosed state, anatomy and angioarchitecture, therapeutic goals and options, therapeutic techniques, complications and recurrence, and prognosis. We found that SDAVF is a rare disabling disease and is often misdiagnosed. SDAVF has a poor natural history, and spontaneous disappearance is uncommon. SDAVF has a complex angioarchitecture, which is the consequence of the arteriovenous shunt and venous medullary outflow impairment or obstruction. SDAVF is a potentially curable cause and thus should be treated aggressively. Surgical and endovascular interventions can be used. Microsurgery appeared to be an efficient method in terms of the clinical effect, radicality, and lower recurrence in comparison with endovascular embolization. However, endovascular embolization is becoming popular due to advances in the techniques. Although there are complications and unsatisfactory prognoses, SDAVF treatments are still recommended; moreover, the sooner the treatment is administered, the better the prognosis.

Keywords

Spinal dural arteriovenous fistula · Microsurgery · Embolization · Complication · Prognosis

8.1 Introduction

A spinal dural arteriovenous fistula (SDAVF) is a type I spinal vascular malformation in the dura, consisting of an arteriovenous shunt without an intervening capillary network (Fig. 8.1) [1]. SDAVF is often supplied by one or more radiculomeningeal arteries and ends in a single draining vein; therefore, the arterial flow is transferred to engorged spinal venous collaterals in a retrograde manner [2]. SDAVF is rare, with an annual incidence of 5–10 cases/one million persons, accounting for 80–85% of all spinal vascular malformations [3–5]. Patients with SDAVF are typically middle-aged men, and men are affected 5 times more often than women [6]. SDAVF is exceedingly rare in children [7].

The etiology of SDAVF is unknown, although it is most likely an acquired disease after throm-

J. Yu (✉)
Department of Neurosurgery, First Hospital of Jilin University, Changchun, China
e-mail: jlyu@jlu.edu.cn

X. Lv (ed.), *Endovascular and Neurovascular Surgery for Spinal Vascular Malformations*,
https://doi.org/10.1007/978-981-97-4661-3_8

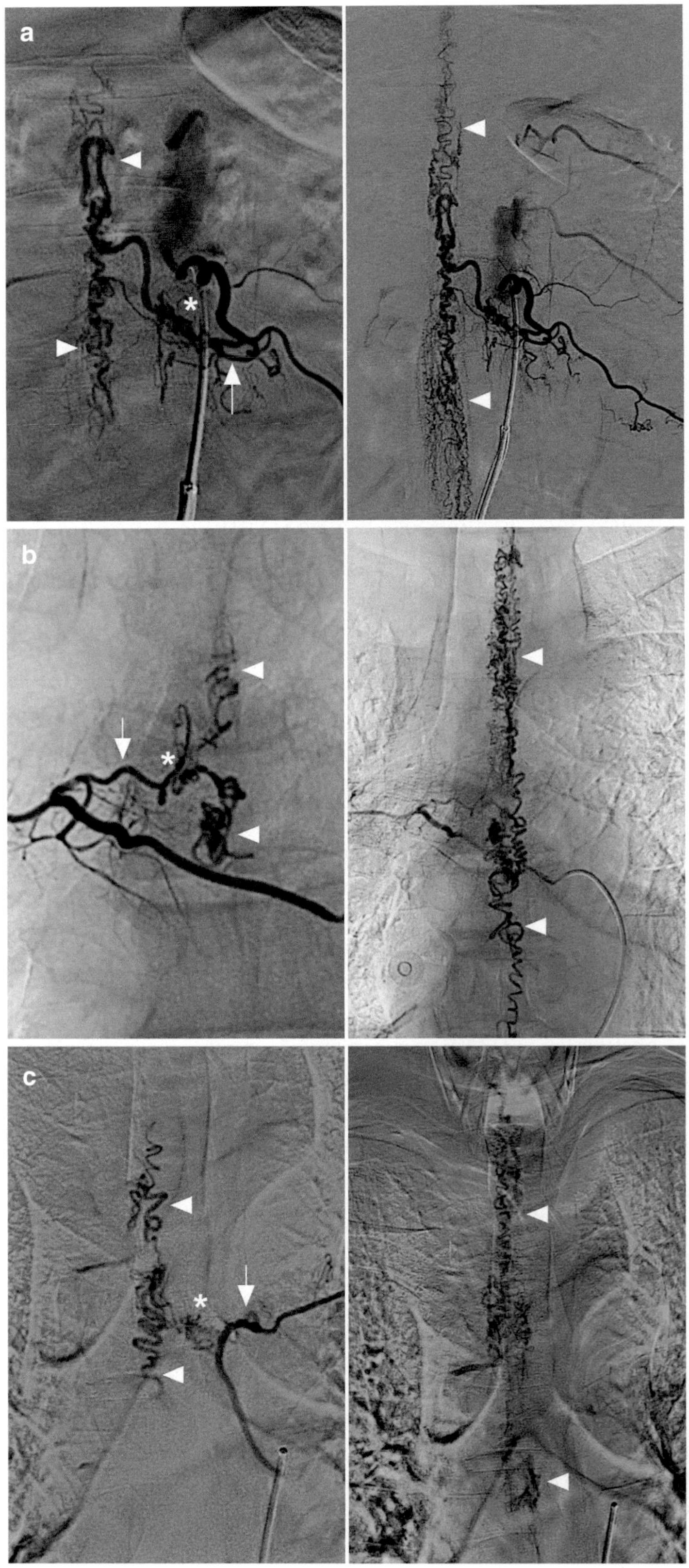

Fig. 8.1 Angiographic features of SDAVF. (**a–c**) Case A was a lumber SDAVF. Cases in B and C were thoracic SDAVFs. The left images in **a–c** are from the arterial phase, and the right images are from the venous phase. Arrows in **a–c** indicate the feeding artery. Asterisks in **a–c** indicate the fistula point. Arrowheads in **a–c** indicate the draining vein. Abbreviation: *SDAVF* spinal dural arteriovenous fistula

bosis or because of a hypercoagulable state [6]. It has been suggested that SDAVF is primarily a venous disease, often presenting with progressive and ascending myelopathy and/or radiculopathy [8, 9]. SDAVF is a potentially curable cause and thus should be treated aggressively; microsurgery and endovascular embolization are the treatment choices [10]. Currently, with the progress in SDAVF treatment, an updated review is still necessary. Additionally, we provide educational images and cases in this review to increase the reading interest. These images and cases are from our hospital, and there are no copyright disputes.

8.2 Natural History and Current Diagnosed State

8.2.1 Natural History

In general, SDAVF has a poor natural history [11]. Spontaneous regression is uncommon [12]. As described by Aminoff and Logue, if left untreated, severe locomotor disability may develop in nearly 20% of patients within 6 months of the onset of functional impairment in the legs; 50% of untreated patients are severely disabled, and nearly 10% are able to walk independently after 3 years [13]. SDAVF is often a slow progressive myelopathy, and a sudden onset of symptoms is rare [4, 14]. Valsalva-like maneuvers can increase venous pressure and compromise venous drainage of SDAVF, and these maneuvers may also change the natural history when there is rapid deterioration of the clinical course [15].

Steroid administration can change the natural history, and acute neurological deterioration in patients with SDAVF receiving steroids has been reported, even after successful obliteration of the fistula. This is because steroids produce hydrostatic retention, hypervolemia, and secondary venous hypertension, which may lead to worsening of spinal cord edema [16–18]. Therefore, steroids should be avoided in patients with SDAVFs.

8.2.2 Diagnosed State

The initial symptoms of SDAVF can be nonspecific, nonlocalizing, and gradual. Therefore, misdiagnoses are frequent and are attributed to aging, stress, or exercise [3, 19, 20]. A diagnostic delay may range from 1 to 2 years, at which time 78% of patients have severe lower limb weakness and 19% are wheelchair bound [21–23]. Currently, in China, SDAVF is also an underdiagnosed disease [24]. In Zhang et al.'s report, the diagnostic time was 14.7 months from symptom onset [25]. Therefore, SDAVFs should be considered in all patients with paraparesis, sensory deficits, or bowel/bladder dysfunction [26].

In addition, a major factor that contributes to a misdiagnosis or a delayed diagnosis of SDAVF is false-negative spinal angiographic imaging findings due to the fistulas having limited shunting owing to the relatively low venous hypertension and technical difficulty of the procedure [27]. Furthermore, SDAVFs can originate far from the areas of visible pathological features seen on the initial MR image or CT scan. The failure to perform angiographic evaluations at every spinal level can lead to false-negative results [27].

8.3 Anatomy and Angioarchitecture

8.3.1 Feeding and Draining Vessels of the Normal Spinal Cord

The spinal artery from the intersegmental artery supplies the spinal cord, dura, and adjacent structures. The spinal artery gives off the radicular artery, which supplies the spinal nerve root, the radiculomeningeal branch (dural artery) of the spinal artery supplies the dura, and the radiculomedullary artery of the spinal artery supplies the spinal cord via the anterior spinal artery and paired posterior spinal arteries [28].

Many arteries can give off spinal arteries, including the vertebral artery, deep cervical artery, ascending cervical artery, intercostal artery, and lumbar and lateral sacral arteries

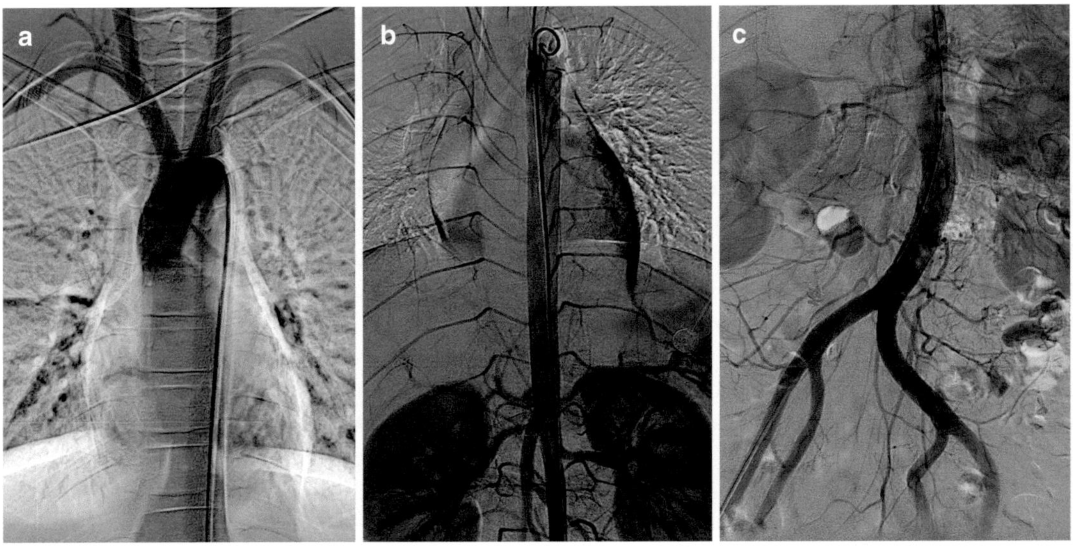

Fig. 8.2 Overview of intersegmental arteries. (**a**) Aorta angiography showing that intersegmental arteries may arise from the aorta, vertebral artery, thyrocervical trunk, and costocervical trunk. (**b** and **c**) Descending aorta angiographies clearly showing the thoracic and lumbar (**b**) and lumbar and sacral (**c**) arteries

(Fig. 8.2) [24]. The venous drainage of the spinal cord is collected by the anterior and posterior longitudinal spinal veins linked together into radicular veins and then via transdural emissaries into intervertebral, longitudinal efferent, and other level-specific venous channels [29, 30].

8.3.2 Angioarchitecture of SDAVF

Approximately 80% of SDAVFs are found along the lower thoracic cord surface between the levels of T5 and L2 [19, 31, 32]. Low cervical DAVFs (below C2 and above T1) are rare (Fig. 8.3) [9]. Most lesions are solitary, double, or multiple and may be present in 0.5–4% of SDAVFs [33–36]. SDAVFs are often located in the dura of the dorsal nerve root sleeve and/or adjacent dura at the intervertebral foramen [3, 37]. However, in the conus/lumbar regions, SDAVFs are not always the dorsal types [38, 39]. SDAVFs are often supplied by adjacent segmental radicular arteries that are not at the same level of the fistula point, and the feeding artery may be single but also uncommonly can be multiple [24, 32].

In SDAVFs, the feeding artery splits into multiple vessels on the outer dural surface and crosses the dura to the inner dural surface; these vessels gather into a single arterialized draining vein, which appears to be the caput medusae [26, 38, 40–42]. Therefore, more arterial blood flow is delivered into the perimedullary vein in a retrograde manner.

Because the normal local radicular venous drainage in SDAVF is often missing, stenosed, or occluded, the blood has to flow over a long distance along the dorsal perimedullary veins, upward, downward, or both to arrive at the outflow into the epidural network, depending on the patent intradural-to-epidural venous connections and the pressure in the epidural space [16, 24, 43, 44]. An insufficient venous outlet plays a significant role in the development and/or persistence of SDAVFs [38]. SDAVF may remain silent if the radicular venous drainage is patent, especially for cervical lesions with abundant collateral venous pathways [45]. However, when the venous drainage system is inadequate to cope with the blood volume, progressive myelopathy will develop, resulting in decreased tissue perfusion with edema and progressive loss of cord function from the venous medullary congestion and increased pressure (Fig. 8.4) [14].

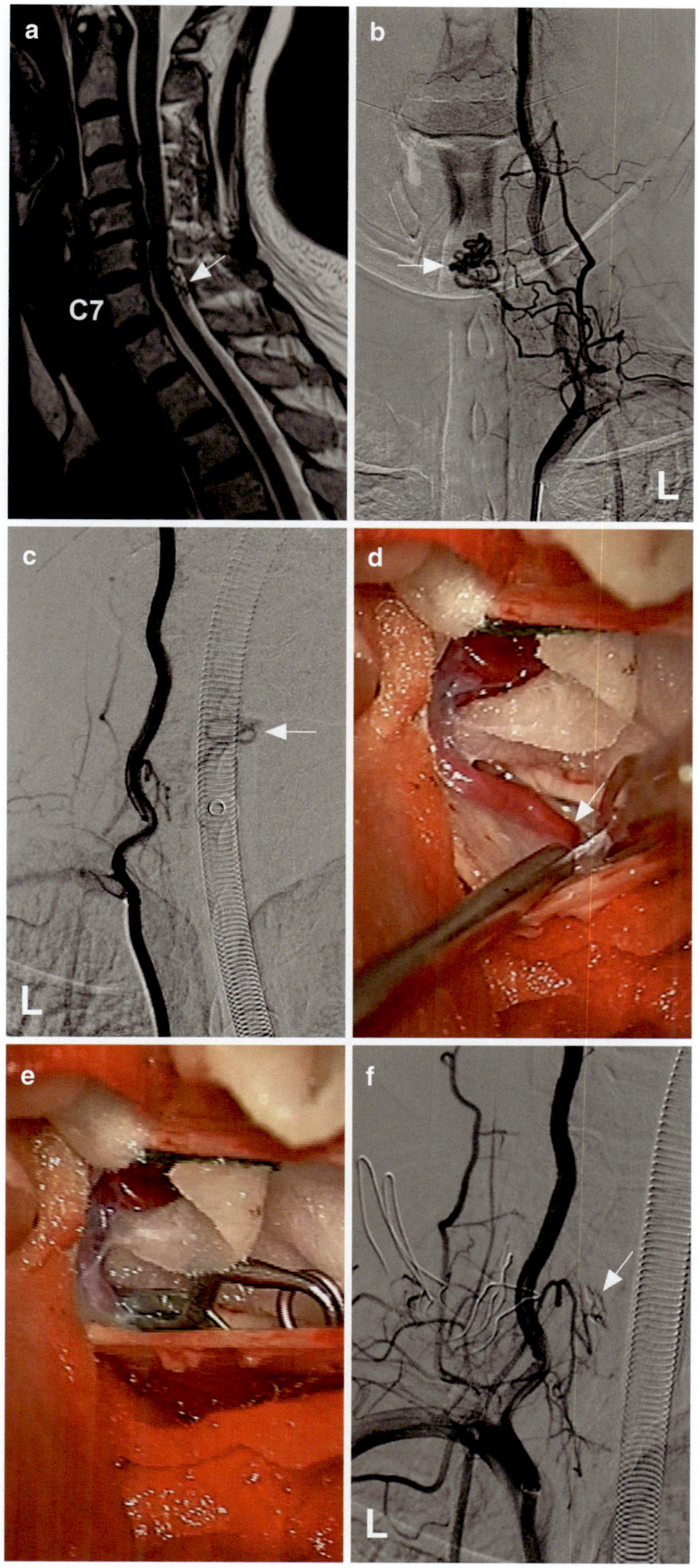

Fig. 8.3 Cervical SDAVF treated by microsurgery. (**a**) MR T2WI showing an intradural mass of vessels (arrow) on the dorsal surface of the spinal cord. (**b**) Angiography of the left subclavian artery showing an SDAVF (arrow) supplied by the thyrocervical trunk. (**c**) Preoperative angiography of the left subclavian artery with the patient in the prone position, and the SDAVF (arrow) is shown. (**d**) Intraoperative image showing an intradural arterialized draining vein (arrow) attached to the inner dura. (**e**) Intraoperative image showing that the arterialized draining vein was clipped temporarily. (**f**) After clipping the arterialized draining vein, intraoperative angiography showed that the SDAVF was completely occluded, and the arrow indicates the temporary clip. Abbreviations: *C7* seventh cervical vertebra, *L* left, *SDAVF* spinal dural arteriovenous fistula

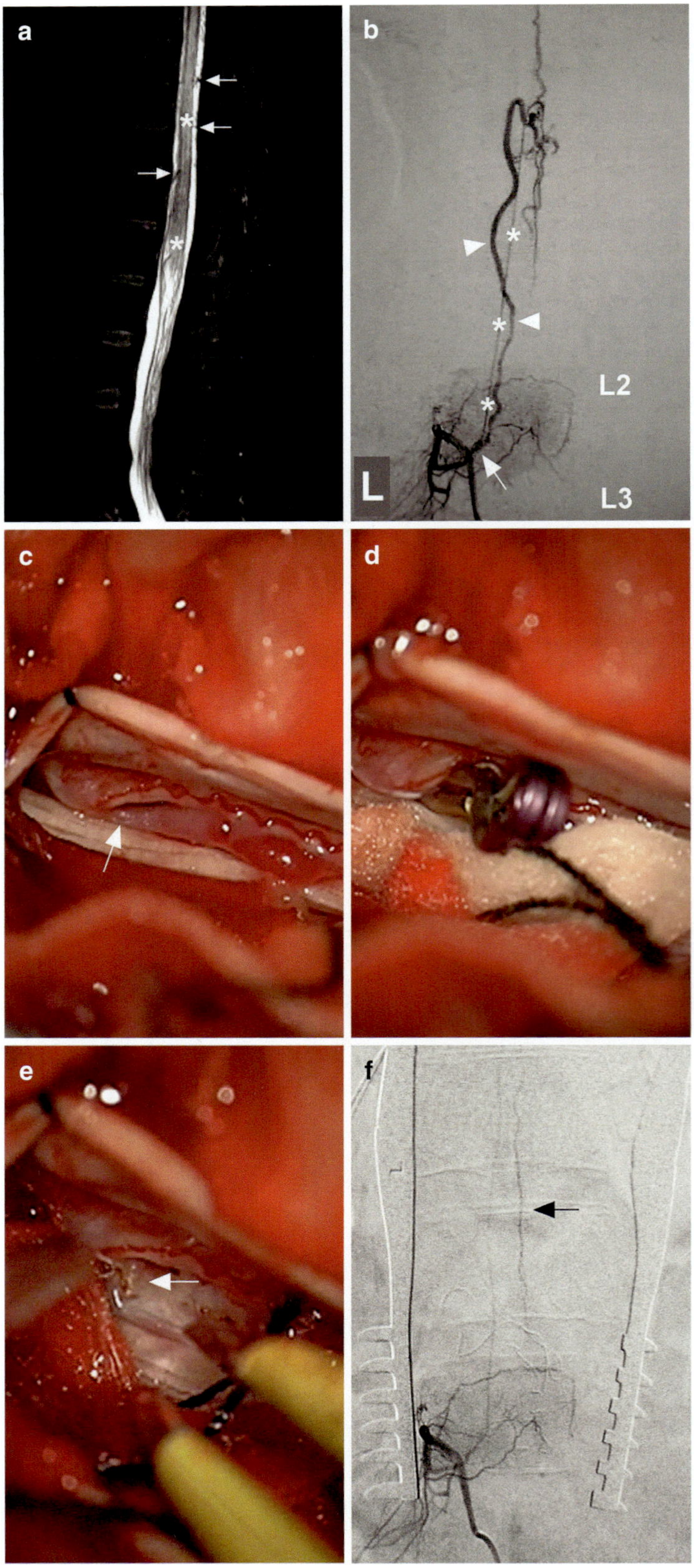

Fig. 8.4 Lumber SDAVF treated by microsurgery. (**a**) MR T2WI showing dilated vessels (arrows) on the ventral and dorsal surfaces of the spinal cord and edema of the spinal cord (asterisks). (**b**) Preoperative angiography of the lumbar artery with the patient in the prone position showing the SDAVF (arrow) between the L2 and L3 vertebral levels. The arrowheads indicate the draining vein, and the asterisks indicate the anterior spinal artery (artery of Adamkiewicz). (**c**–**e**) Intraoperative images showing an intradural arterialized draining vein (arrow in **c**) attached to the inner dura, an arterialized draining vein (arrow in **d**) that is clipped temporarily, and an arterialized draining vein (arrow in **f**) that was cut. (**f**) Postoperative angiography showing complete occlusion of the SDAVF and preservation of the anterior spinal artery (arrow). Abbreviations: *L* left, *L2* second lumbar vertebra, *L3* third lumbar vertebra, *SDAVF* spinal dural arteriovenous fistula

8.3.3 Classification of SDAVF

Similar to intracranial DAVFs, SDAVFs can be classified according to the Cognard subtypes: type I, anterograde outflow into the spinoradicular (dural) vein or extradural venous plexus; type II, retrograde outflow into the extradural venous plexus and pial venous plexus; and type III, retrograde outflow into the pial venous plexus only [46].

8.4 Therapeutic Goal and Options

Based on the poor natural history, the treatment of SDAVF is mandatory and aims at the interruption of the venous side of the SDAVF and restoration of the normal venous drainage of the spinal cord [19, 26]. Even for asymptomatic SDAVF, treatment should be offered [45, 47]. If the patient refuses treatment, aspirin should be recommended to reduce the risk of venous thrombosis to increase the pressure of the spinal cord venous drainage [43]. Surgical and endovascular interventions can be used to treat SDAVFs [48]. For type II SDAVFs, when both intra- and extradural venous drainage are present, complete surgical excision or embolization of all the intra- and extradural venous drainage is recommended [44, 49].

Microsurgery appears to be an efficient method in terms of the clinical effect, radicality, and lower recurrence (Fig. 8.4) [5, 32, 50–52]. In recent years, advances in endovascular techniques have greatly improved the ability to treat a majority of SDAVF patients, especially for those patients with a reduced physical condition (Fig. 8.5) [53, 54]. The increased use of endovascular embolization has led to many recurrent SDAVFs [55]. For SDAVFs in which endovascular embolization does not obtain a cure or recurs, microsurgery can be recommended [56–58]. Endovascular embolization increases the degree of surgical complexity because of the dissection and the identification of vessels and tissues that are filled with embolic material.

In addition, when SDAVF harbors a common segmental artery supplying both the fistula and anterior spinal artery (especially for the artery of Adamkiewicz) (Fig. 8.4) or posterior spinal artery, which can be seen in 14% of SDAVFs, endovascular embolization should not be attempted due to the possibility of developing a dangerous anastomosis to the radiculomedullary arteries, which will result in embolization risks of spinal cord infarction. In these instances, microsurgery can be recommended [3, 19, 26, 38, 59].

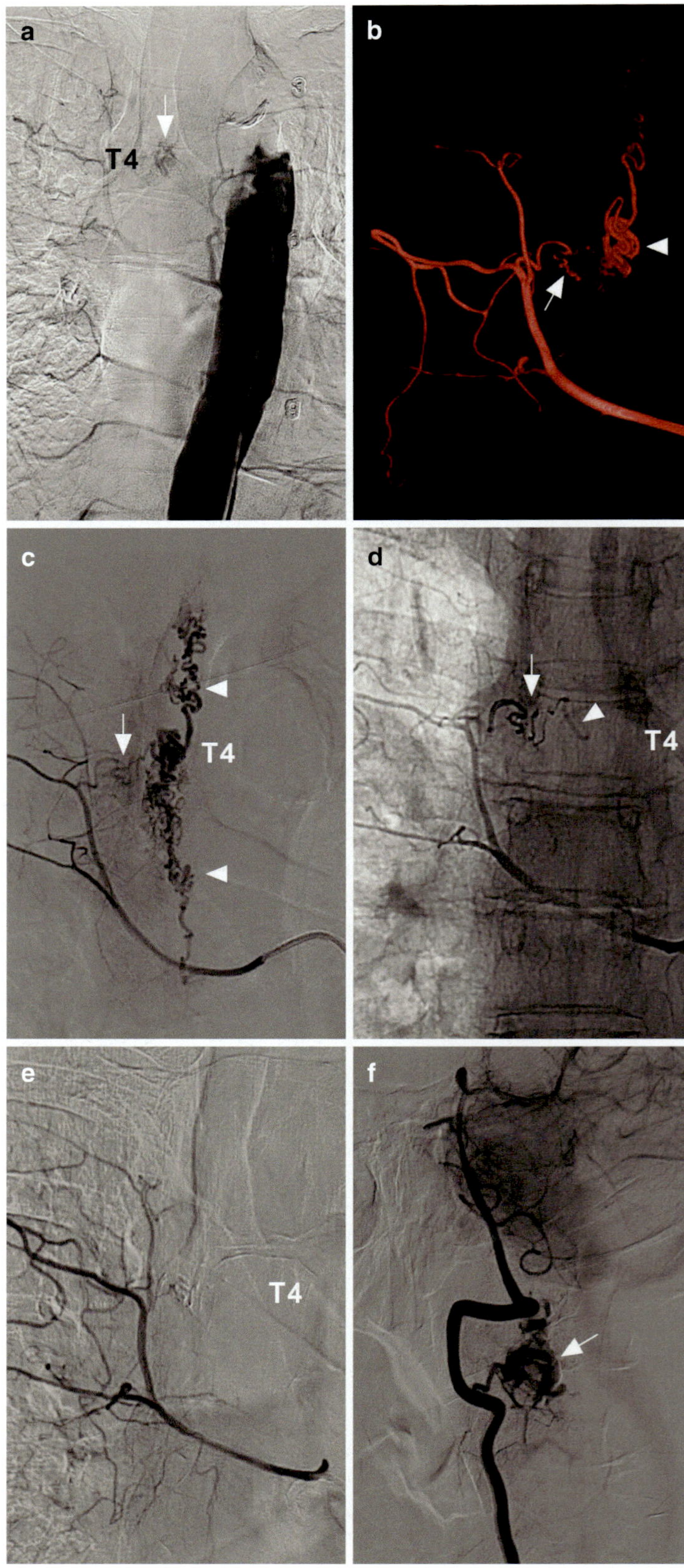

Fig. 8.5 Thoracic SDAVF treated by endovascular embolization. (**a**) Descending aorta angiography showing an SDAVF (arrow) at the T4 vertebral level. (**b** and **c**) Three-dimensional (**b**) and two-dimensional (**c**) angiographies of the intercostal artery showing the fistula point (arrows) and draining vein (arrowheads). (**d**) Unsubtracted angiography showing that the fistula (arrow) had been penetrated by Onyx into the proximal draining vein (arrowhead). (**e**) Six-month follow-up angiography of the intercostal artery showing complete embolization of the SDAVF without recanalization. (**f**) Vertebral artery angiography showing an associated epidural cervical arteriovenous fistula (arrow). Abbreviations: *T4* fourth thoracic vertebra, *SDAVF* spinal dural arteriovenous fistula. Note: The patient was a weak old woman with a reduced physical condition

8.5 Microsurgery Technique

Microsurgery can be performed via posterior laminectomy or hemilaminectomy [3, 46]. A major challenge is determining the accurate preoperative location of SDAVF. Intraoperative DSA can help to confirm the center of the surgical approach to reduce the region of surgical explosion (Fig. 8.6) [55]. After dura opening, the intravertebral foramen region should be sufficiently explored. The fistula is typically located in a dorsal arterialized vein and in a nerve root sleeve [60]. Then, the arterialized vein close to the dura can be coagulated and divided (Figs. 8.3 and 8.4) [41]. It is of utmost importance to preserve the artery of Adamkiewicz; it can share a common trunk with the feeding artery of the SDAVF. At this time, simple surgical interruption of the draining vein is a good choice (Fig. 8.4) [61].

In addition, it is crucial to avoid inadvertent venous sacrifice without disconnection of the fistula, which can lead to catastrophic consequences [62]. For microsurgery of SDAVF, intraoperative identification of the fistula and confirmation of its obliteration are important. Intraoperative DSA is the best choice when a temporary clip can be applied on the arterialized vein before coagulation and division (Fig. 8.3) [63]. In addition, fluorescein and indocyanine green arteriography or microvascular Doppler can provide real-time information about the precise location of SDAVFs [55, 64–67].

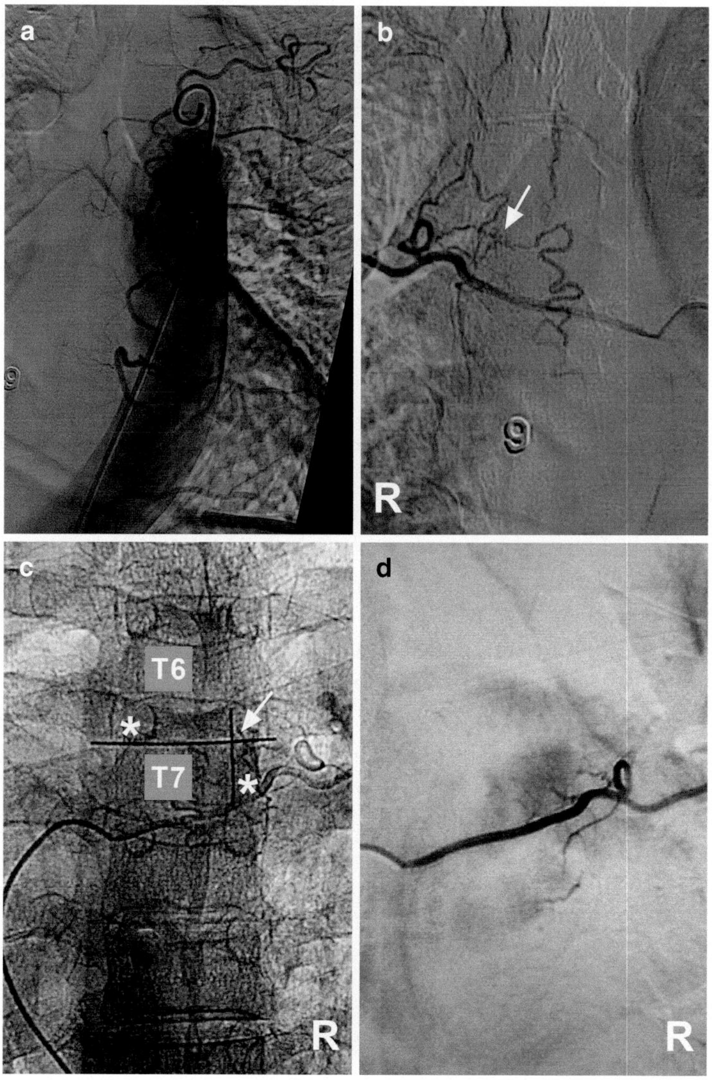

Fig. 8.6 Preoperative location of thoracic SDAVF. (**a**) Descending aorta angiography showing that no SDAVF can be found, which indicated the importance of superselective angiography. (**b**) Right intercostal artery angiography showing an SDAVF (arrow). (**c**) Unsubtracted preoperative angiography of the right intercostal artery with the patient in the prone position showing the fistula between the T6 and T7 vertebral levels at the junction (arrow) of horizontal and vertical lead bars (asterisks). (**d**) Postoperative angiography showing complete occlusion of the SDAVF. Abbreviations: *R* right, *SDAVF* spinal dural arteriovenous fistula, *T6* sixth thoracic vertebra, *T7* seventh thoracic vertebra

8.6 Endovascular Technique

Currently, the liquid embolic agents for endovascular embolization for SDAVFs mainly include N-butyl-2-cyanoacrylate (NBCA) and Onyx (Medtronic, Irvine, CA, USA) [19, 37]. For embolization of SDAVF, occlusion of the proximal draining vein plays an essential role (Fig. 8.5) [68]. Only interruption of the feeding artery with proximal occlusion alone is not considered effective, although it results in a transient improvement of symptoms [57].

Successful endovascular embolization requires a microcatheter to obtain the wedged position; at this time, the vessel lumen of the fistula feeder is blocked with a microcatheter tip, and the blood flow is arrested, which allows better penetration of the liquid embolic agent into the fistula and the proximal draining vein [69]. However, the wedged position cannot be obtained in all cases, especially in SDAVFs with tortuous feeders, and the microcatheter may fail to access the site of the fistula [26].

To improve the curative rate of endovascular embolization, if the feeding artery has a large diameter, the dual-lumen balloon and pressure cooker technique called the induced-wedge technique is helpful when it is not possible to navigate a flow-directed microcatheter to close the fistulous zone [42, 69, 70]. A dual-lumen Scepter C balloon (MicroVention, Tustin, USA) can increase the venous penetration of liquid embolic agents, and the balloon can block the reflux and favor anterograde migration of liquid embolic agents into the fistula [71]. In the pressure cooker technique, after the first microcatheter is placed into the fistula, a second microcatheter is used and is substituted for the balloon by performing coiling of the feeding artery to block the reflux, which can also favor the penetration of liquid embolic agents into the fistula [70].

8.7 Complications and Recurrence

8.7.1 Complications

In a meta-analysis by Goyal et al., the complication rates of microsurgery and endovascular embolization were 7.7% and 6.9%, respectively [51]. Microsurgical complications were associated with wounds, such as infections and hematomas of the surgical field and CSF leaks [38]. Complications with endovascular embolization were technique-related adverse events, such as microcatheter ruptures, spinal cord infarction, and other unintended ischemic complications due to nontarget embolization [70, 72].

In addition, after closure of the vein by microsurgery and embolization, in theory, there is a risk of retrograde venous thrombosis, which could involve veins that participate in the drainage of the normal spinal cord [49, 73]. Therefore, the patient is well hydrated and begins a low-dose heparinization and aspirin regimen for prophylaxis and/or treatment of venous thromboembolism during the immediate postoperative period [73].

8.7.2 Recurrence

Postoperative recurrence or recanalization was defined as the presence of persistent arteriovenous shunting or SDAVF at the time of the first and/or last angiographic follow-up compared with the initial posttreatment angiogram, and there was clinical deterioration or lack of improvement following the intervention [55, 60, 72]. In a meta-analysis by Goyal et al., endovascular embolization was associated with 19.8% of patients having initial residue and 11.2% of patients having late recurrence [51]. The main reason is that SDAVFs are often fed by long arcades and are supplemented by adjacent segments, sometimes with a seemingly complete angiographic occlusion, and recanalization is seen with the opening of new venous drainage [38, 74].

In addition, in some cases of SDAVF, embolic material deposits along the inner walls of draining veins, giving the false radiological impression of complete occlusion while an inner lumen persists, and the persistent shunt often leads to progressive recruitment and growth of secondary arterial feeders [55, 75].

8.8 Prognosis

Microsurgical treatment and endovascular embolization are associated with cure rates of nearly 100% and 25–89.5%, respectively [1, 9, 51, 56, 73, 74]. An anatomical cure of SDAVF can be obtained by either microsurgery or embolization, but the functional outcome is not always satisfactory [49]. The spinal cord neurological function can be assessed and graded according to the Aminoff-Logue disability (ALD) scale and modified Rankin scale (mRS) [13, 74, 76]. In Durnford et al.'s report of 57 patients with SAVDF who underwent occlusion, the ALD scores improved during the 5-year follow-up by a median of 1 point, and 49% of the patients had a 1-point improvement in their mRS score [74]. In the Japanese Registry of Neuroendovascular Therapy 2 and 3 with 172 SDAVFs, postoperative neurological improvement was achieved in 48.3% of the patients, and an mRS score of 0–2 on postoperative day 30 was achieved in 60.5% of the patients [31].

In general, postoperatively, two-thirds of patients have relief and resolution of symptoms [14]. In these patients, the motor symptoms improved more than the sensory disorders, pain, or sphincter impairment [2, 3, 22, 77]. These improvements are preserved over an average of 3 years of follow-up [26]. For the treatment of SDAVFs, one-third of patients had no satisfying recovery. How to predict the treatment outcome of SDAVF is still a matter of dispute [78]. It remains difficult to predict whether patients will obtain clinical improvement or whether the treatment will simply halt the progression of symptoms [20].

It seems that the neurological function status before treatment and the anatomical location of the fistula can predict the postoperative outcome. SDAVFs associated with severe neurological deficits at presentation tend to have worse posttreatment functional outcomes [22]. Preoperative (1 day before treatment) ALD was the strongest predictor of clinical improvement [78]. The lower thoracic area was associated with a favorable outcome, and the middle thoracic and lumbar areas were associated with lower rates of improvement [3, 20, 23, 79]. In lumbosacral SDAVF, the postoperative micturition function recovery was superior to thoracic SDAVF [80].

It is worth noting that postoperatively, approximately 50% of patients suffered late clinical deterioration after temporary recovery, especially at the 72-month follow-up [78]. The main mechanism underlying this phenomenon is a gradual and irreversible decline in spinal function related to hemodynamic modifications induced by SDAVF and to the persistence of a state of deficiency of spinal venous drainage (Fig. 8.7) [81].

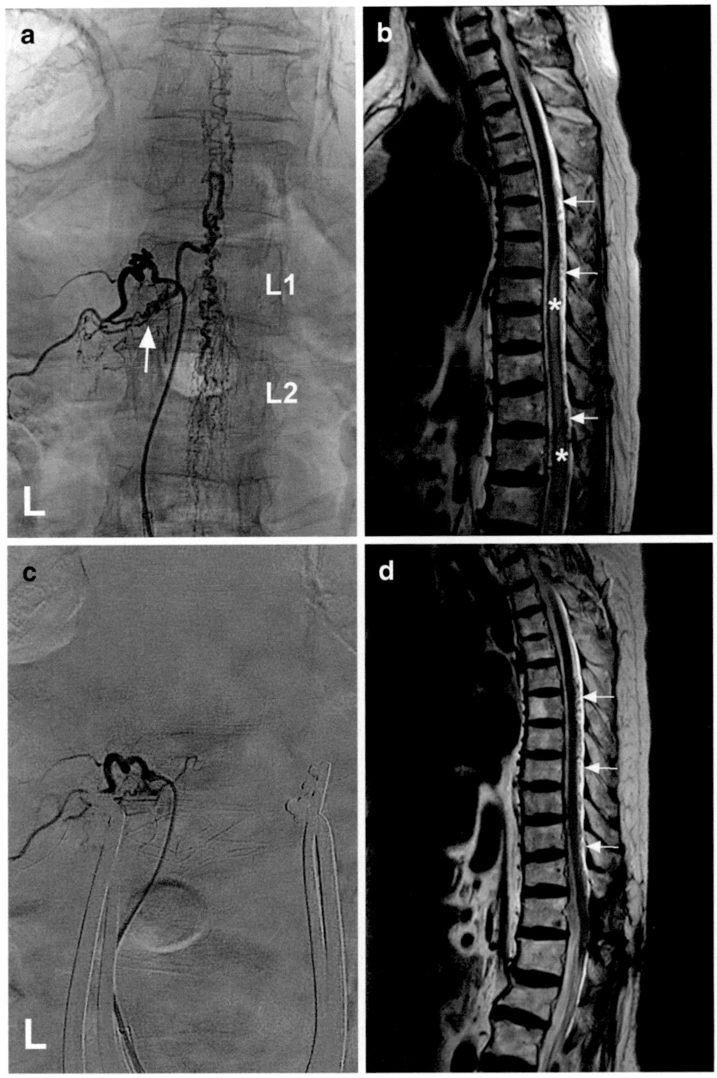

Fig. 8.7 Postoperative state of venous drain age of SDAVF. (**a**) Preoperative angiography of the left lumbar artery showing an SDAVF (arrow) between the L1 and L2 vertebral levels. (**b**) Preoperative MR T2WI showing dilated vessels (arrows) on the ventral and dorsal surfaces of the spinal cord and edema of the spinal cord (asterisks). (**c**) Postoperative angiography showing the SDAVF and the complete occlusion of the SDAVF. (**d**) Postoperative 8-month follow-up MR T2WI showing the regression of spinal cord edema; however, dilated vessels (arrows) on the dorsal surfaces of the spinal cord still exist. Abbreviations: *L* left, *L1* first lumbar vertebra, *L2* second lumbar vertebra, *SDAVF* spinal dural arteriovenous fistula

8.9 Summary

SDAVF is a rare disabling disease and is often misdiagnosed. SDAVF has a poor natural history. The angioarchitecture of the SDAVF is complex. SDAVF is a potentially curable disease and thus should be treated aggressively. Surgical and endovascular interventions can be used. Microsurgery appeared to be an efficient method in terms of the clinical effect, radicality, and lower recurrence in comparison with endovascular embolization. However, endovascular embolization is becoming popular due to the advances in the techniques. Although there are complications and unsatisfactory prognoses, SDAVF treatments are still recommended; moreover, the sooner the treatment is implemented, the better the prognosis.

Acknowledgments The author thanks Dr. Yunbao Guo for providing the educational images in Figs. 8.3 and 8.4 and Xuan Chen for providing the educational images in Fig. 8.5 (other images are provided by the author). The author confirms that the permission from the colleagues who provided the case images to include these in a commercial publication.

Funding None.

Conflicts of Interest The author declares that he has no conflicts of interest.

Ethics Approval Ethics approval is not needed for review articles at our institution.

Informed Consent Informed consent was obtained from all individual participants included in the study or their legal guardians.

References

1. Open and endovascular treatment of spinal dural arteriovenous fistulas: a 10-year experience. J Neurosurg Spine. 2017;26(4):519–23. https://doi.org/10.3171/2016.9.spine16394.
2. Jellema K, Tijssen CC, van Rooij WJ, Sluzewski M, Koudstaal PJ, Algra A, van Gijn J. Spinal dural arteriovenous fistulas: long-term follow-up of 44 treated patients. Neurology. 2004;62(10):1839–41. https://doi.org/10.1212/01.wnl.0000125322.76322.6e.
3. Cenzato M, Versari P, Righi C, Simionato F, Casali C, Giovanelli M. Spinal dural arteriovenous fistulae: analysis of outcome in relation to pretreatment indicators. Neurosurgery. 2004;55(4):815–22; discussion 822-813. https://doi.org/10.1227/01.neu.0000137630.50959.a7.
4. Ogbu II, Tzerakis N, Al-Shamary Z. Sudden-onset paraplegia in a 72-year-old male with a spinal dural arteriovenous fistula: illustrative case. Journal of neurosurgery Case lessons. 2021;2(9):CASE21283. https://doi.org/10.3171/CASE21283.
5. Steinmetz MP, Chow MM, Krishnaney AA, Andrews-Hinders D, Benzel EC, Masaryk TJ, Mayberg MR, Rasmussen PA. Outcome after the treatment of spinal dural arteriovenous fistulae: a contemporary single-institution series and meta-analysis. Neurosurgery. 2004;55(1):77–88. https://doi.org/10.1227/01.neu.0000126878.95006.0f.
6. Koch C. Spinal dural arteriovenous fistula. Curr Opin Neurol. 2006;19(1):69–75. https://doi.org/10.1097/01.wco.0000200547.22292.11.
7. Rajadurai J, Kohan S, Wenderoth J. Management of spinal dural arteriovenous fistula in a child with myelopathy. Surg Neurol Int. 2020;11:91. https://doi.org/10.25259/sni_33_2020.
8. Gailloud P. Spinal vascular malformations: angiographic evaluation and endovascular management. Handb Clin Neurol. 2021;176:267–304. https://doi.org/10.1016/b978-0-444-64034-5.00013-4.
9. Schuss P, Daher FH, Greschus S, Vatter H, Güresir E. Surgical treatment of spinal dural arteriovenous fistula: management and long-term outcome in a single-center series. World Neurosurg. 2015;83(6):1002–5. https://doi.org/10.1016/j.wneu.2015.02.026.
10. Dehdashti AR, Da Costa LB, terBrugge KG, Willinsky RA, Tymianski M, Wallace MC. Overview of the current role of endovascular and surgical treatment in spinal dural arteriovenous fistulas. Neurosurg Focus. 2009;26(1):E8. https://doi.org/10.3171/foc.2009.26.1.e8.
11. Yu JX, Hong T, Krings T, He C, Ye M, Sun LY, Zhai XD, Xiang SS, Ma YJ, Bian LS, Ren J, Tao PY, Li JW, Yang F, Li GL, Ling F, Zhang HQ. Natural history of spinal cord arteriovenous shunts: an observational study. Brain. 2019;142(8):2265–75. https://doi.org/10.1093/brain/awz153.
12. Meder JF, Devaux B, Merland JJ, Frédy D. Spontaneous disappearance of a spinal dural arteriovenous fistula. AJNR Am J Neuroradiol. 1995;16(10):2058–62.
13. Aminoff MJ, Logue V. The prognosis of patients with spinal vascular malformations. Brain. 1974;97(1):211–8. https://doi.org/10.1093/brain/97.1.211.
14. Jablawi F, Mull M. The clinical value of venous drainage in patients with spinal dural arteriovenous fistula. J Neurol Sci. 2019;397:50–4. https://doi.org/10.1016/j.jns.2018.12.024.
15. Koerts G, Vanthuyne V, Delavallee M, Rooijakkers H, Raftopoulos C. Spinal dural arteriovenous fistula presenting with paraplegia following lumbar puncture. J Neurosurg Spine. 2013;19(1):57–60. https://doi.org/10.3171/2013.3.spine12888.
16. Hetts SW, Narvid J, Singh T, Meagher S, Corcoran K, Higashida RT, Dowd CF, Halbach VV. Association between lumbar epidural injection and development of acute paraparesis in patients with spinal dural arteriovenous fistulas. AJNR Am J Neuroradiol. 2007;28(3):581–3.
17. Cabrera M, Paradas C, Márquez C, González A. Acute paraparesis following intravenous steroid therapy in a case of dural spinal arteriovenous fistula. J Neurol. 2008;255(9):1432–3. https://doi.org/10.1007/s00415-008-0943-2.
18. Ma Y, Hong T, Chen S, Peng C, Wang C, Yang K, Yu J, Ren J, Bian L, Liu J, Wang Z, Krings T, Ling F, Zhang H. Steroid-associated acute clinical worsening and poor outcome in patients with spinal dural arteriovenous fistulas: a prospective cohort study. Spine (Phila Pa 1976). 2020;45(11):E656–e662. https://doi.org/10.1097/brs.0000000000003370.
19. Van Dijk JM, TerBrugge KG, Willinsky RA, Farb RI, Wallace MC. Multidisciplinary management of spinal dural arteriovenous fistulas: clinical presentation and long-term follow-up in 49 patients. Stroke. 2002;33(6):1578–83. https://doi.org/10.1161/01.str.0000018009.83713.06.
20. Jablawi F, Schubert GA, Dafotakis M, Pons-Kühnemann J, Hans FJ, Mull M. Long-term outcome of patients with spinal dural arteriovenous fistula: the dilemma of delayed diagnosis. AJNR Am J Neuroradiol. 2020;41(2):357–63. https://doi.org/10.3174/ajnr.A6372.
21. Yen PP, Ritchie KC, Shankar JJ. Spinal dural arteriovenous fistula: correlation between radiological and clinical findings. J Neurosurg Spine.

2014;21(5):837–42. https://doi.org/10.3171/2014.7.spine13797.
22. Fugate JE, Lanzino G, Rabinstein AA. Clinical presentation and prognostic factors of spinal dural arteriovenous fistulas: an overview. Neurosurg Focus. 2012;32(5):E17. https://doi.org/10.3171/2012.1.focus11376.
23. Cenzato M, Debernardi A, Stefini R, D'Aliberti G, Piparo M, Talamonti G, Coppini M, Versari P. Spinal dural arteriovenous fistulas: outcome and prognostic factors. Neurosurg Focus. 2012;32(5):E11. https://doi.org/10.3171/2012.2.focus1218.
24. Schick U, Hassler W. Treatment and outcome of spinal dural arteriovenous fistulas. Eur Spine J. 2003;12(4):350–5. https://doi.org/10.1007/s00586-002-0487-6.
25. Zhang HB, Zhai XL, Li L, Wu DS, Zhuang GL, Xu QW, Guo H, Wang J. Imaging characteristics, misdiagnosis and microsurgical outcomes of patients with spinal dural arteriovenous fistula: a retrospective study of 32 patients. Ann Transl Med. 2022;10(15):832. https://doi.org/10.21037/atm-22-3568.
26. Narvid J, Hetts SW, Larsen D, Neuhaus J, Singh TP, McSwain H, Lawton MT, Dowd CF, Higashida RT, Halbach VV. Spinal dural arteriovenous fistulae: clinical features and long-term results. Neurosurgery. 2008;62(1):159–66; discussion 166-157. https://doi.org/10.1227/01.neu.0000311073.71733.c4.
27. Ronald AA, Yao B, Winkelman RD, Piraino D, Masaryk TJ, Krishnaney AA. Spinal dural arteriovenous fistula: diagnosis, outcomes, and prognostic factors. World Neurosurg. 2020;144:e306–15. https://doi.org/10.1016/j.wneu.2020.08.126.
28. Kona MP, Buch K, Singh J, Rohatgi S. Spinal vascular shunts: a patterned approach. AJNR Am J Neuroradiol. 2021;42(12):2110–8. https://doi.org/10.3174/ajnr.A7312.
29. Geibprasert S, Pereira V, Krings T, Jiarakongmun P, Toulgoat F, Pongpech S, Lasjaunias P. Dural arteriovenous shunts: a new classification of craniospinal epidural venous anatomical bases and clinical correlations. Stroke. 2008;39(10):2783–94. https://doi.org/10.1161/STROKEAHA.108.516757.
30. Flores BC, Klinger DR, White JA, Batjer HH. Spinal vascular malformations: treatment strategies and outcome. Neurosurg Rev. 2017;40(1):15–28. https://doi.org/10.1007/s10143-016-0713-z.
31. Tsuruta W, Matsumaru Y, Iihara K, Satow T, Sakai N, Katsumata M, Hosoo H, Sato M, Ito Y, Marushima A, Hayakawa M, Ishikawa E, Matsumura A. Clinical characteristics and endovascular treatment for spinal dural arteriovenous fistula in Japan: Japanese registry of Neuroendovascular therapy 2 and 3. Neurol Med Chir (Tokyo). 2019;59(12):492–7. https://doi.org/10.2176/nmc.st.2018-0218.
32. Takai K, Endo T, Yasuhara T, Seki T, Watanabe K, Tanaka Y, Kurokawa R, Kanaya H, Honda F, Itabashi T, Ishikawa O, Murata H, Tanaka T, Nishimura Y, Eguchi K, Takami T, Watanabe Y, Nishida T, Hiramatsu M, Ohtonari T, Yamaguchi S, Mitsuhara T, Matsui S, Uchikado H, Hattori G, Yamahata H, Taniguchi M. Neurosurgical versus endovascular treatment of spinal dural arteriovenous fistulas: a multicenter study of 195 patients. J Neurosurg Spine. 2020;34(3):514–21. https://doi.org/10.3171/2020.6.spine20309.
33. El-Serwi A, Maubon A, Vidal J, Chapot R. Double spinal dural arteriovenous fistulas. AJNR Am J Neuroradiol. 2006;27(2):321–3.
34. Foote AM, Bower SP, Danks RA, Chong W. Multiple spinal dural arteriovenous fistulae and deterioration post lumbar puncture. J Clin Neurosci. 2010;17(1):137–8. https://doi.org/10.1016/j.jocn.2009.02.032.
35. Jablawi F, Mull M. Double spinal dural arteriovenous fistulas. J Neuroradiol. 2019;46(3):168–72. https://doi.org/10.1016/j.neurad.2018.09.004.
36. Jellema K, Tijssen CC, van Gijn J. Spinal dural arteriovenous fistulas: a congestive myelopathy that initially mimics a peripheral nerve disorder. Brain. 2006;129(Pt 12):3150–64. https://doi.org/10.1093/brain/awl220.
37. Nogueira RG, Dabus G, Rabinov JD, Ogilvy CS, Hirsch JA, Pryor JC. Onyx embolization for the treatment of spinal dural arteriovenous fistulae: initial experience with long-term follow-up. Technical case report. Neurosurgery. 2009;64(1):E197–8; discussion E198. https://doi.org/10.1227/01.neu.0000335157.90249.97.
38. Takai K, Kin T, Oyama H, Shojima M, Saito N. Three-dimensional angioarchitecture of spinal dural arteriovenous fistulas, with special reference to the intradural retrograde venous drainage system. J Neurosurg Spine. 2013;18(4):398–408. https://doi.org/10.3171/2013.1.spine12305.
39. O'Reilly ST, Hendriks EJ, Brunet MC, Itsekson Z, Shahrani RA, Agid R, Nicholson P, terBrugge K, Radovanovic I, Krings T. Recognition of the variant type of spinal dural arteriovenous fistula: a rare but important consideration. J Neurosurg Spine. 2022;37(4):624–8. https://doi.org/10.3171/2022.3.spine22225.
40. Takai K, Komori T, Taniguchi M. Microvascular anatomy of spinal dural arteriovenous fistulas: arteriovenous connections and their relationships with the dura mater. J Neurosurg Spine. 2015;23(4):526–33. https://doi.org/10.3171/2014.11.spine14786.
41. Sorenson T, Giordan E, Cannizzaro D, Lanzino G. Surgical ligation of spinal dural arteriovenous fistula. Acta Neurochir. 2018;160(1):191–4. https://doi.org/10.1007/s00701-017-3381-z.
42. Trivelato FP, Rezende MTS, Ulhoa AC, Nakiri GS, Abud DG. Dual-lumen balloon to increase onyx venous penetration in the treatment of spinal dural arteriovenous fistulas. J Neuroradiol. 2018;45(2):142–6. https://doi.org/10.1016/j.neurad.2017.09.006.
43. Houdart E, Redondo A, Saint-Maurice JP, Merland JJ. Natural history of an incidentally discovered spinal dural arteriovenous fistula. Neurology. 2001;57(4):742–3. https://doi.org/10.1212/wnl.57.4.742.

44. Gailloud P. Spinal dural arteriovenous fistula (SDAVF) variant with dual perimedullary and epidural drainage. Eur Spine J. 2018;27(Suppl 3):375–9. https://doi.org/10.1007/s00586-017-5298-x.
45. Shimizu K, Takeda M, Mitsuhara T, Tanaka S, Nagano Y, Yamahata H, Kurisu K, Yamaguchi S. Asymptomatic spinal dural arteriovenous fistula: case series and systematic review. J Neurosurg Spine. 2019;31(5):733–41. https://doi.org/10.3171/2019.5.spine181513.
46. Bertuccio A, Robba C, Spena G, Versari PP. Intracranial and spinal dural arterio-venous fistula (DAVF): a surgical series of 107 patients. Acta Neurochir Suppl. 2016;123:177–83. https://doi.org/10.1007/978-3-319-29887-0_25.
47. Sato K, Terbrugge KG, Krings T. Asymptomatic spinal dural arteriovenous fistulas: pathomechanical considerations. J Neurosurg Spine. 2012;16(5):441–6. https://doi.org/10.3171/2012.2.spine11500.
48. Ehresman J, Catapano JS, Baranoski JF, Jadhav AP, Ducruet AF, Albuquerque FC. Treatment of spinal arteriovenous malformation and fistula. Neurosurg Clin N Am. 2022;33(2):193–206. https://doi.org/10.1016/j.nec.2021.11.005.
49. Ushikoshi S, Hida K, Kikuchi Y, Miyasaka K, Iwasaki T, Abe H. Functional prognosis after treatment of spinal dural arteriovenous fistulas. Neurol Med Chir (Tokyo). 1999;39(3):206–12; discussion 212-203. https://doi.org/10.2176/nmc.39.206.
50. Česák T, Adamkov J, Poczos P, Kanta M, Krajina A, Krajíčková D, Herzig R, Vališ M. Multidisciplinary approach in the treatment of spinal dural arteriovenous fistula-results of endovascular and surgical treatment. Acta Neurochir. 2018;160(12):2439–48. https://doi.org/10.1007/s00701-018-3672-z.
51. Goyal A, Cesare J, Lu VM, Alvi MA, Kerezoudis P, Brinjikji W, Nasr D, Lanzino G, Bydon M. Outcomes following surgical versus endovascular treatment of spinal dural arteriovenous fistula: a systematic review and meta-analysis. J Neurol Neurosurg Psychiatry. 2019;90(10):1139–46. https://doi.org/10.1136/jnnp-2019-320648.
52. Gemmete JJ, Chaudhary N, Elias AE, Toma AK, Pandey AS, Parker RA, Davagnanam I, Maher CO, Brew S, Robertson F. Spinal dural arteriovenous fistulas: clinical experience with endovascular treatment as a primary therapy at 2 academic referral centers. AJNR Am J Neuroradiol. 2013;34(10): 1974–9. https://doi.org/10.3174/ajnr.A3522.
53. Oh Y, Heo Y, Jeon SR, Roh SW, Park JH. Microsurgery versus endovascular treatment—which is adequate for initial treatment of spinal dural arteriovenous fistula: a case series. Neurospine. 2021;18(2):344–54. https://doi.org/10.14245/ns.2040826.413.
54. Patsalides A, Santillan A, Knopman J, Tsiouris AJ, Riina HA, Gobin YP. Endovascular management of spinal dural arteriovenous fistulas. J Neurointerv Surg. 2011;3(1):80–4. https://doi.org/10.1136/jnis.2010.003178.
55. Rothrock RJ, Haldeman C, Shah A, Lu VM, Lavi ES, Peterson EC, Levi AD. Challenges in diagnosis and management of previously embolized spinal dural arteriovenous fistulae. World Neurosurg. 2021;154:e710–7. https://doi.org/10.1016/j.wneu.2021.07.122.
56. Bretonnier M, Hénaux PL, Gaberel T, Roualdes V, Kerdiles G, Le Reste PJ, Morandi X. Spinal dural arteriovenous fistulas: clinical outcome after surgery versus embolization: a retrospective study. World Neurosurg. 2019;127:e943–9. https://doi.org/10.1016/j.wneu.2019.04.005.
57. Kirsch M, Berg-Dammer E, Musahl C, Bäzner H, Kühne D, Henkes H. Endovascular management of spinal dural arteriovenous fistulas in 78 patients. Neuroradiology. 2013;55(3):337–43. https://doi.org/10.1007/s00234-013-1134-0.
58. Harel R, Kimchi G, Yaniv G, Orion D, Knoller N. Surgical management of failed endovascular treatment for spinal dural arteriovenous fistulas. World Neurosurg. 2021;147:e354–62. https://doi.org/10.1016/j.wneu.2020.12.062.
59. Adrianto Y, Yang KH, Koo HW, Park W, Jung SC, Park JE, Kim KK, Jeon SR, Suh DC. Concomitant origin of the anterior or posterior spinal artery with the feeder of a spinal dural arteriovenous fistula (SDAVF). J Neurointerv Surg. 2017;9(4): 405–10. https://doi.org/10.1136/neurintsurg-2016-012267.
60. Fiaschi P, Prior A, Sbaffi PF, Bizzi F, D'Andrea A, Cagetti B, Badaloni F, Allegretti L, Mavilio N, Padolecchia R, Valsania V, Zona G. Spinal dural arteriovenous fistulas: clinical results and quality of life assessment with surgical treatment as a crucial therapy. The joint experience of two centers. World Neurosurg. 2019;122:e270–8. https://doi.org/10.1016/j.wneu.2018.10.019.
61. Cawley CM, Howard BM, Barrow DL. Microsurgical management of a spinal dural arteriovenous fistula with shared blood supply to the artery of Adamkiewicz: 3-dimensional operative video. Oper Neurosurg (Hagerstown). 2019;16(6):E174–e175. https://doi.org/10.1093/ons/opy293.
62. Albader F, Serratrice N, Farah K, Fuentes S. Minimally invasive microsurgical treatment of spinal dural arteriovenous fistula: how I do it. Acta Neurochir. 2022;164(6):1669–73. https://doi.org/10.1007/s00701-022-05200-2.
63. Kienzler JC, Schoepf S, Marbacher S, Diepers M, Remonda L, Fandino J. Intraoperative spinal angiography during microsurgical occlusion of spinal dural arteriovenous fistula within the hybrid operation room. J Neurol Surg A Cent Eur Neurosurg. 2022;83(5):486–93. https://doi.org/10.1055/s-0041-1736634.
64. Hanel RA, Nakaji P, Spetzler RF. Use of microscope-integrated near-infrared indocyanine green videoangiography in the surgical treatment of spinal dural arteriovenous fistulae. Neurosurgery. 2010;66(5):978–84; discussion 984-975. https://doi.org/10.1227/01.neu.0000368108.94233.22.

65. Colby GP, Coon AL, Sciubba DM, Bydon A, Gailloud P, Tamargo RJ. Intraoperative indocyanine green angiography for obliteration of a spinal dural arteriovenous fistula. J Neurosurg Spine. 2009;11(6):705–9. https://doi.org/10.3171/2009.6.spine09315.
66. Bretonnier M, Morandi X, Le Reste PJ. Fluorescein-guided surgery for spinal dural arteriovenous fistulas: a short series. J Clin Neurosci. 2019;70:226–8. https://doi.org/10.1016/j.jocn.2019.08.036.
67. Xing XZ, Guan BL, Jie LX. Directional multistage intraoperative microvascular Doppler in the hemilaminectomy surgical obliteration of spinal dural arteriovenous fistular. Clin Neurol Neurosurg. 2019;176:61–6. https://doi.org/10.1016/j.clineuro.2018.11.014.
68. Jellema K, Sluzewski M, van Rooij WJ, Tijssen CC, Beute GN. Embolization of spinal dural arteriovenous fistulas: importance of occlusion of the draining vein. J Neurosurg Spine. 2005;2(5):580–3. https://doi.org/10.3171/spi.2005.2.5.0580.
69. Suh DC, Cho SH, Park JE, Liu H, Jung SC. Induced-wedge technique to improve liquid embolic agent penetration into spinal dural arteriovenous fistula. World Neurosurg. 2016;96:309–15. https://doi.org/10.1016/j.wneu.2016.09.002.
70. Clarençon F, Stracke CP, Shotar E, Wallocha M, Mosimann PJ, Boch AL, Sourour N, Chapot R. Pressure cooker technique for endovascular treatment of spinal arteriovenous fistulas: experience in 15 cases. AJNR Am J Neuroradiol. 2021;42(7):1270–5. https://doi.org/10.3174/ajnr.A7078.
71. Lebovitz J, Storey C, Sweid A, Tjoumakaris S, Gooch MR, Rosenwasser R, Jabbour P. Onyx embolization of spinal arteriovenous fistula via scepter balloon. World Neurosurg. 2020;134:62–6. https://doi.org/10.1016/j.wneu.2019.10.112.
72. Ruiz-Juretschke F, Perez-Calvo JM, Castro E, García-Leal R, Mateo-Sierra O, Fortea F, Iza B, Garbizu JM, Villoria F. A single-center, long-term study of spinal dural arteriovenous fistulas with multidisciplinary treatment. J Clin Neurosci. 2011;18(12):1662–6. https://doi.org/10.1016/j.jocn.2011.03.008.
73. Jablawi F, Schubert GA, Hans FJ, Mull M. Anticoagulation therapy after surgical treatment of spinal dural arteriovenous fistula. Effectiveness and long-term outcome analysis. World Neurosurg. 2018;114:e698–705. https://doi.org/10.1016/j.wneu.2018.03.061.
74. Durnford AJ, Hempenstall J, Sadek AR, Duffill J, Mathad N, Millar J, Sparrow OC, Bulters DO. Degree and duration of functional improvement on long-term follow-up of spinal dural arteriovenous fistulae occluded by endovascular and surgical treatment. World Neurosurg. 2017;107:488–94. https://doi.org/10.1016/j.wneu.2017.07.140.
75. Adamczyk P, Amar AP, Mack WJ, Larsen DW. Recurrence of "cured" dural arteriovenous fistulas after onyx embolization. Neurosurg Focus. 2012;32(5):E12. https://doi.org/10.3171/2012.2.focus1224.
76. Suh DC, Song Y, Park D, Han M, Lim YM, Park JE, Lee SH, Jeon SR, Kim KK. New grading system for the clinical evaluation of patients with spinal vascular lesions. Neuroradiology. 2018;60(10):1035–41. https://doi.org/10.1007/s00234-018-2076-3.
77. Behrens S, Thron A. Long-term follow-up and outcome in patients treated for spinal dural arteriovenous fistula. J Neurol. 1999;246(3):181–5. https://doi.org/10.1007/s004150050331.
78. Yang C, Ma Y, Tian A, Yu J, Chen S, Peng C, Yang K, Li G, He C, Ye M, Hong T, Bian L, Wang Z, Ling F, Zhang H. Long-term outcomes and prognostic factors in patients with treated spinal dural arteriovenous fistulas: a prospective cohort study. BMJ Open. 2022;12(1):e047390. https://doi.org/10.1136/bmjopen-2020-047390.
79. Safaee MM, Clark AJ, Burkhardt JK, Winkler EA, Lawton MT. Timing, severity of deficits, and clinical improvement after surgery for spinal dural arteriovenous fistulas. J Neurosurg Spine. 2018;29(1):85–91. https://doi.org/10.3171/2017.11.spine17988.
80. Endo T, Kajitani T, Inoue T, Sato K, Niizuma K, Endo H, Matsumoto Y, Tominaga T. Clinical characteristics of lumbosacral spinal dural arteriovenous fistula (DAVF)-comparison with thoracic DAVF. World Neurosurg. 2018;110:e383–8. https://doi.org/10.1016/j.wneu.2017.11.002.
81. Cecchi PC, Musumeci A, Rizzo P, Faccioli F, Bricolo A. Late deterioration of neurologic function in patients surgically treated for spinal dural arteriovenous fistulas. Surg Neurol. 2009;72(3):257–61; discussion 261-252. https://doi.org/10.1016/j.surneu.2009.03.010.

Paraspinal Arteriovenous Malformations

9

Huachen Zhang, Shikai Liang, and Xianli Lv

Abstract

Arteriovenous malformations (AVMs) of the spine and spinal cord can be categorized as intradural AVMs, epidural AVMs, paraspinal AVMs, and mixed intradural/extradural AVMs. The term "paraspinal AVM" summarizes an inhomogeneous variety of rare vascular disorders. Bruit, thrill, vascular murmur, intradural or epidural hemorrhage, and acute progressive myelopathy are common symptoms of paraspinal AVMs. Paraspinal AVMs occur isolated or associated with genetic syndrome. Isolated paraspinal AVMs are either acquired, due to trauma. Congenital paraspinal AVMs are associated with systemic genetic background or metameric link. The route of venous drainage, either extraspinal or intraspinal, is mainly responsible for the symptoms. Endovascular treatment is considered as the first choice of treatment for most cases of paraspinal AVMs based on individual clinical and anatomical criteria. In this chapter, the etiology, clinical features, treatment options, and outcomes are discussed for paraspinal AVMs.

Keywords

Paraspinal · Arteriovenous malformation · Cobb syndrome · Klippel · Trénaunay syndrome · CLOVES syndrome

9.1 Introduction

Spinal vascular malformations affect all age groups from neonates to the elderly in connection with different entities [1]. They can be classified on the basis of their location: intradural arteriovenous malformations (AVMs), epidural AVMs, paraspinal AVMs, and mixed intradural/extradural AVMs [2, 3]. Paraspinal AVMs are located outside the spine and are responsible for neurological symptoms because of spinal cord compression by ectatic veins, venous congestion, or arterial steal. Epidural AVMs are located in the epidural space and drain in epidural veins with secondary intradural congestion. Dural AVMs are embedded in the dura and produce a congestive venous myelopathy after draining through radicular veins piercing the dura or accompanying a nerve root. Intradural shunts affect the cord, the roots, or the filum. Angioarchitecture dictates the clinical presentation as intradural AVMs are more likely to present with hemorrhage and acute onset myelopathy, while dural and extradural AVMs presented as either incidental lesions or gradually progressive congestive myelopathy [4, 5]. In this

H. Zhang · S. Liang · X. Lv (✉)
Department of Neurosurgery, Beijing Tsinghua Changgung Hospital, School of Clinical Medicine, Tsinghua University, Beijing, China

X. Lv (ed.), *Endovascular and Neurovascular Surgery for Spinal Vascular Malformations*,
https://doi.org/10.1007/978-981-97-4661-3_9

chapter, the etiology, clinical features, treatment options, and outcomes are discussed for paraspinal AVMs.

9.2 Etiology and Classifications

On the embryonic basis of the vascular insult, Rodesch et al. divided spinal AVMs into three categories: genetic hereditary, genetic nonhereditary, and single lesions [6]. Paraspinal AVMs are congenital or post-traumatic vascular malformations [7]. Congenital paraspinal AVMs are usually diagnosed in children during clinical examination and drained by paraspinal and epidural ectatic veins, which caused massive erosion of the vertebral bodies and may be associated with multicystic kidney [8, 9]. In a systematic review, 3/4 paraspinal AVMs are of the isolated and 1/4 paraspinal AVMs are a part of a genetic syndrome [4]. In Stuttgart classification of paraspinal AVMs, isolated paraspinal AVMs are subdivided into "acquired," "traumatic," and "congenital" without an identifiable genetic hereditary disorder. According to the route of venous drainage, the subgroups are differentiated as exclusively extraspinal or involving intraspinal veins (Table 9.1) [10]. Congenital paraspinal AVMs are divided into hereditary genetic mutations and nonhereditary genetic mutations. Several genetic hereditary conditions are known to be associated with paraspinal AVMs, most notably neurofibromatosis type 1, hereditary hemorrhagic telangiectasia (Rendu–Osler–Weber syndrome), and Parkes Weber syndrome (Table 9.2) [11, 12, 14]. Neurofibromatosis type 1 is one of the most common autosomal dominant hereditary genetic disorders with an incidence of approximately 1:3500 caused by a mutation in the NF1 gene on chromosome 17q11.2 that results in inactivation or downregulation of neurofibromin [15]. Rendu–Osler–Weber syndrome is an autosomal dominant

Table 9.1 Classification of paraspinal AVMs, mainly divided into their origins (isolated or associated with a metameric link or genetic syndrome) and their drainage pathways [10]

Stuttgart classification of paraspinal AVMs		
Isolated	Acquired	Extraspinal venous drainage
		Intraspinal venous drainage
	Traumatic	Extraspinal venous drainage
		Intraspinal venous drainage
	Congenital	Extraspinal venous drainage
		Intraspinal venous drainage
Associated	Metameric link	Extraspinal venous drainage
		Intraspinal venous drainage
	Genetic syndrome	Extraspinal venous drainage
		Intraspinal venous drainage

Table 9.2 Genetic syndromes associated with paraspinal AVMs [11–13]

Types	Nonhereditary genetic vascular disorder		Hereditary genetic vascular disorder	
Genetic syndromes	Cobb syndrome	CLOVES syndrome	HHT (Rendu–Osler–Weber) syndrome	Parkes Weber syndrome
Metameric spinal AVM	100%	100%	2.5% in ENG-HHT and 1.0% in ACVL1-HHT	12.5%
Genetic mutation	KRAS	PIK3CA	ENG, ACVRL1, and SMAD4	RASA1
Vascular anomalies	CM + AVM	CM + VM + LM + lipomatous overgrowth+AVM	Nasal/mucosal telangiectasia+brain AVM/spinal AVM/lung AVM/liver AVM/small intestine AVM	CM + VM + LM + limb overgrowth+AVM

CLOVES congenital lipomatous overgrowth, vascular malformations, epidermal nevi and spinal/skeletal anomalies and/or scoliosis, *HHT* hereditary hemorrhagic telangiectasia, *CM* capillary malformation, *LM* lymphatic malformation, *VM* venous malformation, *AVM* arteriovenous malformation disorder caused by mutations of either the endoglin (ENG) or the activin A receptor-like type 1 (ACVRL1) gene in more than 80% of cases [12, 16]. Parkes Weber syndrome is due to an RASA1 mosaic pathogenic variant [11, 13]. Paraspinal AVMs of nonhereditary genetic metameric origin affect the spinal cord as well as other tissues originating from the same metamere. The most important representative of this group is the Cobb syndrome, an association of a cutaneous hemangioma with spinal AVMs at the level corresponding to the respective dermatome. Moreover, overgrowth syndromes such as CLOVES syndrome, which also seem to have a metameric link, can be accompanied by spinal AVMs [10]. The phosphatidylinositol 3-kinase catalytic subunit alpha (PIK3CA) gene mutation is identified in the patients with CLOVES [17, 18].

9.3 Electrophysiological Changes

Electrophysiological abnormalities are described in most patients with spinal AVMs presenting with lower motor neuron clinical deficits [19]. These abnormalities depended on the duration of symptoms, on the caudal extension of the AVM, and on an arterial supply at T10 or below. In addition to the expected abnormalities in the distribution of the AVM location, electrophysiological changes at a distance may be due to venous stasis [19]. Electrophysiological changes in the corticospinal tract and/or lower motor neurons are found in patients with spinal dural AVM and are classified into three types: upper motor neuron sign, lower motor neuron sign, and mixed sign categories [20]. In 88% of patients with spinal AVMs, the electrophysiological changes are found, including abnormal nerve conduction in 43%, needle electromyography in 77%, and tibial somatosensory evoked potentials in 88% [19]. The patterns of involvement are of scattered, multiple, bilateral thoracolumbosacral radiculopathies, associated with paraspinal fibrillations or abnormal activation of motor unit potentials, consistent with axonal or neuronal destruction [19].

9.4 CT, MRI, and DSA

CT and MRI scans allow identification of four types of spinal AVMs: paraspinal, epidural, dural, and intradural ones [21]. MRI is usually the first examination performed when a spinal cord lesion is suspected. The level of hypoesthesia in the patient's physical examination helps with the planning of the angiographic procedure as well as MRI examination. MRI demonstrates vertebral erosion, flow void signal on T1- and T2-weighted imaging, partial enhancement after gadolinium injection, and signs of congestive myelopathy [22]. MRI and MRA are able to visualize spinal AVMs early after the onset of clinical symptoms. Small isolated paraspinal AVMs, despite their extraspinal location and small size, can cause hypertension of the intradural venous system and produce symptoms that are similar to those of spinal dural AVM. Contrast-enhanced MRI is helpful to detect such a small lesion [23]. The type of shunt and its localization may remain difficult to be precise. Digital subtraction angiography (DSA) remains the gold standard for analysis of the anatomical, morphological, and architectural features necessary for therapeutic decisions in both pediatric and adult populations. The imaging hallmark of paraspinal AVMs on DSA is the presence of a dilated epidural venous pouch [24]. Forty percent of paraspinal AVMs have multiple feeders, and 22% paraspinal AVMs have intradural venous involvement [4]. Understanding properly the lesional and regional vascular anatomy is mandatory to plan an appropriate therapeutic strategy and obtain good clinical outcomes stable at long-term follow-up [25]. One potentially useful imaging modality in the evaluation of paraspinal AVMs is XperCT or DynaCT. These cone beam CT techniques allow for exquisite anatomic characterization of paraspinal AVMs and can allow interventionalists and surgeons to pinpoint the site of the paraspinal AVMs. Typically, in cases of paraspinal AVMs, the venous pouch is very well visualized as well as its location in relation to the vertebral body and nerve root sleeve. Bridging veins can be seen with high definition [26].

9.5 Facial Paraspinal AVM

Facial paraspinal AVMs are usually iatrogenic or related to trauma. In the facial region, these AVMs involve exclusively the metameric arteries: maxillary, ascending pharyngeal, occipital, and vertebral arteries [27]. Signs and symptoms are variable, depending on the characteristics of the feeding vessel and the draining pathway.

9.6 Cervical Paraspinal AVMs

Cervical paraspinal AVMs are fed by the radicular arteries, the ascending cervical arteries, and the deep cervical arteries in the intervertebral foramen and drain into the epidural venous plexus with or without reflux into the intradural venous system causing myelopathy due to direct compression of the spinal cord by a large varix (Fig. 9.1) [27]. MRI at the cervical level can disclose remarkable compression of the spinal cord by a large venous pouch. Lhermitte–Duclos disease is associated with cervical paraspinal AVM and mutation of the phosphatase and tensin homolog deleted on chromosome ten (PTEN) gene [28]. Lhermitte–Duclos disease is a rare dysplastic cerebellar gangliocytoma manifesting as a slowly growing mass and is usually asymptomatic [29].

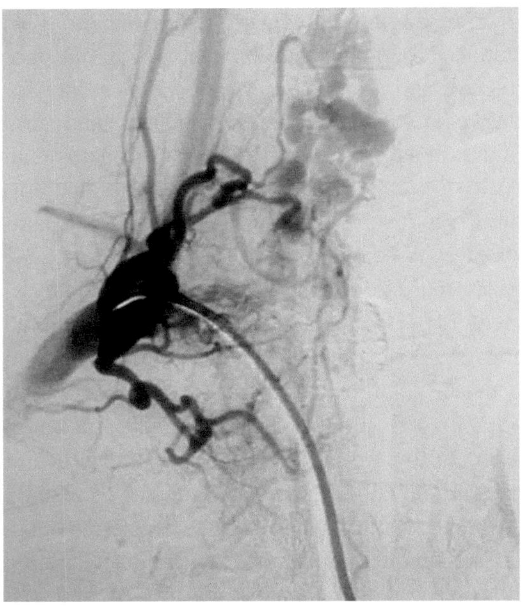

Fig. 9.1 A 37-year-old female presented with intraspinal hemorrhage caused by a paraspinal metameric AVM. A subclavian artery angiography confirmed a paraspinal AVM with arterial supply from the right ascending cervical artery and the right deep cervical artery in the intervertebral foramen and draining into the epidural venous plexus with reflux into the intradural venous system causing a large varix

9.7 Vertebral Arteriovenous Fistulas

Vertebral arteriovenous fistulas (VAVFs) include arterial contributions from the upper and lower vertebral artery (VA), with venous drainage into a variety of spinal and paraspinal collectors [29]. Most VAVFs occur as a result of direct trauma during accidents as well as iatrogenic origin [29]. VAVFs draining to the spinal epidural venous plexus presented with limb weakness and walking instability [30]. Most VAVFs are located at the first cervical metamere [31]. MRI showed that the dilated ventral epidural veins as well as the dilated paraspinal veins compressed the spinal cord. DSA demonstrated high-flow VAVF between the VA and the surrounding venous plexus at the cervical level. The fistulas also can be fed by backward flow from the contralateral VA and ascending cervical arteries. The endovascular treatment of direct VAVF with combination of detachable coils and Onyx (ev3 Inc., Irvine, California) is feasible, safe, and highly effective with low morbidity and mortality [32]. VAVF can rarely occur in patients with neurofibromatosis type 1 [14].

9.8 Presacral AVMs

Presacral AVMs drain through the ascending lumbar vein to the epidural plexuses and perimedullary veins [7]. Presacral AVMs present with paralysis of both lower extremities, bladder and sphincter dysfunction, gluteal and perineal pain, or a local sensation of hyperesthesia (Fig. 9.2). CT scan of the lumbosacral spine may

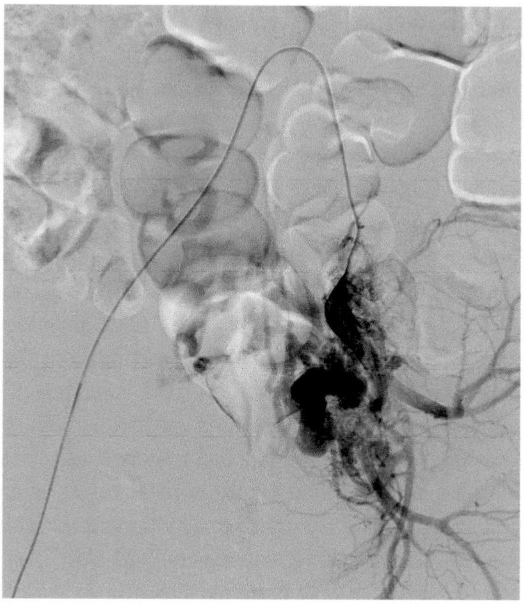

Fig. 9.2 A 40-year-old male presented with a sudden onset of the paralysis of both lower extremities and bladder and sphincter dysfunction. The selective left internal iliac arteriography demonstrated a paraspinal AVM in the sacral ventral pelvis

be normal. MRI discovers unidentified mass in the sacral spinal canal, spinal cord edema, and paraspinal vasodilatation [33]. DSA reveals high-flow AVMs anterior to the sacrum fed by internal iliac arteries. Numerous ectactic high-flow intra- and extraspinal shunts are typically presented with extremely rapid antegrade drainage via the often dilated intra- and extraspinal venous pathways [34]. Endovascular embolization should be performed, and open surgery should be avoided [33].

9.9 Spinal Epidural Arteriovenous Malformations

Spinal epidural arteriovenous malformations (SEAVMs) are rare complex lesions often presenting with protean clinical manifestations secondary to compressive symptoms or congestive myelopathy [24]. Patients with exclusively extradural venous drainage can present incidentally or with a compressive myelopathy in the setting of a large venous varix, whereas those with intradural venous drainage generally present with a congestive myelopathy. The fistulous site of SEAVMs locates in the epidural space and not at the level of the nerve root sleeve. SEAVMs are more likely to be located in the lumbosacral spine, more likely to be associated with prior spinal surgery, and more likely to be associated with neural tube defects [26]. SEAVMs have a preferred location at L4 and L5. SEAVMs at lumbosacral spine are supplied from branches of the iliac arteries, and these AVMs can be missed if an angiogram of iliac system is not performed [26].

Venous drainage route of SEAVMs may be intradural, via bridging veins from the epidural to the intradural space and into perimedullary veins, extradural, or combined [35]. SEAVMs can be classified on the basis of their variable venous drainage. Type A SEAVMs are characterized as having both an epidural venous plexus and a vein that pierces the dura, travels intradurally, and drains into the venous plexus surrounding the spinal cord. Type B SEAVMs have venous drainage only into the Batson plexus (vertebral venous plexus). Type B SEAVMs can be further divided by means of clinical correlation into type B1 if the epidural venous plexus causes compression of the thecal sac and myelopathy and type B2 if they have no radiographic and clinical mass effect [36].

Surgical treatment of SEAVMs can be challenging because of the common location ventral to the dural sac and the presence of arterialized venous lakes. The embolization with Onyx for SEAVMs and intradural venous drainage is effective [35]. The draining veins of SEAVMs are located in the azygos venous system. These veins contain valves as well as numerous metameric connections in paraspinal longitudinal veins. These features make transvenous embolization technically difficult and often times anatomically impossible. Nevertheless, successful fistula obliteration via transvenous embolization with glue and coils has been reported and is considered to be a more effective treatment, especially when multiple arterial feeders are present [37]. There were two modes of treatment, in which transarterial embolization was used for nonosseous SEAVMs and transvenous embolization for osseous SEAVMs [38]. The “osseous type” was defined as SEAVMs with bone involvement, such as bone erosion, osteolytic destruction, or compression fracture [38]. An osseous SEAVM shows bone involvement and compression of the nerve root or the spinal cord by bulging with cortical erosion. A nonosseous SEAVM shows engorgement (fistulous sac or pouch) of the epidural vein within the spinal canal compressing the spinal cord.

9.10 Cerebrospinal Fluid–Venous Fistula

Cerebrospinal fluid–venous fistula (CSF-VF) is increasingly recognized as a cause of spontaneous intracranial hypotension [2]. The exact pathogenesis of these lesions is unclear, with hypotheses that they represent aberrant connections between the nerve root sleeve and paraspinal veins or are secondary to increased CSF drainage via spinal arachnoid granulations that rupture into adjacent radicular veins. Digital subtraction myelography and decubitus CT myelography have been used to diagnose this lesion with increasing frequency [2]. Surgical ligation has been shown to be effective in treating CSF-VF by means of disconnecting the venous outflow pathway from the thecal sac. Transvenous Onyx embolization of the paraspinal and radicular veins draining the fistula is emerging as an efficacious minimally invasive treatment [3].

9.11 Spinal Metameric AVMs

The term "spinal metameric AVMs" is relatively new and is derived from craniofacial metameric AVMs 1, which was introduced to designate a rare form of vascular malformation involving both the brain and face. Spinal metameric AVMs include all spinal vascular malformations of nonhereditary genetic metameric origin, affecting not only the central nervous system (spinal cord) but also other tissues originating from the same metamere, such as the bony spine, paraspinal tissues, and skin [34]. Spinal metameric AVMs are the least common type of spinal AVMs, with estimated frequencies between 5.4% and 9%. Most cases involve the thoracic spine, followed by the cervical spine [34]. Because spinal metameric AVMs are most commonly present in children or young adults, they are so-called "juvenile" malformations and are characterized by voluminous, high-flow lesions and possessing normal cord tissue within their interstices (Fig. 9.3) [39].

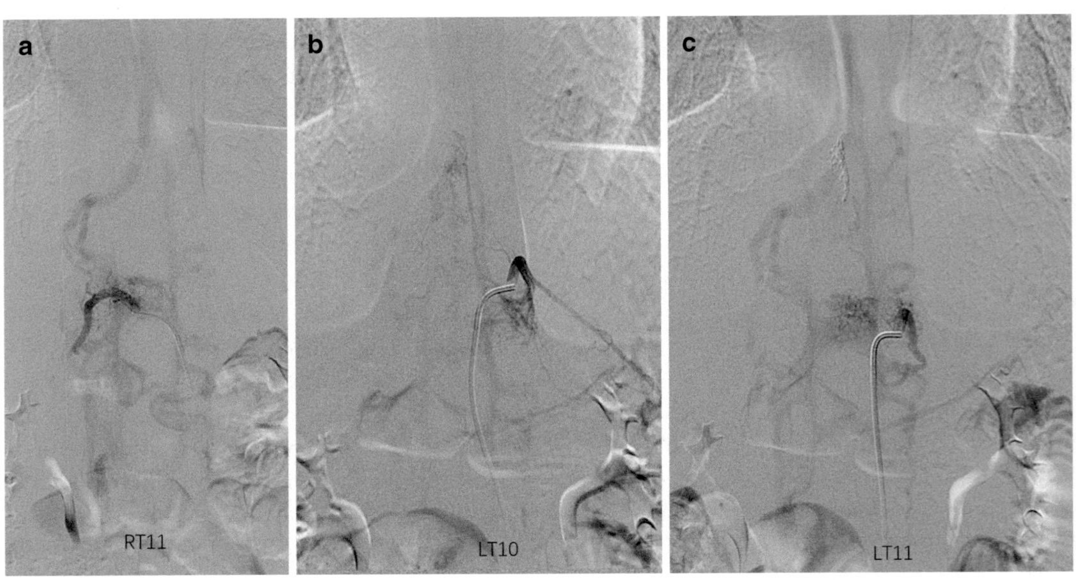

Fig. 9.3 A 13-year-old boy presented with gradual onset of the paralysis of both lower extremities and bladder and sphincter dysfunction caused by a spinal metameric AVM. (**a**) Selective catheterization of the right T4 intercostal artery. (**b**) Selective catheterization of the left T10 intercostal artery. (**c**) Selective catheterization of the left T11. Spinal cord and vertebral AVMs draining into the medullary, epidural, and paraspinal veins are shown

The typical presentation age is younger than 15 years, with a slight male predominance (male/female ratio = 1.7:1) [40]. In a 2014 meta-analysis of 51 cases of spinal metameric AVMs [40], the most common presentation was a progressive neurologic deficit in 35%, followed closely by acute hemorrhage (31%) and an acute neurologic deficit without hemorrhage (22%). Twelve percent of cases were incidental discoveries. Cardiac output may be increased significantly by this so-called "juvenile" malformation, and a bruit is commonly noted [41]. However, in the study of Niimi et al., 79% of spinal metameric AVM patients suffered hemorrhage, either subarachnoid hemorrhage or hematomyelia. Coexisting aneurysms were found in nearly 50% of cases of spinal metameric AVMs, which is a much higher number of associated aneurysms compared with isolated spinal AVMs [42]. Retroperitoneal hemorrhage due to rupture of thoracolumbar artery aneurysms has previously been described in association with a spinal metameric AVM [43].

Because the basic vascular anatomy of the spinal cord consists of many intradural and extradural anastomoses, a spinal metameric AVM is often supplied by many direct and indirect arterial pedicles. This complex angioarchitecture adds to the difficulty of treating such lesions. Endovascular embolization with or without a combination of surgical excision of the AVM can result in neurological improvement in selected spinal metameric AVMs (juvenile spinal AVMs) [44].

9.12 Cobb Syndrome

Cobb syndrome refers to the clinical manifestations of spinal metameric AVM involving all tissues of the involved metamere, including the spinal cord, bone, and skin [34]. It is first described in 1915 by Stanly Cobb, who was a resident of Harvey Cushing at that time [45]. Thus, this syndrome has long been called Cobb syndrome. Cobb syndrome is an extension of the craniofacial arteriovenous metameric syndrome. However, the phenotypic presentation may be less complete, and, therefore, Cobb syndrome is usually defined as the association of at least two AVMs in a metameric distribution. Though the majority of spinal AVMs in Cobb syndrome represent high-flow AVMs, spinal low-flow vascular malformations associated with cutaneous vascular lesions occurring in the same metamere are also defined as Cobb syndromes [46].

Cobb syndrome is rare and its intradural lesions in most cases are spinal cord AVM [46]. The prevalence of Cobb syndrome in patients with spinal intradural AVM varies from 12% to 19% in the series published. There is no significant gender difference. The onset age is usually younger than in patients with sporadic intramedullary AVM. Hematomyelia and SAH are the most frequent clinical presentation (occurring in 65% of patients). The rate of recurrent hemorrhages is high in this population, with a poor long-term functional prognosis [47]. Bilateral optic disc pits as an unusual finding were reported in association with Cobb syndrome [48].

Managing such cases is a challenge for the interventionalists and neurosurgeons as the results are often suboptimal [49]. Historically, surgical excision carried a high morbidity, and conservative management without intervention was preferred. More recently, endovascular embolization has been performed with good success [39]. Cobb syndrome is recently reported to have somatic KRAS mutations suggesting potential for treatment with mitogen-activated protein kinase inhibitors, such as trametinib. In a report, treatment with trametinib resulted in a substantial decrease in blood flow to the AVM, with a > 75% reduction in arterial inflow at 6 months [50].

9.13 CLOVES Syndrome

The occurrence of intraspinal or extraspinal high-flow AVMs within or adjacent to the truncal overgrowth or a cutaneous birthmark can be found in CLOVES syndrome (Fig. 9.4) [51]. Its intraspinal and extraspinal extension causes neurologic sequelae. Scoliosis and other musculoskeletal, neurologic, renal, and cutaneous malformations are encountered. Acral deformities included large, wide feet and hands, macrodactyly, and a wide sandal gap. The uniform and highly characteristic features of the truncal lipomatous mass, in combination with vascular, acral, and other

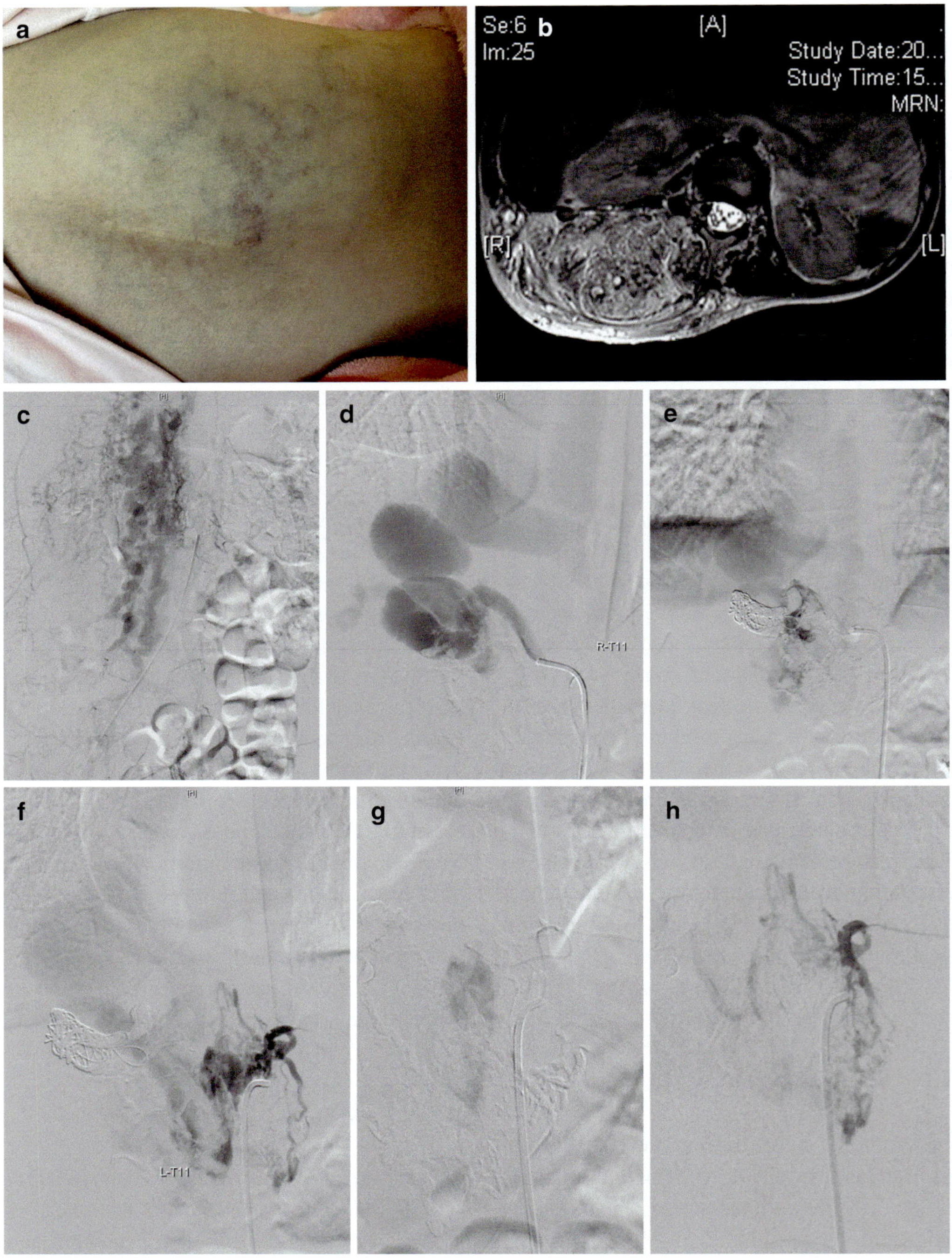

Fig. 9.4 An 11-year-old girl presented with 3 years of bilateral lower limb paralysis caused by CLOVES syndrome. (**a**) Physical examination showed large cutaneous stains on the right side of the back associated with a truncal mass. (**b**) MRI, T2-weighted, showed a giant mass with clear borders and mixed high signal inside on the right to the spine. (**c**) Abdominal aorta angiography showed corresponding vascular blush and delayed contrast pooling in the affected regions. (**d**) The right T11 intercostal artery demonstrated a high-flow fistula at the level of the neural foramen, with drainage to the azygos vein. (**e**) Endovascular treatment from the feeding artery was provided using coils and Onyx. (**f**) The left T11 intercostal artery angiography showed an epidural AVM. (**g**) Superselective angiograms through the microcatheters. (**h**) The left T11 intercostal artery showed the fistula was embolized with Onyx. (**i**) Onyx cast after endovascular embolization

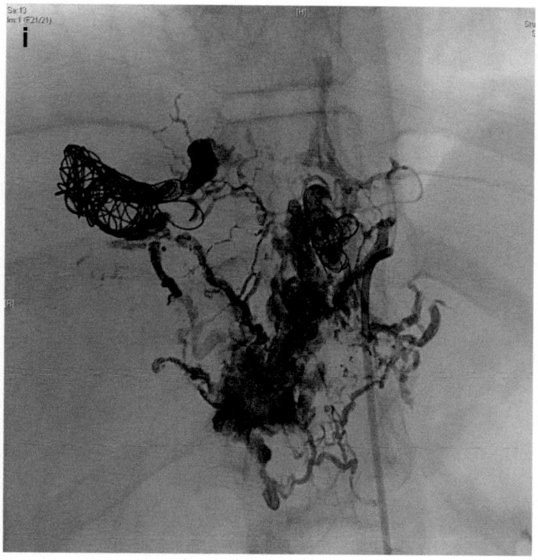

Fig. 9.4 (continued)

anomalies, provide evidence of this distinct clinical entity. Neurologic sequelae of the truncal involvement in CLOVES syndrome can be deforming and disabling; hence, prompt diagnosis and multidisciplinary care are necessary [52]. Capillary malformations and high-flow AVMs are commonly encountered. Variable portion of the truncal masses observed in CLOVES syndrome is lymphatic malformation. The lipomatous mass infiltrated the adjacent anatomic spaces and was associated with capillary, lymphatic, venous, and AVMs.

CLOVES syndrome is a rare congenital overgrowth disorder caused by mutations in the PIK3CA gene. Therefore, research into pharmacological treatments capable of blocking the PIK/AKT/mTOR pathway has increased over the past decade because its surgical treatment is challenging. The results have been promising and suggest that compassionate use of these treatments, such as alpelisib (BYL719) or taselisib, in patients with PIK3CA-related overgrowth syndrome could have clinical benefits [17, 18]. Spinal/paraspinal AVM has been proved to be associated with CLOVES syndrome and Parkes Weber syndrome (PWS) [53], but not with Klippel–Trénaunay syndrome (KTS) [54].

9.14 Parkes Weber Syndrome

Spinal AVM has not been reported to be a feature of PWS because spinal AVMs are only reported in 12.5% of PWS patients [54]. Distributions of spinal AVMs in PWS by locations are as follows: thoracolumbar, lumbosacral, and unspecified. There is no significant gender predominance (female–male ratio: 1:0). All patients have lower limb involvement with progressive myelopathy (paraparesis and sensory deficit with/without bladder and bowel dysfunction) or subarachnoid hemorrhage.

PWS is a congenital vascular malformation, which consists of capillary malformation (CM), venous malformation (VM), lymphatic malformation (LM), and arteriovenous malformation (AVM). PWS is frequently misdiagnosed as KTS that consists of the triad CM, VM, and LM [55]. The misconception that KTS is associated with spinal AVM has been uncontested in the literature for decades since Den Hartog Jager in 1949, René Djindjian (1918–1977), and Pierre Lasjaunias (1948–2008) [56–59]. Although their patients had vascular anomalies, there is no evidence that any met the basic clinical description for KTS. Both PWS and KTS have CM, VM, and LM, but PWS has in addition AVM, which is substantial when planning a treatment strategy [54, 55]. A diagnosis of PWS should be made on the presence of CM, VM, LV, and AVM (as main defect) in overgrowth extremity.

PWS is a widespread and weak staining of capillaries on excessively growing limbs, accompanied by diffuse and slow progression of multiple arteriovenous microfistulas, ulcers, and heart failure. In contrast to KTS, the vascular malformations in PWS are fast-flow and involve arterial malformations; lymphatic involvement is rare. PWS is thus not a type of KTS with AVM because these two conditions are clinically and radiologically distinct. Recently, some patients with a clinical pattern of PWS are reported to be caused by a mutation in the RASA1 gene (CM-AVM) [53, 54].

AVM presents the criterion for distinguishing PWS from KTS, which is substantial for treatment strategy. The main management goal should be to improve the quality of life of patients and reduce complications. Embolization alone/combined with surgical resection targeting occlusion or removal of AVM "nidus" reliably leads to clinical improvement [55].

9.15 Endovascular Treatment

The indication for paraspinal AVM treatment is based on individual circumstances (e.g., myelon compression, vascular bruit, high volume output cardiac failure) [10]. Endovascular embolization rather than surgery is the treatment of choice for such lesions. High-quality angiographic equipment and fluoroscopy added to the safety of the procedure [60]. Provocative test and electrophysiological monitoring were explored in spinal AVM embolization [61]. Approximately 20% of the incomplete obliteration is noted. The unsatisfactory result in a case of paraspinal AVM was due to the etiology of systematic genetic dysplasia and multiple feeders (Figs. 9.5, 9.6, 9.7, 9.8, 9.9, 9.10, 9.11, and 9.12) [4, 62]. Clinical follow-up with repeated spinal MRI is mandatory [63, 64]. The CyberKnife image-guided robotic radiosurgery is the latest in a series of radiation advancements that may improve the treatment of paraspinal AVMs [65].

Isobutyl 2-cyanoacrylate, deposited with a calibrated leak balloon microcatheter, has given satisfactory short-term improvement in spinal AVMs since the 1970s [66]. Current treatment

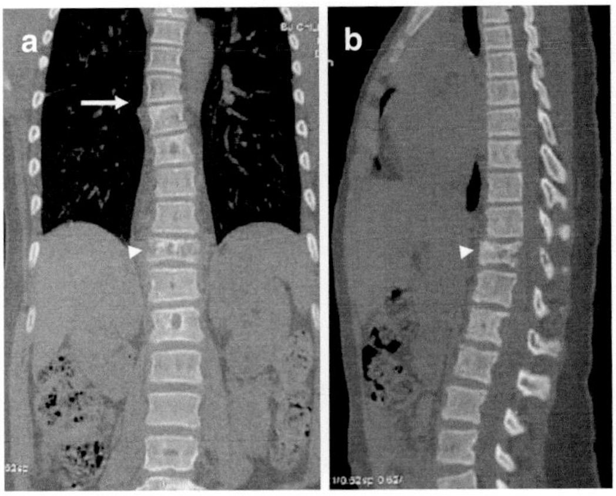

July-2020

Fig. 9.5 A 9-year-old girl presented with 4 months of lumbar pain, urinary retention, and paraplegia prior to admission. CT scanning, anteroposterior view (**a**) and lateral view (**b**), showing thoracic scoliosis (arrow) and multiple vertebral body destruction (arrowheads)

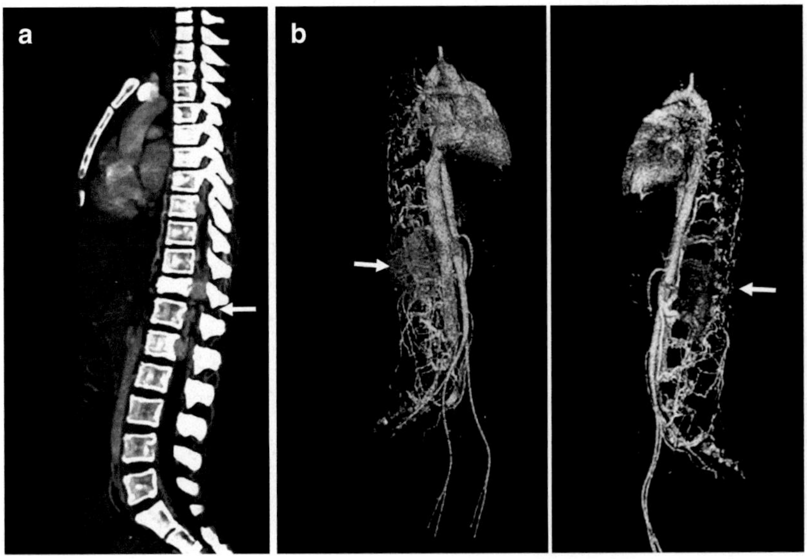

15th-Sep-2020

Fig. 9.6 Enhanced CT scanning, lateral view (**a**), showing multiple vertebral body destruction and multiple high-density lesions in the spinal canal. CT angiography (**b**) showing a giant vascular lesion from T7 to L1 levels

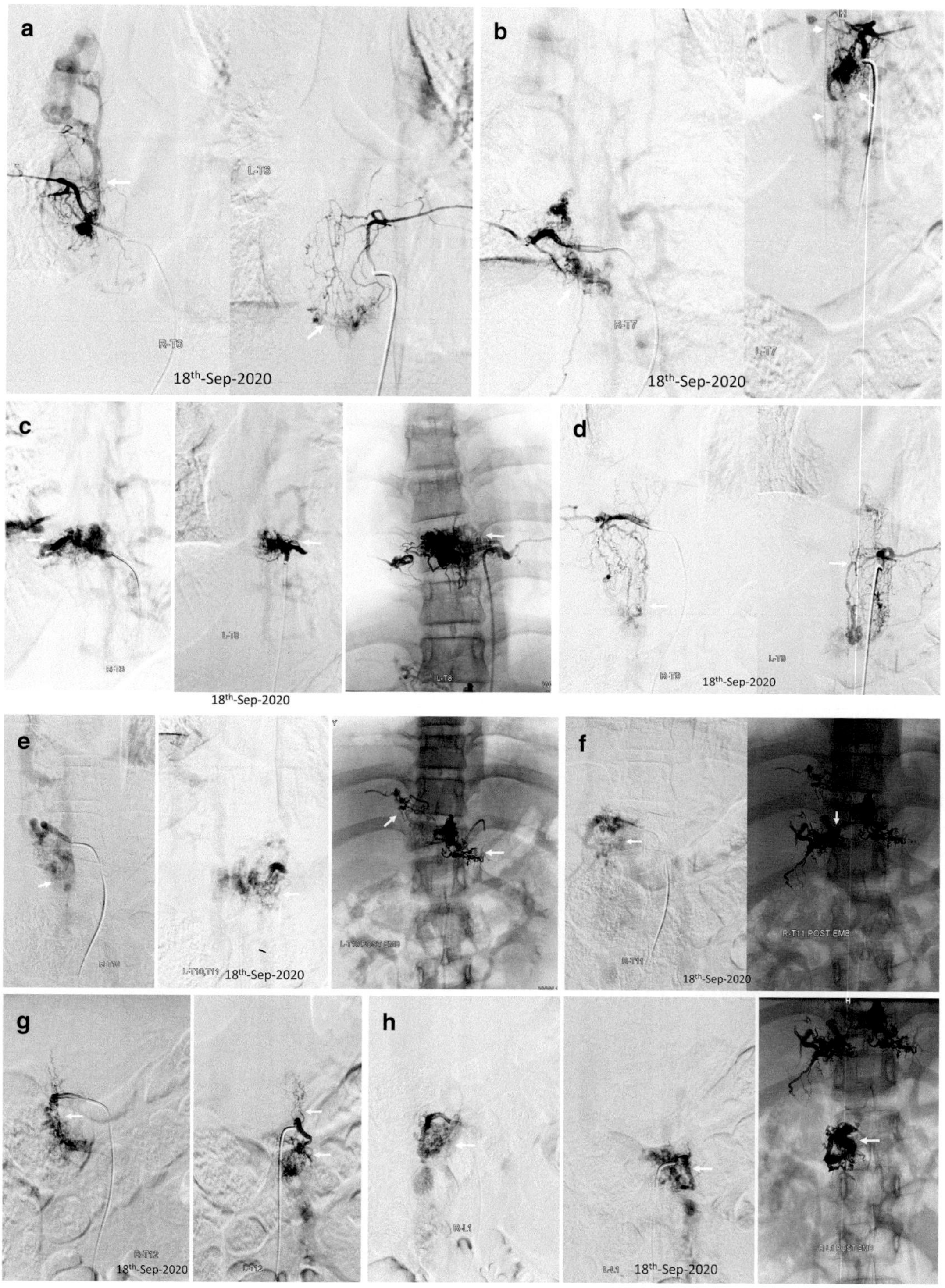

Fig. 9.7 (**a–k**) Spinal angiograms showing a giant spinal arteriovenous fistula from T6 to L4. The artery of Adamkiewicz arised at the left T7. T10, T11, and L2 were embolized using Onyx in other hospital. And the paraplegia deteriorated gradually

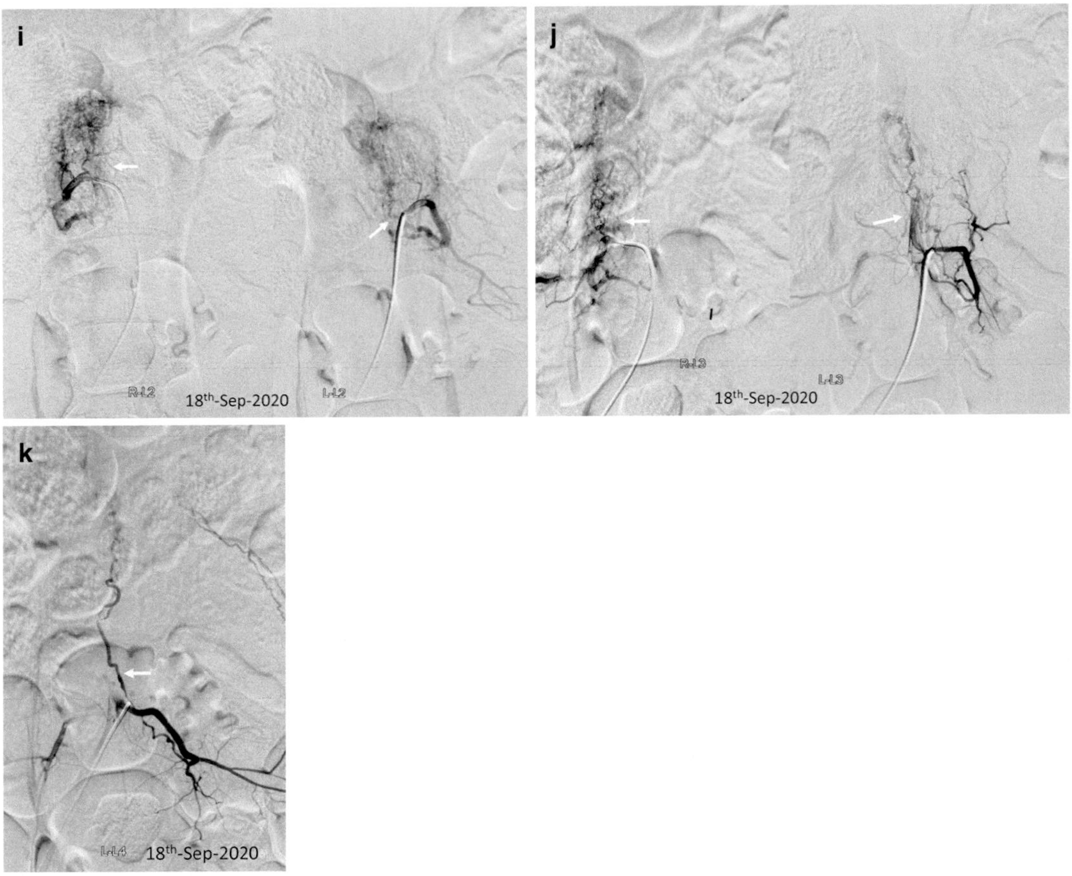

Fig. 9.7 (continued)

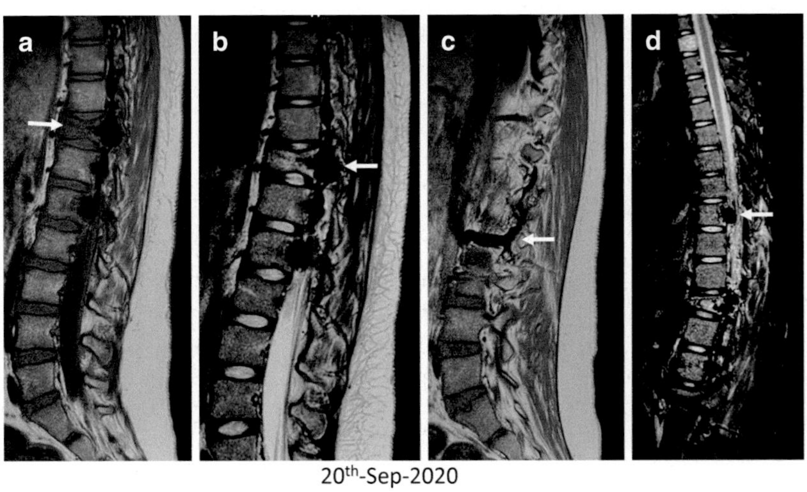

Fig. 9.8 MR images (**a**–**d**) showed multiple large flow void signals from T8 to L1. Sagittal MR images of the spine demonstrated four masses with flow voids from the level of T8 to L1 depicting the spinal AVM with venous aneurysms. Additionally, at the level of L1/L2, there is a flow void corresponding to the venous drainage of intervertebral vein, which demonstrates venomegaly

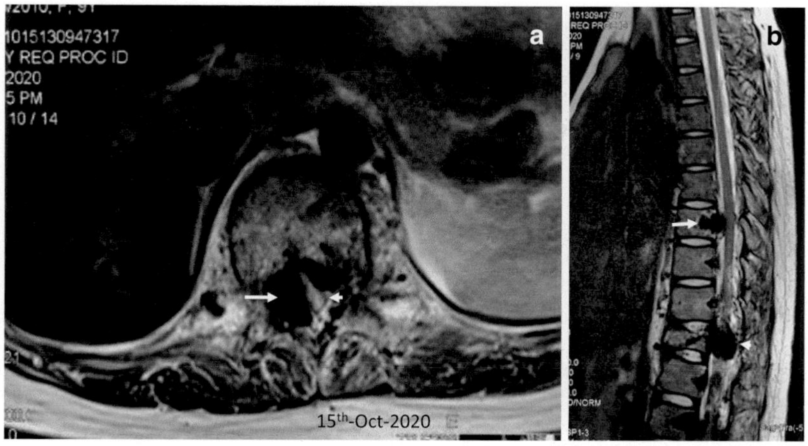

Fig. 9.9 (**a**) Axial T2-weighted image at T11 level showing the flow void of the AVM venous aneurysm occupying nearly the entire spinal canal and compressing the spinal cord from right to left. (**b**) MRI, sagittal view, showing multiple flow void signals in the intraspinal canal and extramedullary from T8 to L1

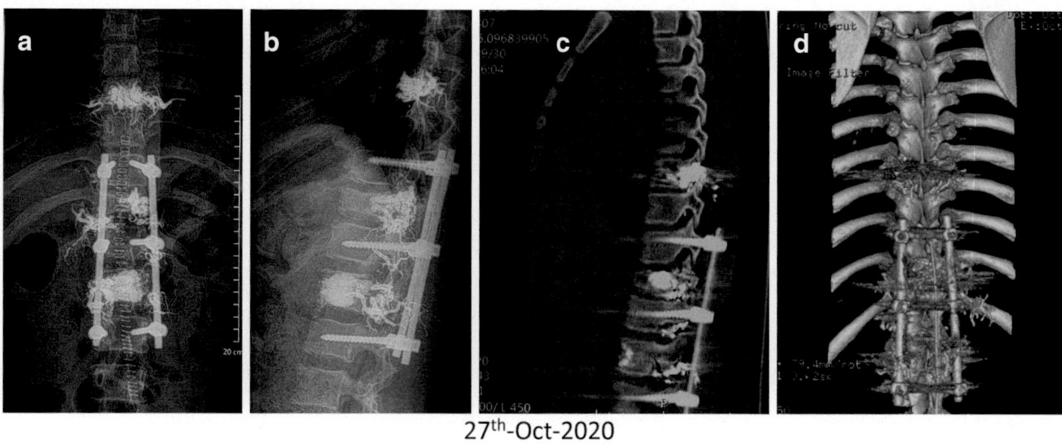

Fig. 9.10 The patient's paraplegia gradually worsened to completely paralyzed, and muscle tone increased. The diagnostic X-ray (**a** and **b**) and CT (**c** and **d**) images showing the local hospital performed L1 vertebroplasty and T10 to L2 vertebral fixation operation. There was no improvement after the operation. The patient was transferred to our hospital for further management on December 24, 2020. She was able to move her upper but not her lower extremities at presentation to our clinic

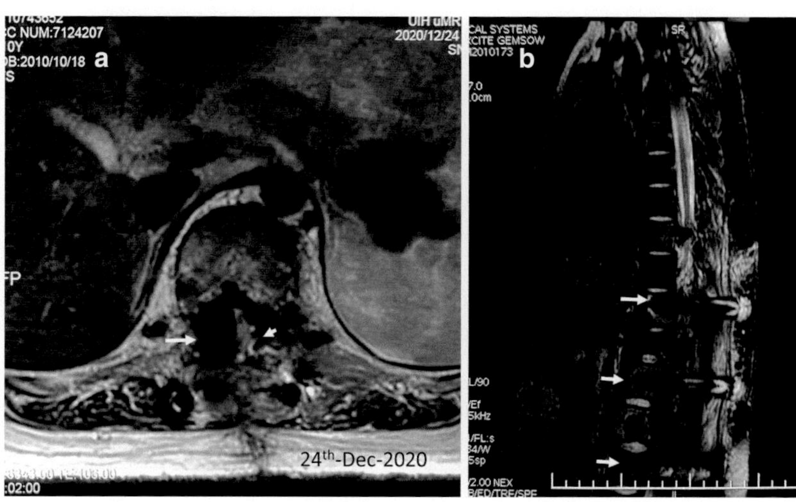

Fig. 9.11 (**a**) Axial T2-weighted image at T11 level showing the flow void of the AVM venous aneurysm occupying nearly the entire spinal canal. (**b**) MRI, sagittal view, showing flow void signals in the intraspinal canal and extramedullary from T8 to L1. She also had perimedullary dilated veins that compressed the spinal cord at T11, displacing it from right to left

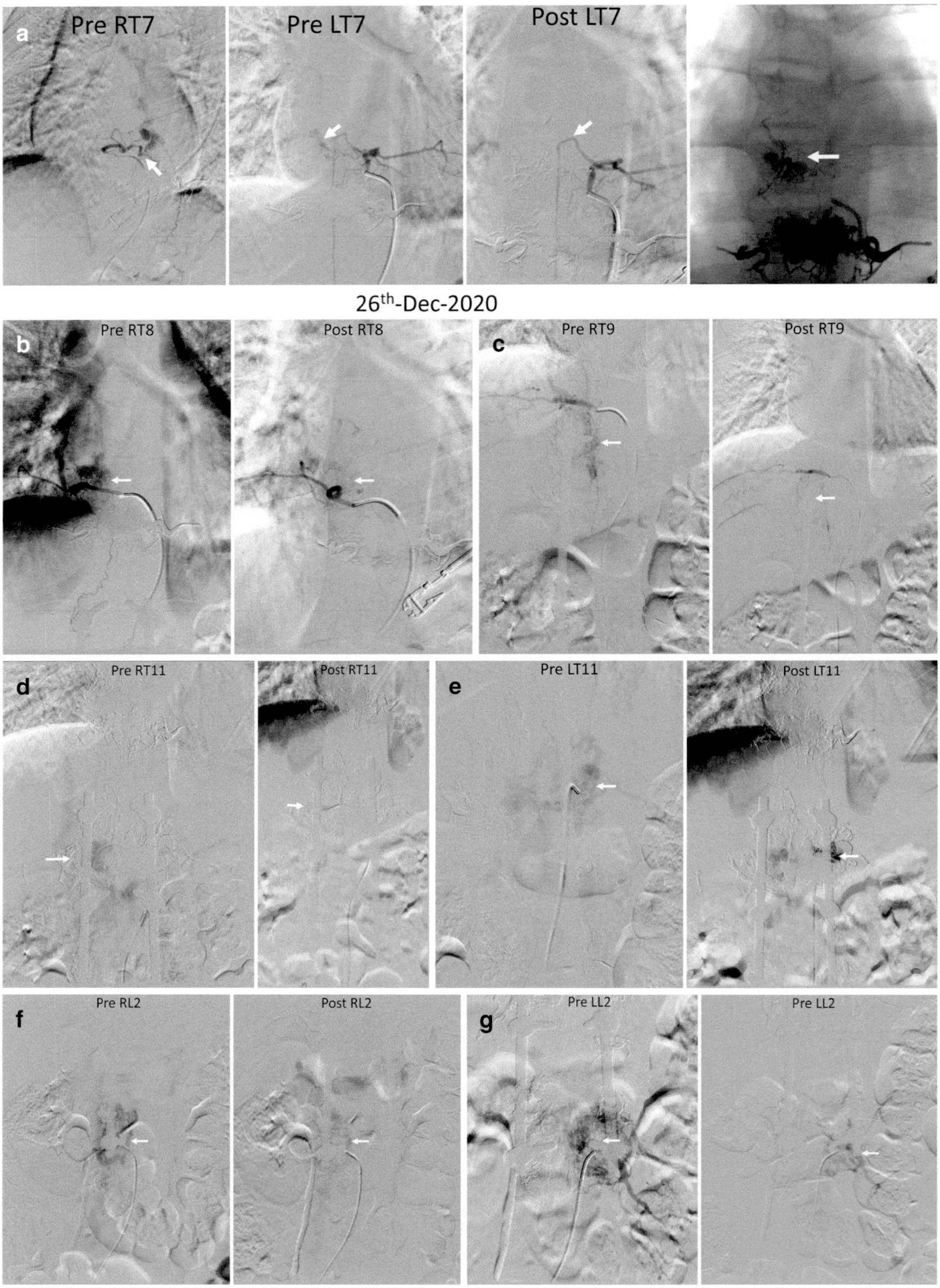

Fig. 9.12 (**a**–**j**) The angiogram and endovascular embolization procedures were performed under general anesthesia. The patient was found to have complex arteriovenous fistulas from the spinal dural and vertebrate branches of T7–L4 radicular arteries. The artery of Adamkiewicz arised at the left T7. The dural and vertebrate suppliers at T7–T9, T11, and L2 and L3 were embolized with Onyx. The patient remained paraplegic postoperatively. The patient is currently followed up. She has some sensation in the lower legs but remains paraplegic with neurogenic bowel and bladder syndrome

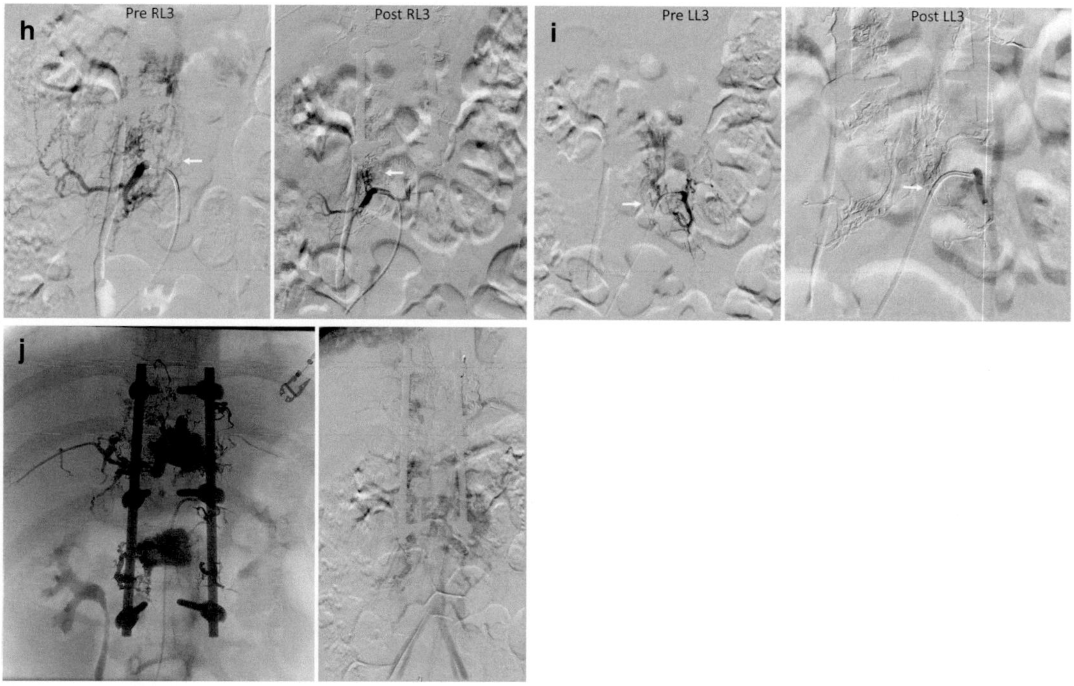

Fig. 9.12 (continued)

options include transarterial or transvenous endovascular embolization with liquid embolic agents (NBCA and Onyx) or coils and surgical resection [24, 67]. The "antegrade drifting Onyx injection technique," which has been promoted from 2017, can prevent reflux of Onyx and encourage Onyx distal penetration, and it has been used for embolization of brain AVMs with excellent results [68]. This technique has prevented serious bleeding complications and elevated complete embolization rate in cerebral nidal AVMs [69]. The drawbacks of conventional Onyx embolization include the time needed to create a proximal plug that allows forward flow of the agent into the lesion [70]. Another drawback is the proximal reflux of Onyx, which may damage the normal vasculature and lead to microcatheter retention [68]. There have been previous reports of a balloon-assisted Onyx embolization technique for paraspinal AVM embolization [49, 71]. Inflation of a proximal balloon creates a "plug," increasing the proximal resistance in the feeder, encouraging Onyx to penetrate more distally into the lesion.

9.16 Conclusions

Paraspinal AVMs occur isolated or associated with genetic syndrome. Isolated paraspinal AVMs are either acquired, due to trauma. Congenital paraspinal AVMs are associated with metameric link or systemic genetic background. The main route of venous drainage that causes symptoms is either extraspinal or intraspinal. The indications and techniques for endovascular therapy are based on individual clinical and anatomical standards.

References

1. Meisel HJ, Lasjaunias P, Brock M. Modern management of spinal and spinal cord vascular lesions. Minim Invasive Neurosurg. 1995;38(4):138–45.
2. Parizadeh D, Vasconcelos AHC, Miller DA, Fermo OP, Huynh TJ. Dual microcatheter and coil/balloon pressure cooker technique for transvenous embolization of cerebrospinal fluid-venous fistulas. J Neurointerv Surg. 2022;15(6):614. https://doi.org/10.1136/neurintsurg-2022-019005.

3. Brinjikji W, Garza I, Whealy M, Kissoon N, Atkinson JLD, Savastano L, Madhavan A, Cutsforth-Gregory J. Clinical and imaging outcomes of cerebrospinal fluid-venous fistula embolization. J Neurointerv Surg. 2022;14(10):953–6.
4. Kim JH, Yoon SH, Park SQ, Ban SP, Cho BK. Clinical features and treatment strategy of paraspinal arteriovenous shunt (PAVS): a systematic review with individual participants data meta-analysis. Eur Spine J. 2021;30(8):2385–400.
5. Toi H, Matsubara S, Watanabe S, Yamashita T, Uno M. Paraspinal arteriovenous fistula presenting with subarachnoid hemorrhage and acute progressive myelopathy–case report. Neurol Med Chir (Tokyo). 2011;51(12):846–9.
6. Rodesch G, Hurth M, Alvarez H, Tadié M, Lasjaunias P. Classification of spinal cord arteriovenous shunts: proposal for a reappraisal–the Bicêtre experience with 155 consecutive patients treated between 1981 and 1999. Neurosurgery. 2002;51(2):374–9; discussion 379-80.
7. Cognard C, Semaan H, Bakchine S, Miaux Y, Thibault S, Sola Martinez MT, Chiras J. Paraspinal arteriovenous fistula with perimedullary venous drainage. AJNR Am J Neuroradiol. 1995;16(10):2044–8.
8. Fotso A, Aubert D, Saltoun K, Galli G, Bonneville JF, Bracard S. Congenital paravertebral arteriovenous fistula: a case report. J Pediatr Surg. 2006;41(3):e21–3.
9. Szajner M, Weill A, Piotin M, Moret J. Endovascular treatment of a cervical paraspinal arteriovenous malformation via arterial and venous approaches. AJNR Am J Neuroradiol. 1999;20(6):1097–9.
10. Wendl CM, Aguilar Pérez M, Felber S, Stroszczynski C, Bäzner H, Henkes H. Paraspinal arteriovenous fistula: Stuttgart classification based on experience and a review of the literature. Br J Radiol. 2018;91(1088):20170337.
11. Diociaiuti A, Rotunno R, Pisaneschi E, Cesario C, Carnevale C, Condorelli AG, Rollo M, Di Cecca S, Quintarelli C, Novelli A, Zambruno G, El Hachem M. Clinical and molecular spectrum of sporadic vascular malformations: a single-center study. Biomedicines. 2022;10(6):1460.
12. Kitayama K, Ishiguro T, Komiyama M, Morisaki T, Morisaki H, Minase G, Hamanaka K, Miyatake S, Matsumoto N, Kato M, Takahashi T, Yorifuji T. Mutational and clinical spectrum of Japanese patients with hereditary hemorrhagic telangiectasia. BMC Med Genet. 2021;14(1):288. https://doi.org/10.1186/s12920-021-01139-y.
13. Eerola I, Boon LM, Mulliken JB, et al. Capillary malformation-arteriovenous malformation, a new clinical and genetic disorder caused by RASA1 mutations. Am J Hum Genet. 2003;73:1240–9.
14. Hughes DG, Alleyne CH Jr. Rare giant traumatic cervical arteriovenous fistula in neurofibromatosis type 1 patient. BMJ Case Rep. 2012;2012:bcr1220115354.
15. Hauck EF, Nauta HJ. Spontaneous spinal epidural arteriovenous fistulae in neurofibromatosis type-1. Surg Neurol. 2006;66(2):215–21.
16. Gaetani E, Peppucci E, Agostini F, Di Martino L, Lucci Cordisco E, Sturiale CL, Puca A, Porfidia A, Alexandre A, Pedicelli A, Pola R. Distribution of cerebrovascular phenotypes according to variants of the ENG and ACVRL1 genes in subjects with hereditary hemorrhagic telangiectasia. J Clin Med. 2022;11(10):2685.
17. Garreta Fontelles G, Pardo Pastor J, Grande MC. Alpelisib to treat CLOVES syndrome, a member of the PIK3CA-related overgrowth syndrome spectrum. Br J Clin Pharmacol. 2022;88(8):3891–5.
18. Luu M, Vabres P, Devilliers H, Loffroy R, Phan A, Martin L, Morice-Picard F, Petit F, Willems M, Bessis D, Jacquemont ML, Maruani A, Chiaverini C, Mirault T, Clayton-Smith J, Carpentier M, Fleck C, Maurer A, Yousfi M, Parker VER, Semple RK, Bardou M, Faivre L. Safety and efficacy of low-dose PI3K inhibitor taselisib in adult patients with CLOVES and Klippel-Trenaunay syndrome (KTS): the TOTEM trial, a phase 1/2 multicenter, open-label, single-arm study. Genet Med. 2021;23(12):2433–42.
19. Armon C, Daube JR. Electrophysiological signs of arteriovenous malformations of the spinal cord. J Neurol Neurosurg Psychiatry. 1989;52(10):1176–81.
20. Nakanishi K, Tanaka N, Fujimoto Y, Nishikawa K, Kamei N, Nakamae T, Kotaka S, Adachi N. Electrophysiological assessment and classification of motor pathway function in patients with spinal dural arteriovenous fistula. J Clin Neurophysiol. 2019;36(1):45–51.
21. Condette-Auliac S, Boulin A, Roccatagliata L, Coskun O, Guieu S, Guedin P, Rodesch G. MRI and MRA of spinal cord arteriovenous shunts. J Magn Reson Imaging. 2014;40(6):1253–66. https://doi.org/10.1002/jmri.24591. Erratum in: J Magn Reson Imaging. 2015 Feb;41(2):555.
22. Schmidt C, Lonjon J, Costalat V, Menjot De Champfleur N, Seris C, Brunel H, Bourbotte G, Bouillot P, Teissier JM, Martinat P, Bonafe A. Paraspinal arteriovenous malformations with perimedullary venous drainage. J Neuroradiol. 2008;35(3):165–72.
23. Chen CJ, Huang CC, Hsu YY, Hsu WC. Small isolated paraspinal arteriovenous fistula. AJNR Am J Neuroradiol. 1997;18(2):359–61.
24. Brinjikji W, Yin R, Nasr DM, Lanzino G. Spinal epidural arteriovenous fistulas. J Neurointerv Surg. 2016;8(12):1305–10.
25. Consoli A, Coskun O, Di Maria F, Gratieux J, Condette-Auliac S, Smadja S, Boulin A, Rodesch G. Spinal cord arterio-venous shunts: from classification to therapeutic management. Rev Neurol (Paris). 2021;177(5):469–76.
26. Brinjikji W, Colombo E, Cloft HJ, Lanzino G. Clinical and imaging characteristics of spinal dural arteriovenous fistulas and spinal epidural arteriovenous fistulas. Neurosurgery. 2021;88(3):666–73.
27. Yamaguchi S, Hida K, Asano T, Yano S, Kashiwazaki D, Iwasaki Y. Case of cervical paraspinal a5lae with a huge intracanalicular varix successfully treated

with transvenous embolization. No Shinkei Geka. 2008;36(6):547–53.
28. Akiyama Y, Ikeda J, Ibayashi Y, Nonaka T, Asai Y, Houkin K. Lhermitte-Duclos disease with cervical paraspinal arteriovenous fistula. Neurol Med Chir (Tokyo). 2006;46(9):446–9.
29. Ashour R, Orbach DB. Lower vertebral-epidural spinal arteriovenous fistulas: a unique subtype of vertebrovertebral arteriovenous fistula, treatable with coil and penumbra occlusion device embolization. J Neurointerv Surg. 2016;8(6):643–7.
30. Mitchell P, Thomas P, Anderson D. Spontaneous resolution of a non-traumatic vertebro-vertebral arteriovenous fistula in a paediatric patient. J Clin Neurosci. 2018;53:220–2.
31. Emery DJ, Willinsky RA, Burrows PE, Armstrong D, Montanera W, Terbrugge K. Paediatric spinal arteriovenous malformations: angioarchitecture and endovascular treatment. Interv Neuroradiol. 1998;4(2):127–39.
32. Wang Q, Song D, Chen G. Endovascular treatment of high-flow cervical direct vertebro-vertebral arteriovenous fistula with detachable coils and onyx liquid embolic agent. Acta Neurochir. 2011;153(2):347–52.
33. Kähärä V, Lehto U, Sajanti J. Presacral arteriovenous fistula: case report. Neurosurgery. 2003;53(3):774–6; discussion 776–7.
34. Kona MP, Buch K, Singh J, Rohatgi S. Spinal vascular shunts: a patterned approach. AJNR Am J Neuroradiol. 2021;42(12):2110–8.
35. Lanzino G, D'Urso PI, Kallmes DF, Cloft HJ. Onyx embolization of extradural spinal arteriovenous malformations with intradural venous drainage. Neurosurgery. 2012;70(2):329–33.
36. Clarke MJ, Patrick TA, White JB, Cloft HJ, Krauss WE, Lindell EP, Piepgras DG. Spinal extradural arteriovenous malformations with parenchymal drainage: venous drainage variability and implications in clinical manifestations. Neurosurg Focus. 2009;26(1):E5.
37. Ramanathan D, Levitt MR, Sekhar LN, Kim LJ, Hallam DK, Ghodke BV. Management of spinal epidural arteriovenous fistulas: interventional techniques and results. J Neurointerv Surg. 2014;6(2):144–9.
38. Song Y, Cho SH, Lee DW, Sheen JJ, Shin JH, Suh DC. Osseous versus nonosseous spinal epidural arteriovenous fistulas: experiences of 13 patients. AJNR Am J Neuroradiol. 2019;40(1):129–34.
39. Lv X, Wang G, Wang J. Craniospinal vascular diseases and endovascular neurosurgery. NY, USA: Nova Science; 2021.
40. Gross BA, Du R. Spinal juvenile (type III) extradural-intradural arteriovenous malformations. J Neurosurg Spine. 2014;20:452–8.
41. Spetzler RF, Zabramski JM, Flom RA. Management of juvenile spinal AVM's by embolization and operative excision. Case report J Neurosurg. 1989;70(4):628–32.
42. Niimi Y, Uchiyama N, Elijovich L, Berenstein A. Spinal arteriovenous metameric syndrome: clinical manifestations and endovascular management. AJNR Am J Neuroradiol. 2013;34(2):457–63.
43. Santillan A, Zink W, Patsalides A, Gobin YP. Thoracolumbar artery aneurysms associated with a metameric paraspinal lesion presenting with retroperitoneal hemorrhage: endovascular management. Surg Neurol Int. 2011;2:137.
44. Fairhall JM, Reddy R, Sears W, Wenderoth JD, Stoodley MA. Successful endovascular and surgical treatment of spinal extradural metameric arteriovenous malformation. Case report J Neurosurg Spine. 2010;13(6):784–8.
45. Komiyama M, Ishiguro T, Terada A, Watanabe Y, Nakajima H, Ohata Y, Matsusaka Y. Spinal arteriovenous metameric syndrome in a neonate presenting with congestive heart failure: case report. Childs Nerv Syst. 2014;30(9):1607–11.
46. Ibrahim D, Mashhour S. Report of a case of cobb syndrome: multimodality imaging. BJR Case Rep. 2020;7(1):20200145.
47. Lenck S, Nicholson P, Tymianski R, Hilditch C, Nouet A, Patel K, Krings T, Tymianski M, Radovanovic I, Mendes PV. Spinal and paraspinal arteriovenous lesions. Stroke. 2019;50(8):2259–69.
48. Mekonnen B, Richardson Q, Bhisitkul JM, Diab M, Rasool N. Bilateral optic disc pits in a pediatric patient with Cobb syndrome. Am J Ophthalmol Case Rep. 2020;19:100749.
49. Prasad SN, Barman B, Singh V, Das KK. Combined endovascular and surgical management of a case of cobb syndrome. BMJ Case Rep. 2022;15(2):e246821.
50. Edwards EA, Phelps AS, Cooke D, Frieden IJ, Zapala MA, Fullerton HJ, Shimano KA. Monitoring arteriovenous malformation response to genotype-targeted therapy. Pediatrics. 2020;146(3):e20193206.
51. Alomari AI, Chaudry G, Rodesch G, Burrows PE, Mulliken JB, Smith ER, Fishman SJ, Orbach DB. Complex spinal-paraspinal fast-flow lesions in CLOVES syndrome: analysis of clinical and imaging findings in 6 patients. AJNR Am J Neuroradiol. 2011;32(10):1812–7.
52. Alomari AI. Characterization of a distinct syndrome that associates complex truncal overgrowth, vascular, and acral anomalies: a descriptive study of 18 cases of CLOVES syndrome. Clin Dysmorphol. 2009;18(1):1–7.
53. Li ZF, Li Q, Xu Y, Hong B, Huang QH, Liu JM. Spinal arteriovenous malformation associated with Parkes weber syndrome: report of two cases and literature review. World Neurosurg. 2017;107:1043.e7–1043.e13. https://doi.org/10.1016/j.wneu.2017.06.080.
54. Alomari AI, Orbach DB, Mulliken JB, et al. Klippel-Trenaunay syndrome and spinal arteriovenous malformations: an erroneous association. AJNR Am J Neuroradiol. 2010;31(9):1608–12. https://doi.org/10.3174/ajnr.A2167.
55. Banzic I, Brankovic M, Maksimović Ž, Davidović L, Marković M, Rančić Z. Parkes weber syndrome-diagnostic and management paradigms: a systematic

review. Phlebology. 2017;32(6):371–83. https://doi.org/10.1177/0268355516664212.
56. Larson A, Covington T, Anderson K, Tollefson M, Lanzino G, Brinjikji W. Spinal neurovascular malformations in Klippel-Trenaunay syndrome: a single center study. Neurosurgery. 2021;88(3):515–22.
57. Den Hartog Jager WA. About two new forms in the group of the phacomatoses. Folia Psychiatr Neurol Neurochir Neerl. 1949;52:356–64.
58. Djindjian M, Djindjian R, Hurth M, et al. Spinal cord arteriovenous malformations and the Klippel-Trenaunay-weber syndrome. Surg Neurol. 1977;8:229–37.
59. Lasjaunias P, Ter Brugge KG, Berenstein A. Surgical Neuroangiography: clinical and interventional aspects in children, vol. 3. New York: SpringerVerlag; 2006.
60. Kerber CW, Cromwell LD, Sheptak PE. Intraarterial cyanoacrylate: an adjunct in the treatment of spinal/paraspinal arteriovenous malformations. AJR Am J Roentgenol. 1978;130(1):99–103.
61. Niimi Y, Berenstein A, Setton A, Pryor J. Symptoms, vascular anatomy and endovascular treatment of spinal cord arteriovenous malformations. Interv Neuroradiol. 2000;6 Suppl 1(Suppl 1):199–202.
62. Itoh S, Ishiguchi T, Negoro M, Hirose M, Fukazu H, Endo T, Ishigaki T, Sakuma S. Evaluation of transcatheter arterial embolization with coaxial microcatheter and micro-coil for vascular lesions. Nihon Igaku Hoshasen Gakkai Zasshi. 1992;52(4):452–60.
63. Farhat N, Desprechins B, Otto B, Ramaekers V, Seghaye MC. Paraspinal arterio-venous fistula in children: two more cases of an exceptional malformation. Clin Pract. 2015;5(2):707.
64. Niimi Y, Berenstein A, Fernandez PM, Brisman JL, Song JK. Pediatric nonvertebral paraspinal arteriovenous fistulas along the segmental nerve: clinical, imaging, and therapeutic considerations. J Neurosurg. 2005;103(2 Suppl):156–62.
65. Gibbs IC. Spinal and paraspinal lesions: the role of stereotactic body radiotherapy. Front Radiat Ther Oncol. 2007;40:407–14.
66. Lv X. Arteriovenous malformations of the brain. New York: Nova Science, NY, USA; 2020.
67. Toyoshima A, Tokunaga K, Manabe H, Sugiu K, Hiramatsu M, Itami H, Hishikawa T, Date I. A case of a paraspinal arteriovenous fistula presenting with retroperitoneal hemorrhage treated by staged transarterial and transvenous embolization. No Shinkei Geka. 2013 May;41(5):429–35.
68. Lv X. Letter: comparison of N-butyl cyanoacrylate and onyx for the embolization of intracranial arteriovenous malformations-analysis of fluoroscopy and procedure times. Oper Neurosurg (Hagerstown). 2017;13(6):E37–8.
69. Lv X, Liang S. Update onyx embolization for plexiform arteriovenous malformation: ante-grade drifting technique. Neuroradiol J. 2020;33(5):386–92.
70. Rangel-Castilla L, Holman PJ, Krishna C, Trask TW, Klucznik RP, Diaz OM. Spinal extradural arteriovenous fistulas: a clinical and radiological description of different types and their novel treatment with onyx. J Neurosurg Spine. 2011;15(5):541–9.
71. Martínez-Galdámez M, Rodriguez-Arias CA, Utiel E, Arreba E, Gonzalo M, Arenillas JF. Paraspinal arteriovenous malformation onyx embolization via an ascent balloon. J Neurointerv Surg. 2014;6(3):e19.

10 Spinal Vascular Malformations and Endovascular Considerations

Nok Lun Chan and Tak Lap Poon

Abstract

Spinal vascular malformations (SVMs) represent a heterogeneous neurovascular disease entity. The group includes arteriovenous malformations (AVMs), arteriovenous fistulas (AVFs), neoplastic in origin like cavernous malformations (CMs) and haemangioblastomas, and rarely venous malformations and spinal aneurysms. In this chapter, the pathophysiology of each group and the treatment modalities including open surgery and endovascular intervention will be briefly discussed. With the increasing popularity of endovascular intervention, the aspects in consideration including anatomy and patients will be evaluated in clinical practice.

Keywords

Spinal vascular malformations · Arteriovenous malformation · Arteriovenous fistula · Endovascular intervention

N. L. Chan · T. L. Poon (✉)
Department of Neurosurgery, Queen Elizabeth Hospital, Hong Kong, China

10.1 Introduction

Spinal vascular malformations (SVMs) are one of the rare entities in neurovascular diseases. This disease group can be subdivided into arteriovenous malformation (AVMs), arteriovenous fistulas (AVFs) and cavernous malformations (CMs), neoplastic in origin including haemangioblastomas, and rarely venous malformations and spinal aneurysms. The rough estimated incidence ranges from 0.05 to 0.67 per 100,000 population [1]. Among the different disease entities, spinal AVMs and AVFs are the most common pathologies and account for 60–80% of all recognized cases, followed by spinal CMs in 10–20% of cases [1]. SVMs can be diagnosed in any age, but they are more to be seen in adult patients between ages of 30 and 40 [1].

10.2 Pathophysiology

Spinal AVMs/AVFs usually affect cervical and upper thoracic spinal regions. The clinical presentation and subsequent neurological impairments relate to the classification according to the classification system proposed by Barrow Neurological Institute [2]:

1. Type I (dural AVFs) typically causes radiculomyelopathy followed by progressive deterioration of neurological symptoms (Fig. 10.1).

X. Lv (ed.), *Endovascular and Neurovascular Surgery for Spinal Vascular Malformations*,
https://doi.org/10.1007/978-981-97-4661-3_10

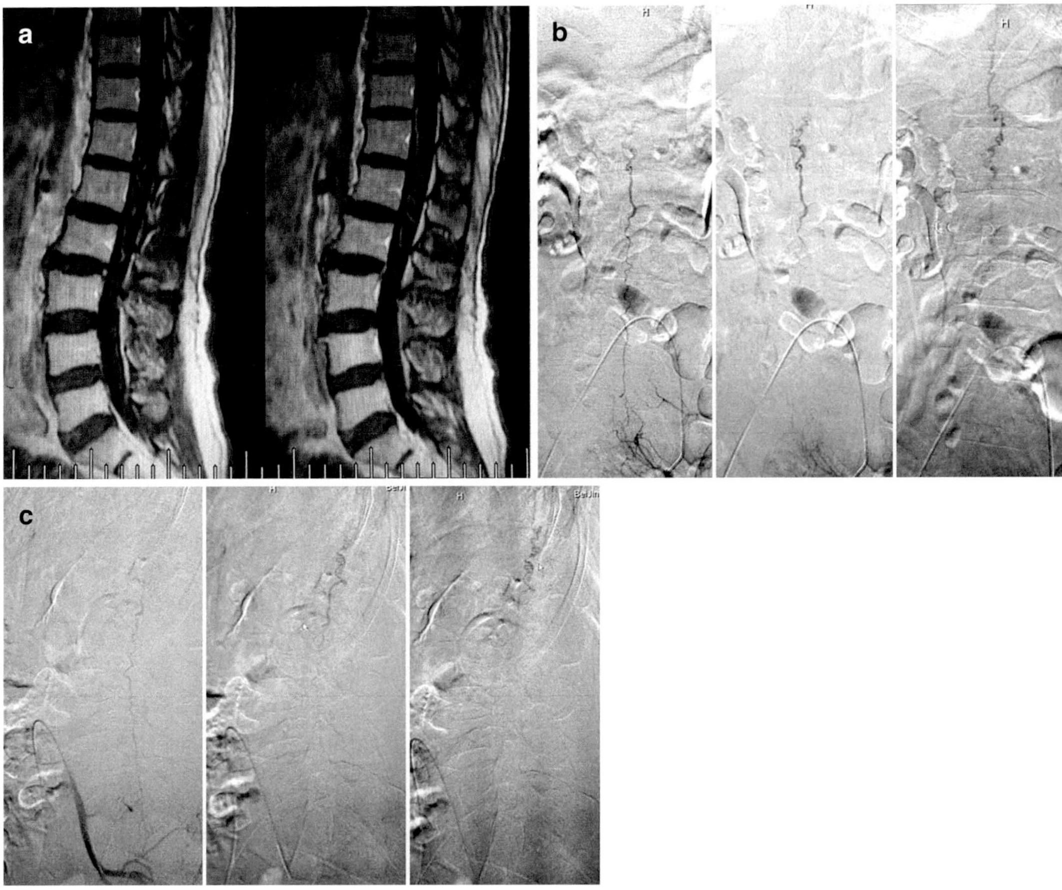

Fig. 10.1 A 51-year-old male patient had weakness in both lower limbs, numbness, and difficulty urinating. (**a**) Lumbosacral MRI, enhanced, showing enhanced vascular image around the cauda equina. (**b** and **c**) The left internal iliac artery angiography, anterior-posterior view (**b**) and lateral view (**c**), showing a sacral dural arteriovenous fistula, which is supplied by the anterior sacral artery and drained upwards from the vein of filum terminale to the thoracolumbar spinal cord veins

Acute bleeding with sudden clinical deterioration is uncommon. The fistula arterial feeders come from the corresponding level of radiculomeningeal artery.

2. Type II (intramedullary glomus AVMs) usually has presentation in progressive and fluctuating myelopathy with long tract sign. Acute neurological deterioration secondary to haemorrhage with AVMs in the forms of subarachnoid haemorrhage or spinal intramedullary haemorrhage is more frequent.
3. Type III (juvenile AVMs) presents similar to type II cases. The neurological deterioration may also be resulted from vascular steal and/or venous hypertension.
4. Type IV (perimedullary AVFs) usually presents gradually progressive neurological changes with occasionally sudden worsening in those patients.

10.3 Natural History of SVMs

Only by knowing the natural history of a disease can you offer the best treatment to patients, especially for those with SVMs.

Type I (spinal dural AVFs): These are the most common type of SVM, accounting for 80–85% of all SVM. There is usually a low-flow fistula between a radicular artery and medullar vein at the dural sleeve of the nerve root, which leads to venous hypertension, cord oedema and subsequently clinical myelopathy. Patients with spinal dural AVF may present with progressive back pain and neurological dysfunction. Acute neurological deterioration due to bleeding is rare. Nearly half of the patients reported back pain as the earliest symptom. One-third of patients had lower limbs weakness as the presenting symptom. Only 10% of patients complained sphincter disturbance or sexual dysfunction. In an observational cohort study, 19% of patients became severely disabled within 6 months after onset of motor symptoms. By 3 years, the number increased to 50%. After 3 years, less than 10% of patients remained physically undisturbed [2].

Type II (intramedullary glomus AVM): These are genuine arteriovenous malformation located completely or partially within the spinal cord. They are composed of nidus supplied by multiple feeding vessels, usually from anterior spinal artery or posterior spinal artery, and drained by medullary veins. In contrast to spinal dural AVFs, they are most likely to have haemorrhage, leading to acute neurological deterioration. Their rebleeding risk is high, at a rate of 10% within 30 days and 40% within the first year [2].

Type III (juvenile AVMs): These are also known as metameric vascular malformation, which are composed of large, high-flow vascular malformation involving structures that are derived from the same spinal metameric segment. They can be localized in the bone, epidural space, spinal cord, paraspinal soft tissue or muscles, subcutaneous tissue and skin. Neurological deficits occur due to mass effect from the AVMs per se, venous congestion, vascular steal phenomenon and haemorrhage. The classical presentation is pain and progressive myelopathy in children and adolescents [2].

Type IV (perimedullary AVFs): These are vascular malformation characterized by the presence of abnormal communication between spinal arteries and veins, on the pial surface of the spinal cord without an intervening nidus. The blood flow with these lesions is usually high, leading to aneurysmal formation and venous ectasia. They usually manifest with either progressive myelopathy due to venous hypertension or acute neurological deterioration secondary to aneurysmal rupture. Natural history is not completely clear, but they typically cause clinical symptoms, and asymptomatic cases are rather rare. Annual rupture risk was estimated as 2.5%, increasing to 5.6% after first haemorrhage in one cohort [2].

To conclude, treatments are recommended for patient with SVMs due to high deterioration and rupture risk. However, the aim of treatment and choice of treatment modalities may vary among these patients. Generally, the aim of treatment for type I and type IV SVMs is complete obliteration of the fistula, to eliminate the venous hypertension, whereas the aim of treatment for type II and type III is usually functional preservation rather than an angiographic cure.

10.4 Treatment Modalities of Choice

Treatment modalities include (1) conservative management, (2) open microvascular surgery, (3) endovascular intervention and (4) radiosurgery/radiotherapy [3–6].

10.4.1 Conservative Management

As discussed, conservative management is generally not recommended due to high risk of deterioration. However, for patient with significant medical comorbidities, or for those with complex malformation that is not amendable with open or endovascular treatment, conservative management may be adopted. Treatment usually focuses on pain management, physiotherapy and general nursing care.

10.4.2 Open Microvascular Surgery

For simple type I dural AVFs, surgical fistula disconnection is not a difficult procedure with reported successful rate as high as 98% [3, 4]. Complication rate is also as low as 1.9%, reported in a meta-analysis. The most challenging part is probably the localization of the spinal level in which the fistula is located. Identification of the fistulous site may be difficult on MRI and spinal angiogram, and preoperative localization with radio-opaque marker, intraoperative fluoroscopy, intraoperative ultrasound and intraoperative neuronavigation are all useful in lesion localization (Fig. 10.2). Clinical results are usually excellent. Previous report showed that over 60% of patients showed clinical improvement in motor function after surgical disconnection. Another report showed favourable result in 77% of their patients. Recurrence rate was reported to be as low as 4%.

However, open microsurgical surgery for type II or type III SMVs is not as effective as for patients with type I SMVs. Previous cohort reported that clinical deterioration could be observed in 20% of patients with spinal AVM treatment with open surgery. Due to the size and complexity of type III SMVs, generally open surgery should not be considered.

Type IV perimedullary AVFs were further classified into three subtypes. Type IVa lesions are small with low-flow single shunting communication. The arterial supply is usually from the anterior spinal artery and small in calibre, which

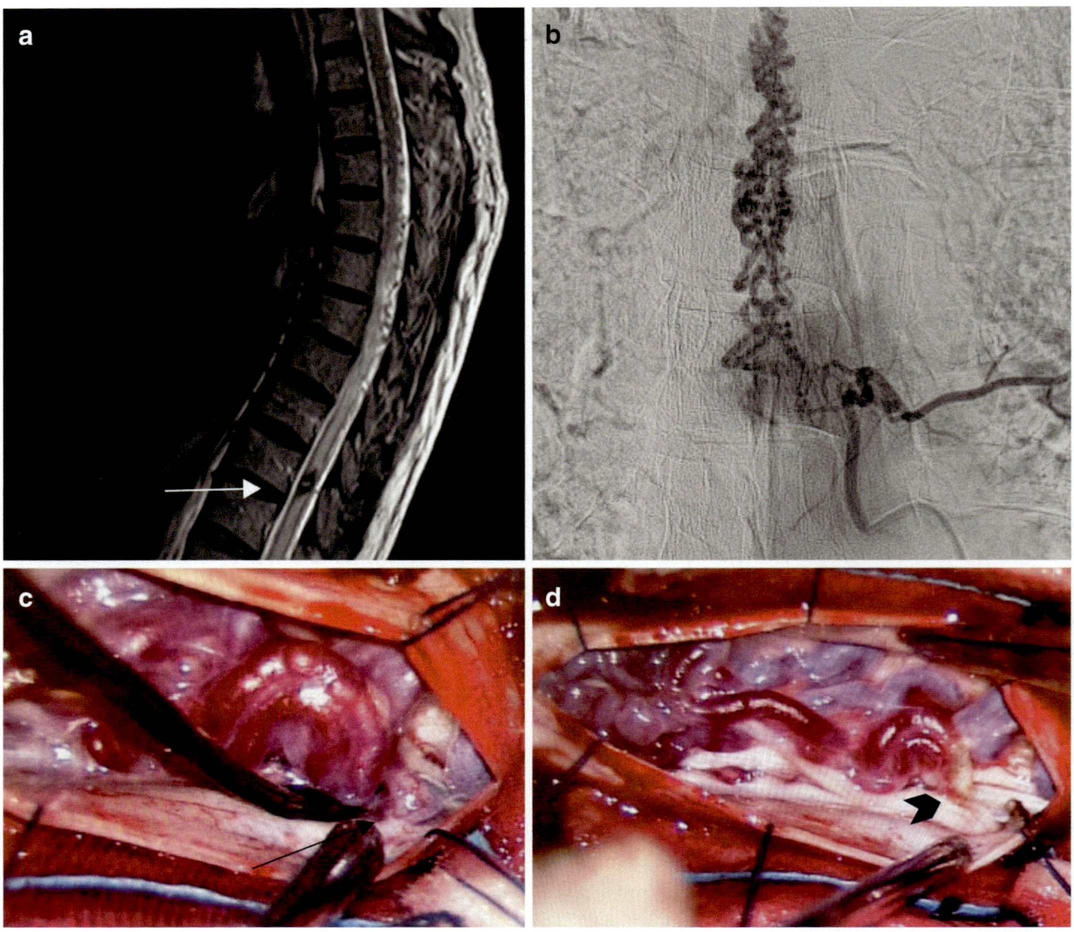

Fig. 10.2 (**a**) A 57-year-old male patient presented with sudden onset of paraplegia. MRI showed serpiginous vessels posterior to the thoracic spinal cord. There was also intra-parenchymal haematoma at T10 (white arrow). (**b**) Spinal angiography showed type I SMV with arterial feeder from left T7 segmental artery. (**c**) Surgical open disconnection. Note the common venous outflow just inferior to the left T7 exiting the nerve root (black arrow). (**d**) The common venous outflow was cauterized and cut (black arrowhead). Note the much less congested vessels on the cord surface after the disconnection

prohibits selective catheterization. Thus, open surgery is usually the choice for treatment. However, the ventral located lesion may pose extra difficulties in the surgical exposure. Type IVb lesions were composed of multiple dilated arterial feeders of intermediate size. Type IVc lesions consist of multiple dilated arterial feeders and ectatic draining veins. These two subtypes were big or even giant in size, making microsurgical dissection difficult. Intraoperative bleeding can be torrential. They were usually tackled with endovascular treatment. Microsurgeries are usually reserved for patient in whom endovascular intervention fails.

The disadvantage of open surgery is obviously the surgical wound. It can lead to significant postoperative pain, haematoma, infection, CSF leakage, etc. Another disadvantage is that intraoperative spinal angiography may be technically difficult, due to patients' prone position. Nowadays, many surgeons prefer intraoperative video angiography using indocyanine green (ICG). Under microscope with appropriate filter, the vasculature can be excellently shown, and the extent of disconnect or resection of AVM can be immediately determined. Twenty per cent of 20 patients with type II AVM with surgery done had worsening of neurological symptoms.

10.4.3 Endovascular Intervention

Advancement in endovascular technology was obviously significant in the past few decades, which made more and more vascular lesions to be tackled with endovascular means. Two major components were new microcatheters and liquid embolic agents.

In order to maximize the effectiveness of trans-arterial embolization, neuro-interventionists should advance the microcatheter as close as possible to the fistulous point. With the newer, extremely fine microcatheters, neuro-interventionists can navigate through small and tortuous vasculatures to the fistulous point. They allow catheterization of previously "inaccessible" arterial route.

Endovascular treatment had been criticized because of its low success rate and high recurrence rate. Previously, commonly used embolic agents were particle-based such as silk and polyvinyl alcohol (PVA). The recurrence rate was reported to be as high as 83%. The use of liquid adhesives such N-butyl-2-cyanoacrylate (NBCA) allows more promising obliteration of the fistula. However, due to its physical properties, complications like non-target embolization and catheter adhesion may occur. Later, the application of Onyx provided further improvement in endovascular intervention. Onyx can be delivered slowly in a more controlled manner and carries lower risk of premature occlusion of draining veins and catheter adhesion. Recently, another new agent called precipitating hydrophobic injectable liquid (PHIL) became more widely used among interventionists [6]. Theoretically, PHIL can be even injected more rapidly than Onyx because of its physical property. It may present an "in-between" agent, which is liquid enough to propagate forward easily but in a controlled manner.

With the advancement in the application of new liquid embolic agent, the endovascular treatment of type I SMVs became more and more acceptable (Fig. 10.3). The obliteration rate increased significantly as long as the embolic penetration into the fistula and proximal draining vein. The latest report showed that endovascular treatment provided durable cure in up to 70–85% of patients when the embolic agent penetrates the proximal draining vein. A meta-analysis reported that the overall complication for embolization was 3.7%, slightly higher than that in open surgery. Overall, both obliteration rate and complication rate are worse when compared with open surgery. However, the non-invasive nature is very attractive and welcomed to some patients. Some interventionists advocated embolization as the first-line treatment as long as there is not a common pedicle for the feeder and spinal artery.

Open surgery for type II lesions carries high risk of postoperative morbidities even under best hands. On the other hand, complete obliteration by endovascular treatment is possible. However, it is usually accompanied by morbidities.

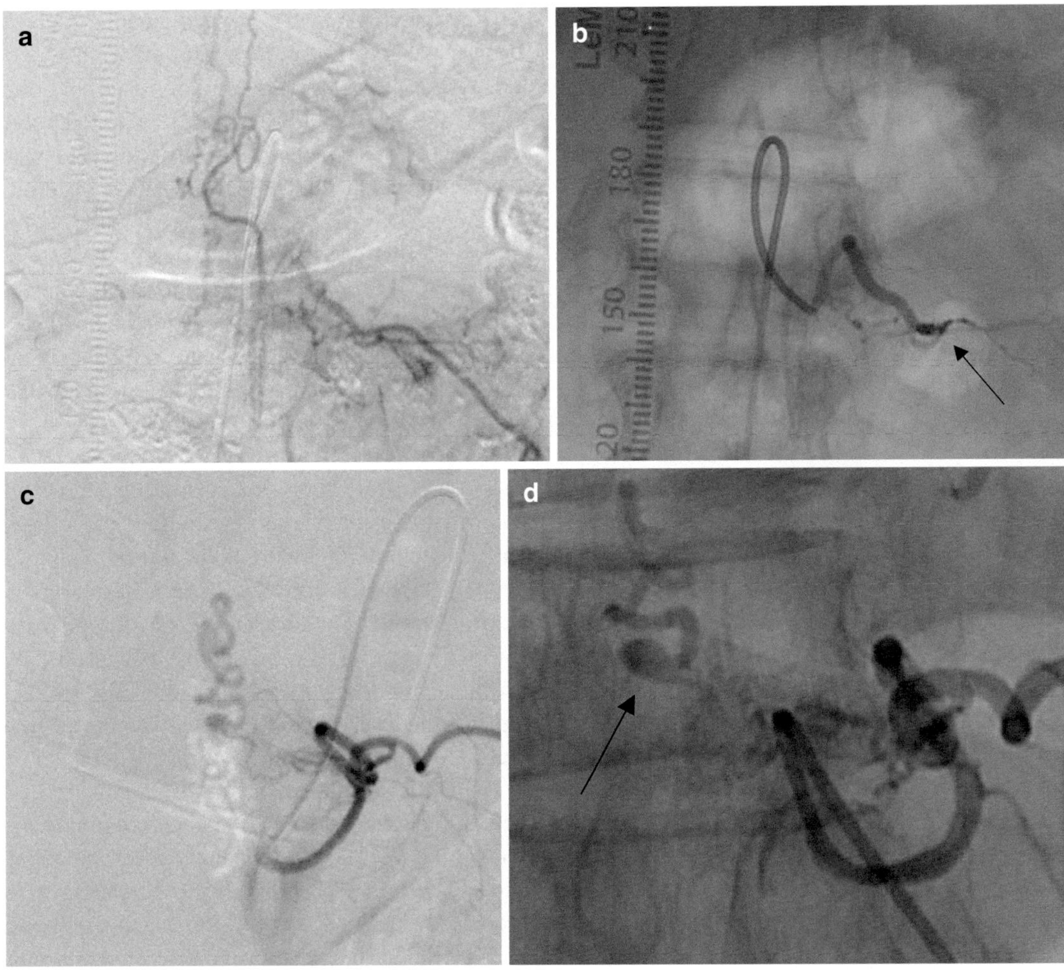

Fig. 10.3 (**a**) Pre-embolization of a patient with type I SMV with arterial feeder from the left T10 segmental artery. (**b**) Post-embolization angiography. Note the coil deployed (arrow) at the left T10 intercostal artery to facilitate forward flow of the liquid embolic agent (25% PHIL) to the proximal drainage vein. (**c**) Pre-embolization angiography of a patient with type I SMV with arterial feeder from left T12 segmental artery. (**d**) Post-embolization angiography. Note the presence of radio-opaque liquid embolic agent at the proximal draining vein (arrow)

Therefore, the general goal in the management of type II lesions is to preserve neurological function rather than to obtain a radiological cure. Partial targeted treatment to obliterate nidal aneurysm, to reduce the size and flow and to decongest the venous drainage may stabilize or even improve the clinical situation. Over 60% of patients exhibited clinical improvement compared with baseline findings in one cohort. Another cohort reported that 9 out of 11 patients with type II SVMs experienced improvement in functional outcome. The reported complication rate is around 8–11%, where the significance of which depends on whether catheterization of the anterior spinal artery is required or not.

Limited case reports of improvement or cure do exist, and treatment of type III SVMs is still largely palliative in nature. Targeting high risk portion of the lesion may benefit some of the patients as described in the management of type II lesion. The involvement and complexity are highly variable, case-by-case basis and multidisciplinary approach are always the best of patients with type III SVMs.

As mentioned, the arterial supply of type IVa DVMs is small in calibre. Catheterization is often technically difficult. Moreover, they usually arise from anterior spinal artery. Embolization may cause ischaemia to the spinal cord and is considered to be contraindicated. Therefore, this type of SMVs is usually managed with open surgery.

Generally, endovascular treatment achieves better result in type IVc lesion than in type IVb. Multiplicity of feeding pedicles is usually present in both types of lesions, making cure more difficult after embolization. However, the larger calibre of the feeding arteries allows more endovascular manoeuvres, which improve the obliteration rate. These manoeuvres include balloon occlusion, formation of anti-reflux plug by coiling, etc. In the literature, endovascular cure in type IVb lesions is usually considered as improbable. Endovascular treatment, nevertheless, remains as a therapeutic alternative for patients who are not good surgical candidates. On the other hand, the obliteration rate for type IVc lesion is generally high (Fig. 10.4). Reports showed that the obliteration rate can be up to 68–83%. Overall good clinical outcome could be seen in 86% of patients after endovascular treat-

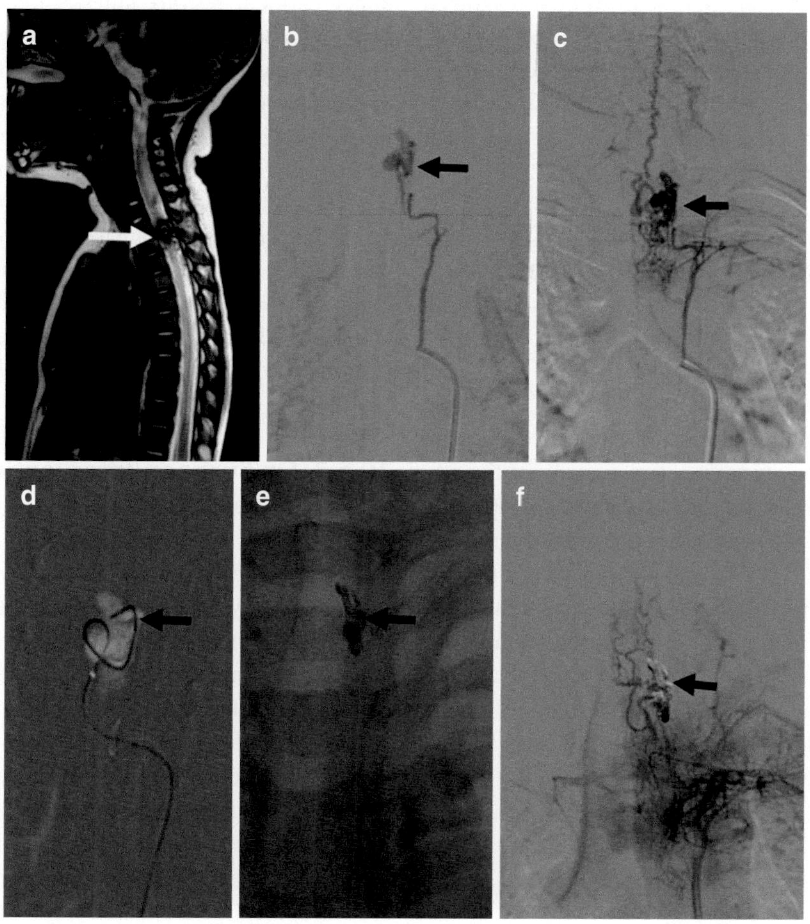

Fig. 10.4 A 2-year-old female patient had paralysis in both lower limbs and weakness in urination. (**a**) Cervicothoracic MRI, T2-weighted, sagittal view, showing a haemorrhagic lesion in the spinal cord at the level of T1. (**b**) The left T5 posterior intercostal artery angiography, early (**b**) and late (**c**) arterial phase, showing T1 level type IVc perimedullary arteriovenous fistula (AVF) supplied from the posterior spinal artery, drained from the spinal surface veins with aneurysmal dilation at the proximal end of the drainage vein. (**d**) Road map visualization of a microcatheter reaching the fistula site. (**e**) Non-subtractive image showing the Onyx casting. (**f**) Post-embolization angiography showing complete embolization of the perimedullary AVF

ment. Type IVc lesions can generally benefit from initial embolization, and open surgery can always be reserved for those in whom endovascular treatments fail.

10.4.4 Radiosurgery/Radiotherapy

Stereotactic radiosurgery and fractionated radiotherapy are used in patients with SMVs as in they are used in cerebral AVMs. Their non-invasiveness and reasonable effectiveness attract popularities. However, they take years to become effective. In a systematic review, over a mean follow-up time of 46.8 months, angiographic follow-up showed the nidus to be obliterated in 16%, decreased in 44.6% and unchanged in 39.3%. Overall good outcomes were reported in 92.2% of patients. Further details of radiotherapy for SMVs are out of scope of this chapter [5].

10.5 Endovascular Considerations

10.5.1 On Patient Aspects

Patient age and medical comorbidity determine whether a patient is a good surgical candidate. Poor cardiorespiratory function significantly increases the risk of general anaesthesia. Patients with poor cardiac and lung condition may be better treated with radiosurgery/radiotherapy or conservative management. Some medical conditions and medication use may lead to poor wound healing. These include, for example, previous radiotherapy, immunosuppressants, steroids, poor skin condition, etc. These patients may carry higher risk after open surgeries.

10.5.2 On Pathology Aspects

The most important consideration is surely the angioarchitecture of the SVMs [6]. All patients with suspected SMVs should have a spinal DSA to determine the types of SMVs. As mentioned, different types of SMVs should be treated with different strategies accordingly. For complex lesions, combined modalities may be necessary to maximize the treatment effectiveness and functional preservation. Another very important angiographic pattern is whether the target arterial feeders share the same pedicle with anterior spinal artery. Catheterization of these arterial feeders may carry risk of spinal cord ischaemia and should be generally avoided.

Lesion location determines the risk and difficulties for open surgery. Open surgery for upper cervical lesions carries the risk of tetraplegic and phrenic nerve palsy. Less aggressive management plan should be adopted for patient with upper cervical lesions unless there is repeated bleeding and deteriorating neurological deficit. Ventral located lesions are usually more difficult to be approached by open surgery, especially for those at the thoracic and lumbar regions. Joint operation with cardiothoracic surgeons and general surgeons may be needed. Moreover, corpectomy and discectomy are needed to expose the ventral dura and subsequently the lesions. Fusion and instrumentation are usually required to maintain the mechanical stability. All these procedures significantly increase the surgical risk.

10.5.3 On Surgeon/Interventionist Aspects

The choice of treatment is inevitably affected by the availability of expertise and facilities. For example, although the successful rate of open surgery for type I SMVs is higher, embolization may be offered as the first-line treatment in some centres with readily available expertise and facilities. In these centres, embolization is attempted immediately after spinal DSA. Open surgery is offered as a second-line treatment only if embolization failed or the lesions are considered not angiographically suitable for embolization. Nevertheless, every patient with SMVs should be individually assessed, and it is undoubtedly the best for them to be managed in specialized centres with both expert neurosurgeons and neuro-interventionists.

References

1. Dehdashti AR, Da Costa LB, terBrugge KG, Willinsky RA, Tymianski M, Wallace MC. Overview of the current role of endovascular and surgical treatment in spinal dural arteriovenous fistulas. Neurosurg Focus. 2009;26(1):E8. https://doi.org/10.3171/FOC.2009.26.1.E8.
2. da Costa L, Dehdashti AR, terBrugge KG. Spinal cord vascular shunts: spinal cord vascular malformations and dural arteriovenous fistulas. Neurosurg Focus. 2009;26(1):E6. https://doi.org/10.3171/FOC.2009.26.1.E6.
3. Medel R, Crowley RW, Dumont AS. Endovascular management of spinal vascular malformations: history and literature review. Neurosurgical Focus FOC. 2009;26(1):E7. Retrieved Apr 28, 2023
4. Klopper HB, Surdell DL, Thorell WE. Type I spinal dural arteriovenous fistulas: historical review and illustrative case. Neurosurg Focus. 2009;26(1):E3. https://doi.org/10.3171/FOC.2009.26.1.E3.
5. Zhan PL, Jahromi BS, Kruser TJ, Potts MB. Stereotactic radiosurgery and fractionated radiotherapy for spinal arteriovenous malformations—a systematic review of the literature. J Clin Neurosci. 2019;62:83–7. https://doi.org/10.1016/j.jocn.2018.12.014.
6. Prashar A, Butt S, Shaida N. Introducing PHIL (precipitating hydrophobic injectable liquid)—a new embolic agent for the body interventional radiologist. Diagn Interv Radiol. 2020;26(2):140–2. https://doi.org/10.5152/dir.2019.19063.

11 Surgical Management of Craniocervical Dural Arteriovenous Fistula

Ivan Ng

Abstract

DAVFs of the craniocervical junction (CCJ) along the first spinal nerve are rare and a unique subtype of DAVFs at the CCJ. These fistulas account for 1–2% of all intracranial and spinal DAVFs. SAH is the major manifestation of DAVFs at C1 spinal nerve that may be overlooked on routine initial DSA. Rotational CT angiography is useful for clarification of the angioarchitecture of these fistulas, including small feeding artery and venous varix. Surgical treatment by interruption of the intradural draining vein should be the treatment of choice for C1 spinal nerve DAVF.

Keywords

Craniocervical junction · Dural arteriovenous fistula · Subarachnoid hemorrhage · Surgery

I. Ng (✉)
Department of Surgical Neurology, Duke-NUS Graduate Medical School, Mount Elizabeth Novena Hospital and National Neuroscience Institute, Singapore, Singapore
e-mail: ivan@neuro-surg.com

Abbreviations

DAVF	Dural arteriovenous fistula
CT	Computed tomography
GCS	Glasgow coma scale
GOS	Glasgow outcome scale
DWI	Diffusion-weighted imaging
PICA	Posterior inferior cerebellar artery
MRA	Magnetic resonance angiography
CTA	Computed tomography angiography
ASA	Anterior spinal artery

11.1 Introduction

Dural arteriovenous fistula (DAVF) accounts for a total of 10–15% of all cerebral vascular anomalies [1–4]. It is defined as an abnormal arteriovenous shunt or connection that occurs within the leaflets of the dura mater, usually within or near the walls of a dural sinus, with drainage into either the former or into the cerebral pial veins [5]. The commonest location of the posterior fossa DAVF is the transverse-sigmoid sinus area [1, 6–8]. Among the less commoner forms are the deep DAVFs residing in the straight sinus and the vein of Galen, as well as DAVFs in association with torcular and marginal sinuses [5, 9]. Dural arteriovenous fistulas (DAVFs) of the craniocervical junction (CCJ) are relatively rare lesions accounting for 1–2% of all patients with intracranial or spinal AVFs [9]. Due to the propensity of

X. Lv (ed.), *Endovascular and Neurovascular Surgery for Spinal Vascular Malformations*,
https://doi.org/10.1007/978-981-97-4661-3_11

significant associated leptomeningeal venous drainage and cortical venous reflux, the course of the natural history for this category of DVAF is largely regarded as aggressive. Patients may present with subarachnoid hemorrhage (SAH), myelopathy, or brainstem dysfunction. From a total of 127 patients in a review, 46 (37.1%) presented with myelopathy, 53 (43.1%) with SAH, and 4 (3.3%) with brainstem dysfunction [10]. These fistulas are usually less than one square inch or less [1] and located at the ventrolateral or dorsolateral at the foramen magnum, C1, and C2 and are characterized by predominantly intracranial or spinal venous drainage [8], in contradistinction to the commoner supratentorial DAVFs, which mainly drain via sinus channels, either in a craniofugal or a craniopedal fashion [1].

Craniocervical junction DAVF derives its main blood supply from the feeders originating from the intradural as well as the extracranial vertebral artery and/or the anterior spinal artery [11]. In addition, there is not uncommon recruitment of the external carotid and the ascending cervical muscular branches [1]. Impaired venous outflow leading to establishment of direct arterial-to-venous communication via the opening of indigenous pre-existing microarteriovenous fistulas in the sinus walls has been postulated as the pathogenesis of DAVF [12].

More recently, Hiramatsu [13] has divided the angioarchitecture of the CVJ DAVF into five subtypes based on the feeding arteries, the presumed location of the AV shunts, and the draining veins:

Type 1 dural AVF (37%): radiculomeningeal arteries of the VA with fistulous connection that drains into intradural veins through AV shunts located on the dura mater (Figs. 11.1 and 11.2).

Type 2 radicular AVF (RAVF) (29%): the AVF was fed by the radiculomeningeal artery that drains into radicular veins through an AV shunt on the spinal nerve (Fig. 11.3). The pial branch of the anterior spinal artery (ASA) can also join the same radicular artery and drains retrogradely into the same intradural vein.

Type 3 epidural AVF with pial feeders (14%): the AVF was fed by a radiculomeningeal artery

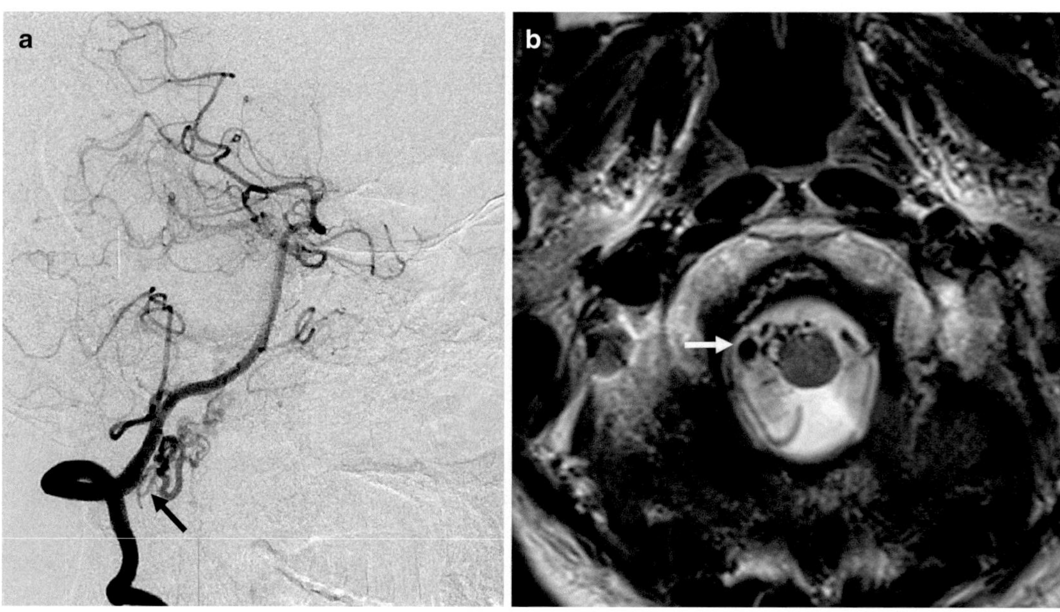

Fig. 11.1 A 56-year-old man with a CCJ-DAVF (type 1) presented with no symptoms. Right VA angiogram (**a**), oblique view, and MR image (**b**) showing a dural AVF (type 1). The AVF is fed by the right C1 radiculomeningeal artery (black arrow in **a**). The feeder drains into the intradural vein (white arrow in **b**). The AV shunt was presumed to be located on the inner surface of the dura mater

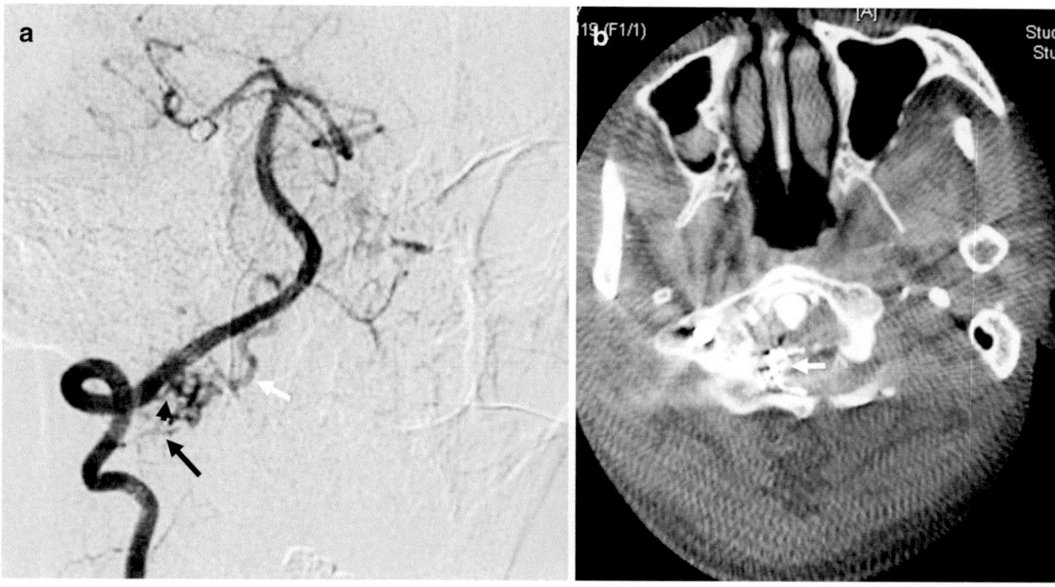

Fig. 11.2 A 68-year-old man with a CCJ-DAVF (type 1) presented with no symptoms. Right VA angiogram (**a**), anteroposterior view, and slab maximum intensity projection (MIP) image (**b**) showing a dural AVF (type 1). The AVF is fed by the right C1 (black arrowhead in **a**) and C2 (black arrow in **a**) radiculomeningeal arteries. The feeder drains into the intradural vein (white arrow in **a**). The AV shunt was located on the inner surface of the dura mater (white arrow in **b**)

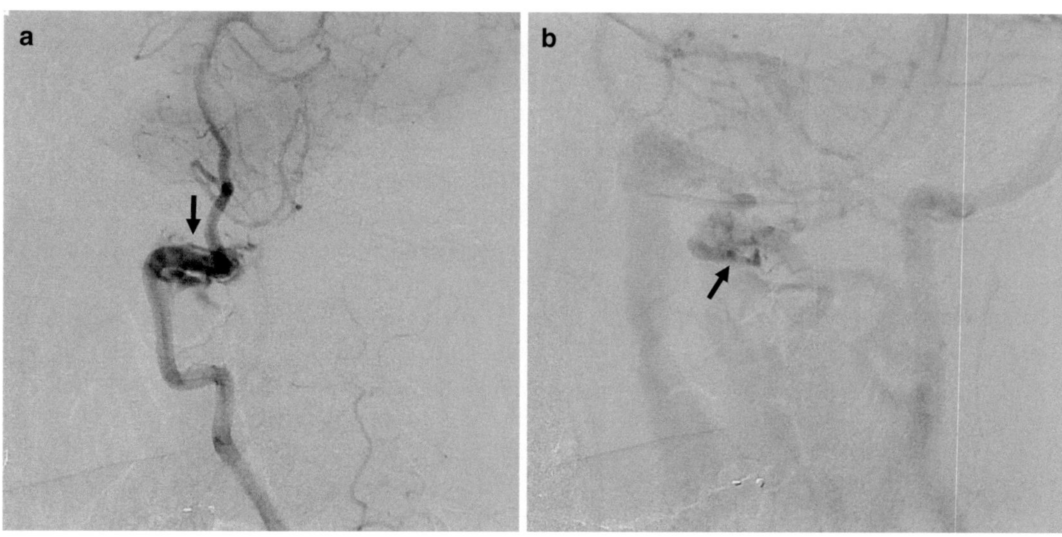

Fig. 11.3 A 58-year-old woman with a CCJ-RAVF (type 2) presented with subarachnoid hemorrhage (SAH). Right vertebral artery (arterial phase, **a**, and venous phase, **b**) angiograms, oblique view, showing a RAVF of the right C1 radiculomeningeal artery. The AVF is fed by the right C1 radiculomeningeal artery (black arrow in **a**) that drains into an intradural vein (black arrow in **b**). The AV shunt was presumed to be located on the left C1 nerve root

that drained into an epidural vein and by the pial branch of the ASA that drained into the same epidural vein. The shunt is therefore outside the dura mater.

Type 4 epidural AVF (EDAVF) (10%): fed by radicular and/or meningeal arteries that drain into epidural veins through AV shunts located outside the dura mater.

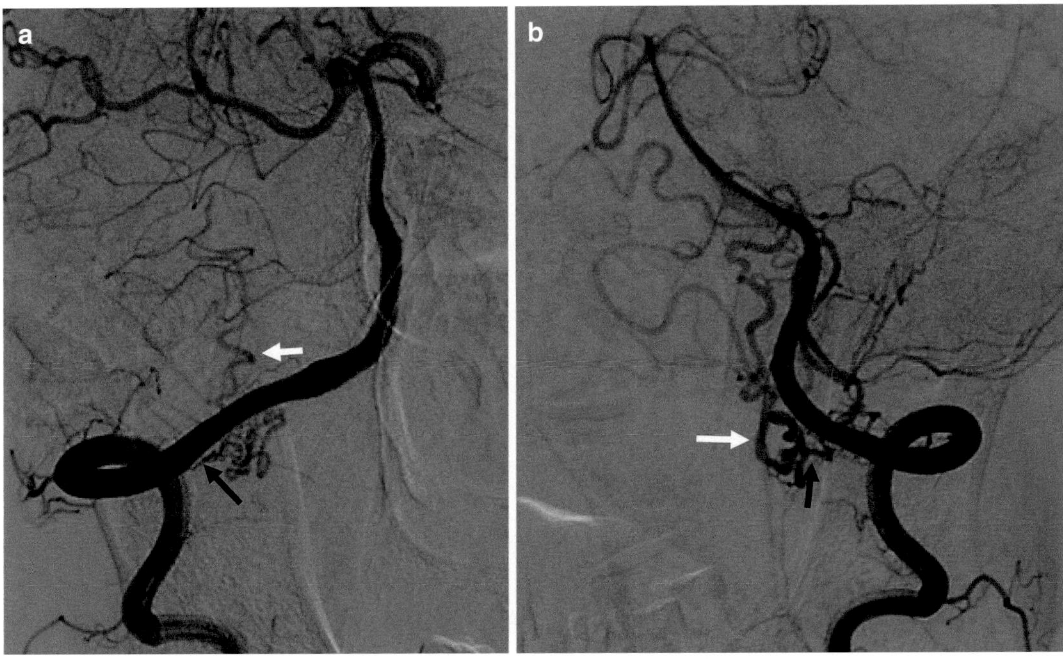

Fig. 11.4 A 64-year-old man had an accidentally discovered CCJ-PAVF (type 5). Right VA (**a**) and left VA (**b**) angiograms, oblique views, showing a PAVF. The AVF is fed by the right C1 radiculomeningeal artery (black arrow in **a**) and the ASA (black arrow in **b**). Both feeders drain into the same intradural vein (white arrows in **a** and **b**). The AV shunt was presumed to be located on the surface of the spinal cord

Type 5 perimedullary AVF (PAVF) (10%): fed by ASA with or without radiculomeningeal artery that drains into intradural veins through AV shunts located on the surface of the spinal cord (Fig. 11.4).

Locations of the AV shunts were presumed to be on the dura mater, on the spinal cord, or on the spinal nerves, based on the change in caliber between the feeding arteries and the draining veins.

11.2 Clinical Presentation and Angiographic Types

The clinical symptoms of DAVFs are dependent on the venous-related manifestations in the forms of mechanical, ischemic, and hydrodynamic effects [1]. When the drainage is into a large venous dural sinus, the sinus easily accepts the additional flow, minimal increases in venous pressure ensue, and symptoms are absent of minimal. When drainage into pial veins occurs, increased venous pressure is transmitted retrogradely into the pial veins, causing engorgement and enlargement. These enlarged veins potentially may rupture with hemorrhagic manifestations or as mass lesions and compression of adjacent neural structures. The venous hypertension causes parenchymal edema and swelling with venous infarction with its attendant neurological deficits.

Patients harboring craniocervical junction fistula may present with protean manifestations, which include headache, subarachnoid hemorrhage, vascular congestive myeloradiculopathy, and cranial nerve dysfunction [8, 11, 14, 15].

Hemorrhagic presentations are the most common of clinical presentations, and they manifest largely as subarachnoid hemorrhage although intraparenchymal hemorrhages have also been reported [10, 16]. Aviv et al. reviewed that intracranially directed drainage as opposed to caudal drainage pathways and presence of venous varix were significant determinants of the occurrence of subarachnoid hemorrhage [14]. The presence of anterior spinal artery feeders, aneurysmal dilatation on the feeder, exclusion of ECA as a feeder, and the SVJ type 2 and RAVF were more likely to present with hemorrhage [13].

Lanz described the occurrence of transient brainstem ischemia resulting in dysarthria, dysphagia, syncope, and respiratory failure as a result of intermittent increase in pressure of the engorged drainage veins [12]. Others have even reported on the rare association of paraparesis with craniocervical junction DAVF as a result of dilation of dependent lower medullary veins [17]. Oda et al. discovered the postmortem cervical cord tissue to be edematous with necrosis and parenchymal hemorrhages [18]. Chronic venous hypertension leads to stagnation of blood flow and hence resultant tissue hypoxia and necrosis [19]. Several authors have reported the uncommon observation of enhancement of the cervicomedullary junction on contrasted MRI as a result of engorged intramedullary veins or breakdown of the blood-brain barrier [18–21]. The presence of cord enhancement denotes a poorer outcome [19]. Hence, it should remain an important but rare differential diagnosis of T2 brainstem/upper medullary cord changes since the condition can be treated with good clinical outcome.

DAVF with leptomeningeal venous drainage with resultant cortical venous reflux is regarded as a high risk entity with dismal natural history [22, 23]. These encompass all types of fistulas except for type 1 based on both Borden and Cognard classifications [24, 25]. The latter author has quoted a rate as high as 50% of progressive myelopathy in patients with type 4 fistula [25]. Based on a study by Fassett, 95% of ruptured cervical DAVF cases fell into Hunt and Hess grade I and II subarachnoid hemorrhages [15]. Fortunately, the SAH resulting from craniocervical DAVF is usually less severe and has better outcomes compared with aneurysmal SAH. The clinical course after hemorrhage also appears to be benign with no cases of vasospasm [15, 26].

11.3 Diagnostic Challenge

Half of the patients in our series had negative cerebral catheter angiography during the first attempt. Modern MRA and CTA may have limited sensitivity for diagnosis of craniocervical DAVF [27]. While catheter angiography is the gold standard in diagnosis, the probability of picking up craniocervical junction fistula depends very much on the thoroughness as well as the astuteness of the interventionist. A lesion is preferably captured from the ultra-early arterial phase until late into the venous phase to visualize the exact architecture of the fistula, including the anterior and posterior medullary venous plexus involved in the drainage of the DAVF [1]. Failure to identify a craniocervical junction DAVF after injection of both vertebral arteries warrants a complete evaluation of the thyrocervical, costocervical, ascending pharyngeal, and occipital arteries in search of an alternative segmental supply [14]. In other words, all trunks arising from the subclavian and the axillary arteries, which may give rise to potential ascending cervical muscular supply, ought to be selectively injected [1]. The presence of distended perimedullary and spinal veins at the craniocervical junction on MRI should prompt a repeat angiography, which may unveil these elusive fistulous lesions. This explains why some centers have made it a protocol to carry out MRI of the cervical spine following an angiographically negative subarachnoid hemorrhage [15]. In unruptured scenarios, the presence of predominant myelopathic manifestations may lead to misdiagnosis as a result of normal noninvasive screening tests of the spinal cord or even a comprehensive spinal angiography [28]. The presence of long serpentine venous dilation within the subarachnoid space of the cervical and thoracic cords may well hint the likelihood of DAVF although this finding adds little information to the localization of the lesion [28–30]. In the presence of thoracic/lumbar spinal cord changes with serpiginous flow void, it is important to consider detailed intracranial/craniocervical/cervical spinal angiogram in the event of normal thoracic/lumbar spinal angiography [28].

11.4 Treatment

The ultimate goal in the treatment of DAVF is the complete and permanent obliteration of the fistula. The main options of treatment include endovascular embolization, surgical extirpation, and stereotactic radiosurgery [31–34]. The latter had been tried as an adjunctive treatment of DAVF although the efficiency is yet to be established.

11.5 Embolization

Proponents of endovascular intervention have hailed embolization as the first-line treatment of the craniocervical junction DAVF [9, 23]. Nevertheless, the role of endovascular treatment is to a great extent limited by the accessibility of the DAVF. The plethora of recruited arterial supply may render safe and complete obliteration of the fistula rather difficult. So does the diminutive size and the tortuosity of arterial twigs, which oftentimes preclude transarterial embolization as a treatment option. Furthermore, the substantial rate of recurrence following a seemingly complete embolization reflects the propensity of recruitment of new arterial feeders as well as recanalization of previously embolized feeders [35]. Similarly, the predominance of leptomeningeal venous drainage as opposed to dural sinus venous outflow prevents adequate transvenous embolization [36–39]. It has been postulated that transvenous embolization alone may redirect arterial supply to subarachnoid veins, thus aggravating intramedullary venous hypertension leading to infarction or hemorrhage [23]. Transvenous embolization also runs the risk of occlusion of normally functioning cortical veins, thus leading to catastrophic venous infarction or hemorrhage [35].

Various studies on the endovascular management managed to achieve barely 50% of complete embolization [23, 39–43].

11.6 Surgery

General surgical principles in the approach of arteriovenous fistula apply to the treatment of those located at the craniocervical junction. We routinely use the far lateral approach to the craniovertebral junction DAVF. The patients were placed in a modified park-bench position, and their heads were pinned with the Mayfield head holder. Frameless stereotaxy was deployed to assist the planning of craniotomy and localization of the involved sinus and the dural nidus [22]. An inverted hockey-stick incision from the mastoid prominence to the midline under the superior nuchal line down until C3 and C4 was made. Awareness of potential massive hemorrhage due to inadequate hemostasis of the heavily arterialized scalp and bone and down to the dura should always be kept in mind. Following subperiosteal dissection of suboccipital as well as upper cervical paraspinous muscles, the key attention is the exposure of the extracranial vertebral artery (V3 segment) from the C1 transverse foramina to its entry into the dura at the foramen magnum. Bleeding from the enveloping arterialized venous plexuses is coagulated, hemostased with Gelfoam and thrombin. Skeletonization of the segment of V3 artery for the purpose of proximal control is performed. The ipsilateral C1 arch and suboccipital bone are then removed. The posteromedial aspect of the occipital condyle and C1 lateral mass should be preserved whenever possible to avoid injury to the hypoglossal nerve and atlanto-occipital instability (Fig. 11.5).

Durotomy is performed painstakingly using the serial clip technique [1] and with each incision preceded by coagulation of the dural leaflets. Some authors advocate temporary clipping of the exposed leptomeningeal venous connections before permanent clips are placed as to allow the detection of stasis and thrombosis of the medullary venous plexuses [1, 8]. More importantly, the brainstem and spinal cord are noted for the slightest evidence of swelling during the course of temporary clipping [1]. Some authors advocate leaving the dural nidus behind, while others demand the complete excision of nidus to avoid the possibility of leaving epidural drainage veins behind [1, 8] As a rule, we skeletonize the vertebral artery to arrest the radiculomeningeal feeders in addition to ligating the fistula if possible to minimize recurrence. The terminal portion of the V3 segment of the vertebral artery enters the vertebral canal by passing anterior to the lateral border of the atlanto-occipital membrane. The adventitia of the V3 artery merges into the dural

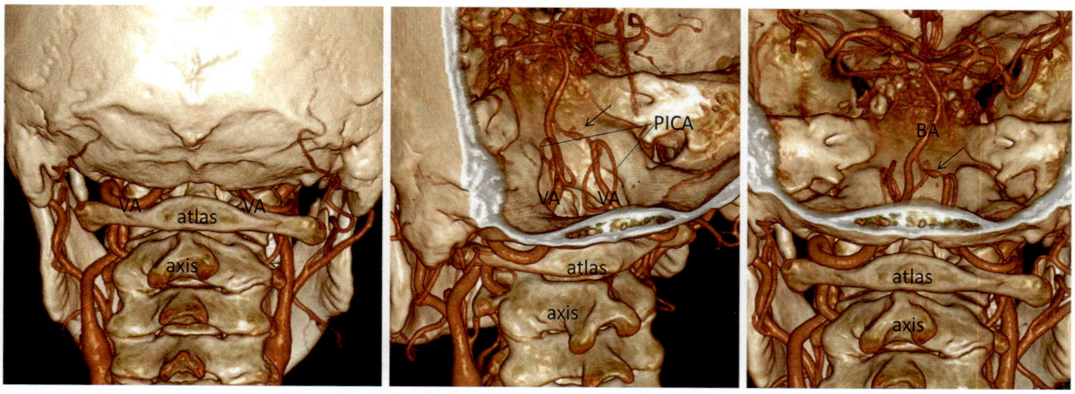

Fig. 11.5 Head and neck CTA images show the anatomical structure of the craniocervical junction area. Paired vertebral arteries (VA) originate from the first part of the subclavian arteries, and they then run superiorly through the transverse foramina of the C6 to C2 vertebrae. After the VA passes through the transverse foramen of the axis (C2), it is subdivided into two parts: vertical and horizontal. Vertical part courses superiorly, crossing the root of the C2 spinal nerve and entering the transverse foramen of the atlas (C1). After passing through the transverse foramen of the atlas, the horizontal part begins. The VA curves medially and posteriorly, passing behind the superior articular process of the atlas, and reaches the groove on the upper surface of the posterior arch of the atlas. From there, it passes under the posterior atlanto-occipital membrane and enters the vertebral canal. After entering the vertebral canal, the VA pierces the dura mater and courses superiorly over the anterior surface of the medulla oblongata originating the posterior inferior cerebellar artery (PICA). At the lower border of the pons, it merges with the opposite VA and forms the basilar artery. The basilar artery ascends along the ventral surface of the pons in its basilar groove within the pontine cistern (the arrow points to a VA aneurysm)

cuff. The key emphasis would be to fully isolate the dural cuff around the artery. The intradural segment of vertebral artery begins at the funnel-shaped dural foramina just inferior to the lateral edge of the foramen magnum [4]. Together with the posterior spinal artery, it passes just superior to the dorsal and ventral roots of the first cervical nerve and anterior to the dentate ligament and the spinal portion of the accessory nerve before it ascends from the lower lateral to the upper anterior surface of the medulla [4]. At its entry point into the posterior fossa proper, the vertebral artery makes an almost 90-degree turn forward and upward at the dural foramina, which serves as the guiding landmark of the localization of DAVF. After temporary clipping of any exposed leptomeningeal venous connections and observations to ensure there is no brainstem and spinal cord swelling, the fistulous point or points are divided, and the dural cuff around the vertebral artery is incised circumferentially to disrupt the radiculomeningeal feeders from the vertebral artery.

Intraoperative angiography is invaluable in ensuring complete obliteration of DAVF [1, 22]. Recently advancement of intraoperative indocyanine green video angiography has been performed as a substitute for intraoperative catheter angiography with good results [44–47]. Nevertheless, a formal postoperative angiography is still indispensible as not all feeding vessels are able to be injected and visualized intraoperatively to exclude accessory feeders and hence residual nidus conclusively. Watertight closure of dura is needed to prevent cerebrospinal fluid leak prior to closure of the muscles and skin.

11.6.1 Clinical Series

There were six patients who were diagnosed to have craniocervical junction DAVF over a time span of 10 years (2005 to 2015) admitted to our institution. There were five males and one female with the age range from 50 to 74; mean age was 61.3 years. Four patients presented with acute spontaneous subarachnoid hemorrhage as the main feature of clinical manifestation (two patients with Hunt and Hess grading I and one with grades IV and II, respectively). Two patients

Table 11.1 Case series summary of craniocervical junction arteriovenous fistula

Age/gender	Presentation	Arterial feeders	Venous drainage	Treatment	GOS
58/male	Headache due to SAH	Left VA, posterior SA (type 2)	Left ASV and perimedullary venous plexus	Surgery	5
62/male	Unresponsiveness due to SAH; quadriparesis and pseudobulbar palsy	Left VA, APA, and OA	Perimesencephalic and perimedullary and vertebral venous plexus	Partial transarterial embolization and surgery	Improved to 3
50/female	Headache due to SAH	Left VA (type 1)	Perimedullary and vertebral venous plexus	Surgery	5
70/male	Progressive quadriparesis	Left VA-radicular artery at C1 (type 2)	Perimedullary vein at cervicomedullary junction and venous reflux inferiorly to posterior spinal vein and posterior fossa vein	Surgery	3
74/male	Tetraparesis	Epidural AVF with pial feeders (type 3)	Drained through an epidural vein	Surgery	4
54/male	SAH with GCS 5	Vertebral artery (type 1)	Perimedullary veins	Surgery	2

SAH subarachnoid hemorrhage, *GOS* Glasgow outcome scale, *VA* vertebral artery, *SA* spinal artery, *APA* ascending pharyngeal artery, *OA* occipital artery, *ASV* anterior spinal vein

presented initially with hemiparesis, which progressed over 3 days to spastic quadriparesis with respiratory hypoventilation. None of the patients had past history of head injury.

Two patients (Cases 2 and 3) underwent cerebral CT angiography as a preliminary diagnostic tool for aneurysmal subarachnoid hemorrhage. One of which was negative (Case 3). All patients ultimately underwent catheter digital subtraction angiography. Two (Cases 1 and 3) had to be repeated in view of inconclusive angiographic results with high suspicion based on clinical grounds. The last patient was initially diagnosed to have a medullary brainstem infarct based on restricted DWI changes. It was on repeat MRI review that anterior medullary serpiginous flow void was detected. Diagnosis was subsequently confirmed on catheter angiography.

All patients harbored type 5 craniocervical junction DAVF as characterized by direct spinal venous drainage on top of direct cortical venous drainage with venous ectasia based on the Cognard classification [25]. All DAVFs in our study belong to Borden classification type 3 in view of the paucity of dural sinus or meningeal venous drainage [24].

All six patients underwent surgery via a far lateral approach with ligation of the fistulous connection as well as a circumferential division of the dura as close to the involved vertebral artery as possible. All did not encounter major complication perioperatively, and postoperative check angiography confirmed complete removal of the offending fistula. The clinical outcomes of these patients are shown in Table 11.1.

11.7 Case Illustrations

Case 1 (Fig. 11.6)

A 58-year-old man came to our attention following a sudden onset of bitemporal and occipital headache for 2 weeks. He was lucid during consultation with paucity of physical sign. Brain CT revealed subarachnoid hemorrhage over the right cerebral hemisphere and the left Sylvian fissure. A repeat cerebral catheter angiography following an initial inconclusive study

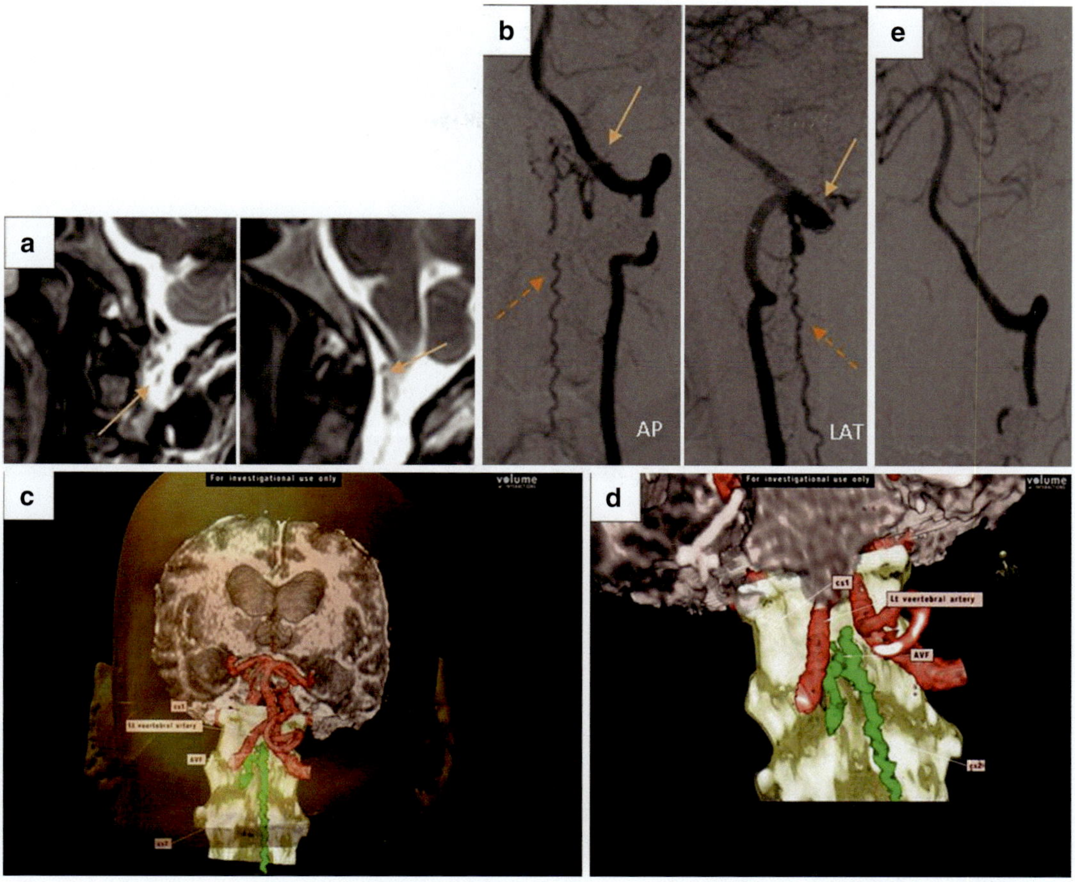

Fig. 11.6 Case 1. (**a**) Arrows showing flow voids at the prepontine cistern on the T2-weighted MR images of the craniocervical junction. (**b**) Left VA run (AP and LAT views) with DAVF nidus (arrow) draining into the anterior spinal vein (dashed arrow). (**c**) Preoperative planning of 3D imaging depicts posterior arterial circulation (in red) and dilated anterior spinal vein (in green). (**d**) Close-up view of similar anatomy with "skin" subtracted. (**e**) Postoperative angiography shows total obliteration of the DAVF following disconnection of a single arterial feeder from the left VA (*VA* vertebral artery, *AP* anteroposterior, *LAT* lateral)

pinned the diagnosis of arteriovenous fistula at the anterior cervical cord at C1 level with feeding vessels noted to arise from the distal left vertebral and the posterior spinal artery. There was evidence of early filling of the paravertebral venous plexus as well as the spinal veins, which served as the drainage conduits for the fistula.

The lesion was approached via far lateral craniotomy with C1 hemilaminectomy. Complete excision of the DAVF was achieved. Postoperatively, Mr. LSH developed aseptic meningitis associated with a pseudomeningocoele. He underwent exploration and repair of the pseudomeningocoele followed by insertion of a ventriculoperitoneal shunt for evolving hydrocephalus. His condition remained stable upon discharge and physically independent on subsequent outpatient clinic follow-ups.

Case 2 (Fig. 11.7)

A 62-year-old male presented with sudden onset of severe headache followed by progressive drowsiness and unresponsiveness. GCS on arrival was E2V2M5. Brain CT revealed acute hydrocephalus and intraventricular hemorrhage with relative sparing of the lateral ventricles. There was associated acute subarachnoid hemorrhage involving the basal cisterns, bilateral Sylvian fissures, bilateral frontotemporal cortical sulci, and

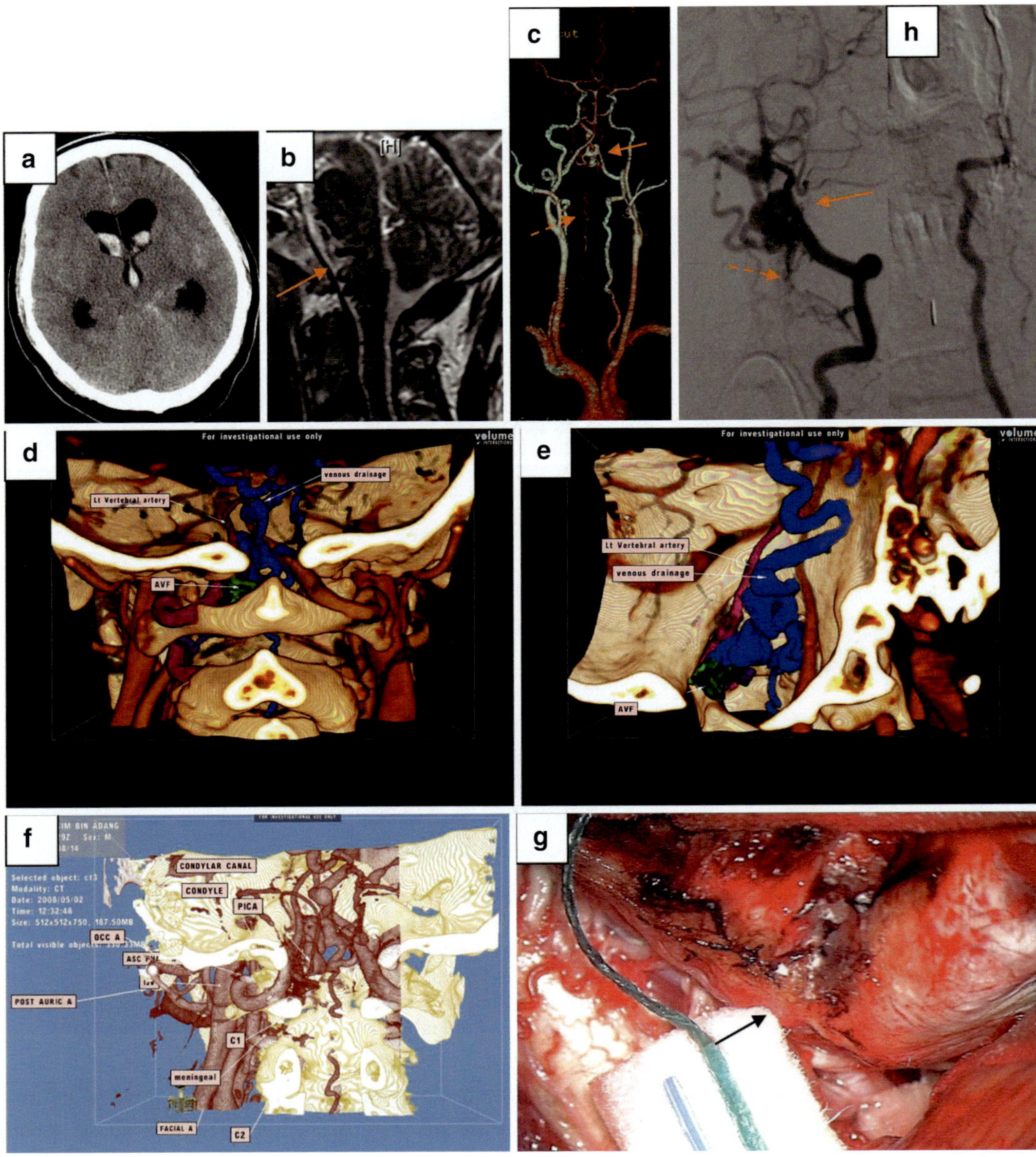

Fig. 11.7 Case 2. (**a**) Brain CT showing intraventricular hemorrhage. (**b**) Flow voids signifying abnormal dilated perimedullary vein on T2-weighted MRI. (**c**) DAVF with venous varix (arrows) draining into perimedullary and spinal venous plexuses (dashed arrows) on CT and catheter angiography. (**d**) Preoperative 3D images of the bony and vascular anatomy (pink, left VA; green, AVF; blue, perimedullary veins). (**e**) Similar image from a different angle, revealing the close proximity of DAVF with the left VA and posterior arch of C1. (**f**) Detailed anatomical delineation on preoperative virtual reality (VR) planning. (**g**) Surgical exposure of cervicomedullary junction and dural penetration site of left VA with adjacent fistula (arrow). (**h**) Postoperative check angiography confirmed total excision of DAVF with ligation of left VA at dural ring

prepontine cistern. CT and digital subtraction angiography confirmed the presence of a type 5 dural arteriovenous fistula at the foramen magnum with multiple meningeal feeders arising from the left vertebral and ascending pharyngeal arteries. Additionally, there was a small contribution from the left occipital artery. There was significant shunting with early venous reflux seen caudally into the dilated spinal venous plexus as well as cranially into the perimedullary and lateral mesencephalic veins before flowing into the straight sinus. The engorged venous varices, which were evident on the scans, were the likely source of hemorrhage.

He underwent emergent insertion of external ventricular drain. Attempt at transarterial embolization was abandoned for fear of untoward upper cervical spinal cord infarction. Two weeks later, he developed pseudobulbar palsy and quadriparesis, which were inexplicable as far as the normal MRI study of the brain and the cervicomedullary junction was concerned. After a lengthy discussion with the patient's family members, a decision was made for surgical excision of the dural arteriovenous fistula. Preoperative partial embolization of the neuromeningeal branch of the left ascending pharyngeal artery with Onyx glue was carried out. The lesion was approached via a far lateral fashion with incorporation of C1 and C2 hemilaminectomy. Intraoperatively, engorged venous varices with multiple dural fistulous connections were found at the left craniocervical junction. The rural cuff with adjacent fistulous shunts was excised, and the adjacent subarachnoid draining veins were extensively coagulated. Postoperative check catheter angiography confirmed the total extirpation of the arteriovenous fistula.

He made a slow neurological recovery albeit in a bed-bound state upon discharge 3 months later. He underwent insertion of a ventriculoperitoneal shunt for persistent hydrocephalus. At 6 months, he managed to ambulate with walking aids but was still dependent on nasogastric tube feeding.

11.8 Conclusion

Despite the rarity and complexity of the disease, craniocervical junction DAVF can be treated surgically with relatively good results. A high index of suspicion is necessary to diagnose these lesions, and a careful study of angiographic images is critical in the successful conduct of the operation.

References

1. Awad IA, Barrow DL, Committee AP. Dural arteriovenous malformations. Park Ridge, Ill: American Association of Neurological Surgeons; 1993.
2. Barrow DL, Committee AP, American Association of Neurological S. Intracranial vascular malformations. Park Ridge, Ill: American Association of Neurological Surgeons; 1990.
3. Partington MD, Rufenacht DA, Marsh WR, Piepgras DG. Cranial and sacral dural arteriovenous fistulas as a cause of myelopathy. J Neurosurg. 1992;76:615–22.
4. Picard L, Bracard S, Moret J, Per A, Giacobbe HL, Roland J. Spontaneous dural arteriovenous fistulas. Semin Intervent Radiol. 1987;4:219–41.
5. Liu JK, Mahaney K, Barnwell SL, McMenomey SO, Delashaw JB Jr. Dural arteriovenous fistula of the anterior condylar confluence and hypoglossal canal mimicking a jugular foramen tumor. J Neurosurg. 2008;109:335–40.
6. Akkoc Y, Atamaz F, Oran I, Durmaz B. Intracranial dural arteriovenous fistula draining into spinal perimedullary veins: a rare cause of myelopathy. J Korean Med Sci. 2006;21:958–62.
7. Graeb DA, Dolman CL. Radiological and pathological aspects of dural arteriovenous fistulas. Case report J Neurosurg. 1986;64:962–7.
8. Kinouchi H, Mizoi K, Takahashi A, Nagamine Y, Koshu K, Yoshimoto T. Dural arteriovenous shunts at the craniocervical junction. J Neurosurg. 1998;89:755–61.
9. Hurst RW, Bagley LJ, Scanlon M, Flamm ES. Dural arteriovenous fistulas of the craniocervical junction. Skull Base Surg. 1999;9:1–7.
10. Wang JY, Molenda J, Bydon A, GP CO, AL CO, Tamargo RJ. Natural history and treatment of craniovertebral junction dural arteriovenous fistulas. J Clin Neurosci. 2015;22:1701–7.
11. Morimoto T, Matsuyama T, Sakaki T. Long-term follow-up of craniovertebral junction arteriovenous fistulas surgically treated by feeder obliteration: report of three cases. J Clin Neurosci. 1998;5(Suppl):5–9.
12. Lanz M, Thiemann U, Grzyska U, Ebke M, Schwendemann G, Kraus JA. Transient brainstem ischemia and recurrent syncope caused by a dural arteriovenous fistula. Neurology. 2003;61:1152–3.
13. Hiramatsu M, Sugiu K, Ishiguro T, Kiyosue H, Sato K, Takai K, Niimi Y, Matsumaru Y. Angioarchitecture of arteriovenous fistulas at the craniocervical junction: a multi-Centre cohort study of 54 patients. J Neurosurg. 2018;128:1839–49.
14. Aviv RI, Shad A, Tomlinson G, Niemann D, Teddy PJ, Molyneux AJ, Byrne JV. Cervical dural arteriovenous fistulae manifesting as subarachnoid hemorrhage: report of two cases and literature review. AJNR Am J Neuroradiol. 2004;25:854–8.
15. Fassett DR, Rammos SK, Patel P, Parikh H, Couldwell WT. Intracranial subarachnoid hemorrhage resulting from cervical spine dural arteriovenous fistulas: litera-

ture review and case presentation. Neurosurg Focus. 2009;26:E4.
16. Zhao J, Xu F, Ren J, Manjila S, Bambakidis NC. Dural arteriovenous fistulas at the craniovertebral junction: a systematic review. J Neurointerv Surg. 2016;8:684–53.
17. Mascalchi M, Scazzeri F, Prosetti D, Ferrito G, Salvi F, Quilici N. Dural arteriovenous fistula at the craniocervical junction with perimedullary venous drainage. AJNR Am J Neuroradiol. 1996;17:1137–41.
18. Oda Y, Konishi T, Suzui H, Fujimoto N, Nakamura K, Matsumoto M, Okumura T, Kang Y, Kikuchi H. Partially thrombosed radiculomeningeal arteriovenous fistula in spinomedullary junction. No Shinkei Geka. 1989;17:63–8.
19. Asakawa H, Yanaka K, Fujita K, Marushima A, Anno I, Nose T. Intracranial dural arteriovenous fistula showing diffuse MR enhancement of the spinal cord: case report and review of the literature. Surg Neurol. 2002;58:251–7.
20. Ernst RJ, Gaskill-Shipley M, Tomsick TA, Hall LC, Tew JM Jr, Yeh HS. Cervical myelopathy associated with intracranial dural arteriovenous fistula: MR findings before and after treatment. AJNR Am J Neuroradiol. 1997;18:1330–4.
21. Hahnel S, Jansen O, Geletneky K. MR appearance of an intracranial dural arteriovenous fistula leading to cervical myelopathy. Neurology. 1998;51:1131–5.
22. Kakarla UK, Deshmukh VR, Zabramski JM, Albuquerque FC, McDougall CG. Spetzler RF: surgical treatment of high-risk intracranial dural arteriovenous fistulae: clinical outcomes and avoidance of complications. Neurosurgery. 2007;61:447–57; discussion 457-449.
23. Kattner KA, Roth TC, Giannotta SL. Cranial base approaches for the surgical treatment of aggressive posterior fossa dural arteriovenous fistulae with leptomeningeal drainage: report of four technical cases. Neurosurgery. 2002;50:1156–60.; discussion 1160-1151,.
24. Borden JA, Wu JK, Shucart WA. A proposed classification for spinal and cranial dural arteriovenous fistulous malformations and implications for treatment. J Neurosurg. 1995;82:166–79.
25. Cognard C, Gobin YP, Pierot L, Bailly AL, Houdart E, Casasco A, Chiras J, Merland JJ. Cerebral dural arteriovenous fistulas: clinical and angiographic correlation with a revised classification of venous drainage. Radiology. 1995;194:671–80.
26. Shinoyama M, Endo T, Takahash T, Shimizu H, Takahashi A, Suzuki M, Tominaga T. Long-term outcome of cervical and thoracolumbar dural arteriovenous fistulas with emphasis on sensory disturbance and neuropathic pain. World Neurosurg. 2010;73:401–8.
27. Hashimoto Y, Kin S, Haraguchi K, Niwa J. Pitfalls in the preoperative evaluation of subarachnoid hemorrhage without digital subtraction angiography: report on 2 cases. Surg Neurol. 2007;68:344–8.
28. Willinsky R, TerBrugge K, Lasjaunias P, Montanera W. The variable presentations of craniocervical and cervical dural arteriovenous malformations. Surg Neurol. 1990;34:118–23.
29. Rosenblum B, Oldfield EH, Doppman JL, Di Chiro G. Spinal arteriovenous malformations: a comparison of dural arteriovenous fistulas and intradural AVM's in 81 patients. J Neurosurg. 1987;67:795–802.
30. Symon L, Kuyama H, Kendall B. Dural arteriovenous malformations of the spine. Clinical features and surgical results in 55 cases. J Neurosurg. 1984;60:238–47.
31. Cifarelli CP, Kaptain G, Yen C-P, Schlesinger D, Sheehan JP. Gamma knife radiosurgery for dural arteriovenous fistulas. Neurosurgery. 2010;67:1230–5.
32. Debrun GM, Vinuela F, Fox AJ, Davis KR, Ahn HS. Indications for treatment and classification of 132 carotid-cavernous fistulas. Neurosurgery. 1988;22:285–9.
33. Lucas CP, Zabramski JM, Spetzler RF, Jacobowitz R. Treatment for intracranial dural arteriovenous malformations: a meta-analysis from the English language literature. Neurosurgery. 1997;40:1119–30.; discussion 1130-1112,.
34. Yang H-c, Kano H, Kondziolka D, Niranjan A, Flickinger JC, Horowitz MB, Lunsford LD. Stereotactic radiosurgery with or without embolization for intracranial dural arteriovenous fistulas. Neurosurgery. 2010;67:1276–85.
35. Irie K, Kawanishi M, Kunishio K, Nagao S. The efficacy and safety of transvenous embolisation in the treatment of intracranial dural arteriovenous fistulas. J Clin Neurosci. 2001;8(Suppl 1):92–6.
36. Halbach VV, Higashida RT, Hieshima GB, Hardin CW, Pribram H. Transvenous embolization of dural fistulas involving the cavernous sinus. AJNR Am J Neuroradiol. 1989;10:377–83.
37. Halbach VV, Higashida RT, Hieshima GB, Mehringer CM, Hardin CW. Transvenous embolization of dural fistulas involving the transverse and sigmoid sinuses. AJNR Am J Neuroradiol. 1989;10:385–92.
38. Halbach VV, Higashida RT, Hieshima GB, Rosenblum M, Cahan L. Treatment of dural arteriovenous malformations involving the superior sagittal sinus. AJNR Am J Neuroradiol. 1988;9:337–43.
39. Halbach VV, Higashida RT, Hieshima GB, Wilson CB, Hardin CW, Kwan E. Treatment of dural fistulas involving the deep cerebral venous system. AJNR Am J Neuroradiol. 1989;10:393–9.
40. Barnwell SL, Halbach VV, Higashida RT, Hieshima G, Wilson CB. Complex dural arteriovenous fistulas. Results of combined endovascular and neurosurgical treatment in 16 patients. J Neurosurg. 1989;71:352–8.
41. Newton TH, Cronqvist S. Involvement of dural arteries in intracranial arteriovenous malformations. Radiology. 1969;93:1071–8.
42. Rodesch G, Hurth M, Alvarez H, Tadie M, Lasjaunias P. Spinal cord intradural arteriovenous fistulae: anatomic, clinical, and therapeutic considerations in a

series of 32 consecutive patients seen between 1981 and 2000 with emphasis on endovascular therapy. Neurosurgery. 2005;57:973–83; discussion 973–983.
43. Wilkins R, Rengachary S. Neurosurgery. New York: McGraw-Hill; 1985.
44. Hanel RA, Nakaji P, Spetzler RF. Use of microscope-integrated near-infrared indocyanine green videoangiography in the surgical treatment of spinal dural arteriovenous fistulae. Neurosurgery. 2010;66:978–84; discussion 984-975.
45. Hanggi D, Etminan N, Steiger HJ. The impact of microscope-integrated intraoperative near-infrared indocyanine green videoangiography on surgery of arteriovenous malformations and dural arteriovenous fistulae. Neurosurgery. 2010;67:1094–103.; discussion 1103-1094,.
46. Hettige S, Walsh D. Indocyanine green video-angiography as an aid to surgical treatment of spinal dural arteriovenous fistulae. Acta Neurochir. 2010;152:533–6.
47. Schuette AJ, Cawley CM, Barrow DL. Indocyanine green videoangiography in the management of dural arteriovenous fistulae. Neurosurgery. 2010;67:658–62; discussion 662.

Open Microsurgery for Spinal Vascular Malformations

12

Timoleon Siempis, George A. Alexiou, Spyridon Voulgaris, Petros Zampakis, and Vasileios Panagiotopoulos

Abstract

Spinal vascular malformations are uncommon. The affected spinal segment and the severity of the abnormality determine clinical presentation. Treatment involves multidisciplinary approach consisting of neurovascular surgeons, interventional radiologists, and radiation therapists. Herewith, we review spinal vascular malformations, their classification, and best treatment options.

Keywords

Spine · Vascular malformation · Dural arteriovenous fistula

T. Siempis · G. A. Alexiou (✉) · S. Voulgaris
Department of Neurosurgery, University of Ioannina, Ioannina, Greece
e-mail: galexiou@uoi.gr

P. Zampakis
Department of Radiology, University Hospital of Patras, Patras, Greece

V. Panagiotopoulos
Department of Neurosurgery, University of Patras, Patras, Greece

Abbreviations

AVM	Arteriovenous malformation
AVF	Arteriovenous fistula
FVA	Fluorescein video angiography
ICG	Indocyanine green
MEP	Motor evoked potentials
SDAVF	Spinal dural arteriovenous fistula
SDAVM	Spinal dural arteriovenous malformation
SSEP	Somatosensory evoked potential

12.1 Introduction

Spinal arteriovenous malformations (AVMs) are rare clinical entities representing 3–4% of all space-occupying lesions that affect the spinal cord. Most information in the literature regarding these lesions comes from case reports or case series. Their clinical presentation depends on the affected spinal segment as well as the extent of the malformation [1].

There is no evidence supporting a standardized approach to the management of these lesions. The treatment approach involves a multidisciplinary team consisting of neurovascular surgeons, interventional radiologists, and radiation therapists, and the options include endovascular embolization and/or surgical obliteration of the shunt. Surgical obliteration of the lesion usually hinders clinical progression and, in

X. Lv (ed.), *Endovascular and Neurovascular Surgery for Spinal Vascular Malformations*,
https://doi.org/10.1007/978-981-97-4661-3_12

some cases, allows for partial or complete recovery. Preoperative planning including neurological, radiographic, and angiographic evaluations is necessary for all the patients undergoing surgery [2].

The first successful surgical treatment of a spinal vascular malformation involved a thoracic laminectomy performed by Charles Albert Elsberg at Mount Sinai Hospital in 1914 [3]. When Kendall and Logue identified the critical pathology of the dural AVF, later corroborated by Symon and Oldfield, microsurgery became the preferred treatment modality for these lesions [4].

12.2 General Principles

Spinal AVM's surgical management is less well defined. The extent of bony removal and the type of surgical approach depend on the anatomical location of the AVM. Most lesions are accessible through a posterior laminectomy and a partial facetectomy. Intradural AVMs that are found ventral or ventrolateral to the spinal cord might require a more extensive arachnoid dissection and dentate ligament resection in order to allow mobilization of the spinal cord medially. Thoracic nerve roots are sometimes sacrificed for further exposure. Electrophysiological monitoring of MEPs (motor evoked potentials) and SSEPs (somatosensory evoked potentials) is a useful adjunct intraoperatively to help guide the extent of resection and therefore minimize the risk of cord injury and vessel sacrifice [5]. A mean arterial pressure of 60 and 80 mmHg is proposed as optimal throughout the procedure in order to prevent hypotension and cord hypoperfusion, which may cause damage to the spinal cord, especially if vascular spasm occurs during dissection [6]. The patient is usually placed in the prone position on a Wilson frame or chest roll.

Spinal vascular malformations are classified into four distinct categories: type I, dural arteriovenous fistulas (AVFs); type II, intramedullary glomus AVMs; type III, juvenile or combined AVMs; and type IV, intradural perimedullary AVFs [7]. A modified classification system for spinal arteriovenous lesions has also been proposed by Kim and Spetzler in 2006. Pathology-specific surgical considerations will be discussed below.

12.3 Type I Spinal Dural Arteriovenous Fistula (SDAVF)

Type I spinal arteriovenous malformations (AVMs), which also refer as spinal dural arteriovenous fistulas (SDAVF) [Fig. 12.1], are the most common type of spinal vascular malformations representing approximately 70% of all spinal AVMs [8]. Treatment options include mainly surgery and endovascular treatment. The gold standard treatment has traditionally been open surgical obliteration. The primary aim of surgery is to disconnect the shunting vein at the point where it emerges from the fistula in order to achieve complete resection. Surgical treatment is superior to endovascular therapy in terms of initial success and late recurrence [8]. The open surgical procedure usually includes opening of the dura via a bilateral laminectomy in order to visualize the origin of the shunting vein. Prior to this step, care must be taken to evaluate for the presence of a nidus within the dura. Preoperative illustration of the level of the fistulous connection is of outmost importance. The laminectomy is often extended at a level above or below the lesion. This allows adequate exposure and ability to open the dura rostral and caudal to the pathology. The fistulous connection is subsequently identified, and either a microsurgical clip is placed between the artery and the vein or alternatively the fistula is coagulated and cut [9].

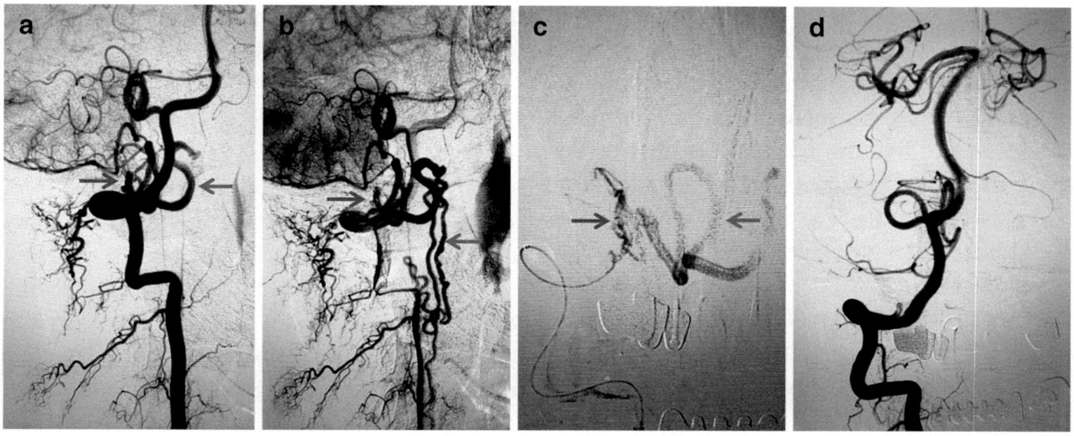

Fig. 12.1 A 67-year-old male patient presented to our outpatient clinic with progressive gait disturbance due to cervical myelopathy. Digital subtraction angiography (**a** early arterial phase and **b** late arterial phase) illustrated a type I intradural dorsal arteriovenous fistula between a radicular artery of the right vertebral artery at the level of C1 (red arrow) and perimedullary venous plexus (blue arrow). A microcatheter was navigated up to the distal part of the radicular artery, and microangiography demonstrated the aforementioned dural fistula (**c** red arrow) and its venous drainage (blue arrow). Subsequently complete embolization of the fistula has been achieved with Onyx infusion as illustrated in post-embolization angiogram (**d**). The patient experienced complete remission of its neurological symptoms

This is considered a safe and highly effective procedure with a reported success rate of up to 98% [10]. In a recent meta-analysis, Bakker et al. compared the success rate of surgical treatment versus endovascular treatment, which was found to be 96.6% and 72.2%, respectively [11]. Open microsurgical obliteration apart from being effective is also considered a safe procedure. In a series of 154 spinal SDAVF patients treated surgically, motor function improved in 82.2% of cases, and none of the patients suffered major neurological complications [12].

Localizing the origin of the shunting vein and verifying the absence of residual shunt postoperatively remains a significant surgical challenge. For this reason, intraoperative angiography technologies and 3D computer graphics have been developed to improve the safety of surgical excision, with indocyanine green (ICG) video angiography being the most commonly used technique [13]. This is a simple and effective technique for intraoperative confirmation of the SDAVF site. The main drawbacks of this technique are that visualization of the surgical field is indirect and magnification is restrained [14–16].

Another method is fluorescein video angiography (FVA) [17]. FVA is usually performed either before the application of a surgical clip or if there is doubt about the location of the shunting vein. It can also be used postoperatively to ensure that there is no residual shunt. The timing is determined by the surgeon. The main drawback of FVA is the extravascular leakage of fluorescein. The occurrence of severe anaphylactic events remains rare and has been reported as low as 1/1900 cases in a large survey of fluorescein retinal angiograms, with 1 death reported for 221,781 injections [18, 19].

There is growing prevalence of initial endovascular treatment for the management of type I AVF. Due to its decreased successful obliteration rate, there are a growing number of patients presenting with recurrent or progressive SDAVF after treatment. Median time to recurrence has been reported to be 5 months. Open surgical ligation continues to provide the most definitive treatment outcomes for these complex cases [20].

With regard to postoperative outcomes, motor symptoms tend to respond better to treatment than sensory. Recovery of sphincteric dysfunction tends to be disappointing, with persisting symptoms postoperatively in the majority of patients [21].

12.4 Open Microsurgery for Type II, III, and IV Spinal AVMs

Surgical removal of intramedullary AVMs is more challenging than that of AVFs. The reason is that these lesions have thin walls and therefore tend to rupture and complicate surgery with bleeding. Type II and III spinal AVMs have an intramedullary nidus that requires excision from within the spinal cord substance. Type IV lesions usually have a component of vascular supply from the anterior spinal artery and multiple dilated perimedullary vessels usually spanning multiple cord segments [22]. The direct involvement of the spinal cord in the type II, III, and IV lesions clinically manifested as an earlier and more rapid onset of symptoms. These lesions usually had multiple feeding and draining vessels and a diffuse nidus of vessels in contrast to the type I AVM. For this reason, endovascular embolization often helps to occlude the primary vascular supply prior to the surgical intervention [23].

Although patient's positioning and incision are similar to AVFs, anterior approach may be used in selected patients [24].

12.5 Type II Intramedullary Glomus AVMs

In Type II intramedullary glomus AVMs, where the AVM manifests as an intramedullary mass lesion, surgical exploration remains the preferred treatment. Operative approach not only alleviates the pressure effects on the cord but also avoids compromising the important feeding vessels common to both the AVM and the spinal cord. Therefore, in contrast to the surgical approach for AVFs, surgical resection does not include obliteration of feeding vessels at their dural entry [6].

Surgery should be reserved for symptomatic cases, especially when embolization is too hazardous or after incomplete obliteration of endovascular treatment [25].

Occasionally, partial resection is performed in some patients. This depends on the part of the AVM that is causing patient's symptoms and whether complete resections involves additional pial dissection or results in changes in spinal monitoring [6].

In rare cases, intramedullary AVMs can be found in the conus medullaris region. They usually have multiple feeders from the anterior spinal artery and posterior spinal artery with direct arteriovenous shunts and large dilated veins. Feeding vessels are identified and embolized, and angiography is used to identify the anterior and posterior spinal arteries and to embolize the feeders from these vessels. Many of these lesions have glomus-type nidus with intramedullary and extramedullary components at the level of the conus. The nidus component is resected with a similar technique used for intramedullary AVMs. Optimal surgical outcomes for this complex pathology are usually after combined endovascular and surgical treatments [26, 27].

12.6 Type III Juvenile AVMs

Optimal treatment strategy for type III juvenile malformations has yet to be established. Complete obliteration of fistulas is rarely possible because of the complexity of this subtype. Treatment options focus mainly on preventing further progression of neurological symptoms, usually by embolization. An important surgical consideration for this subtype of AVM is the proximity of the artery of Adamkiewicz. Damage to this artery can lead to severe spinal cord ischemia similar to anterior spinal artery syndrome, resulting in serious neurological deficits. This artery should be therefore identified early during the operation and preserved [28].

12.6.1 Type IV Intradural or Perimedullary AVF

These lesions are described as extramedullary intradural arteriovenous fistulas with only a simple fistula between the normal arterial supply to the spinal and the draining coronal venous plexus [29]. Type IV lesions can be further classified into three distinct categories on the basis of size and flow: type IVa has a single thin feeding artery, type IVb has multiple dilated arterial feeders with higher flow rates, and type IVc has multiple dilated arteries and ectatic draining veins. This classification affects surgical management [30]. More specifically, type IVa, when found in the ventral cervical spinal cord, can be managed with an anterior approach. Embolization is considered difficult in this case due to the difficulty in catheterizing the small caliber of the feeding vessels. On the other hand, type IVc, being high flow and consisting of large multipediculated feeding arteries, can be managed with endovascular treatment [31, 32].

In type IVb, an optimal treatment has yet to be established. Embolization does not always provide complete obliteration because of multiple feeding arteries and fistulas. Also, there are cases that require open surgery after endovascular interventions [25]. Both endovascular and surgical treatment offer satisfactory obliteration rates of 74% and 88%, respectively [30].

12.7 Spinal Extradural AVFs

Spinal extradural AVFs are not included in the common classification system of spinal vascular malformations. They are described as a communication between an extradural branch of a radicular artery and an epidural venous plexus. Unlike the other DAVFs, fistulous vessels do not directly penetrate the dura at that immediate site but possess an extradural component [33].

Currently, understanding of these lesions is derived from case reports or case series. It is important when managing spinal extradural obliteration and/or excision in order to minimize recurrence [34].

These lesions can be managed with both endovascular and microsurgical techniques, with the combination of these treatments leading to the optimal results. Open approach requires exposure of the dura, and then the fistulous connection is identified and disconnected using a small clip or via electrocautery-assisted ligation [35].

12.8 Conclusions

A summary of the surgical series found in the literature on management of spinal vascular malformations is provided in Table 12.1. Management of spinal vascular malformations requires reducing blood congestion caused by shunting through the aberrant arteriovenous connection. Despite their complexity, most of the patient's neurological symptoms tend to improve postoperatively. These success rates are mostly attributed to the multimodality that combines open microsurgical and endovascular approach.

Table 12.1 Case series on management of spinal vascular malformations

Study	Number of patients	Type	Mean follow-up (years)	Persistence evidence postoperatively (%)	Good outcome (%) (some resolution of symptoms)	Complications
Wojciechowski et al. (2017) [20]	14	SDAVF	0.7 (36 weeks)	0	92.8	Repeat surgery (2)
Bretonnier et al. (2019) [17]	6	SDAVF	0.5–2.4	0	66.6	Cerebrospinal fluid leakage (1)
Rothrock et al. (2021) [36]	6	SDAVF	0.25	0	100	NA
Rosenblum et al. (1987) [37]	14	SDAVM	NA	NA	73	NA
Ronald et al. (2020) [38]	40	SDAVF	1.2	10	62.5	NA
Velat et al. (2012) [6]	20	SDAVM	3.8	NA	70	5%
Wilson et al. (2012) [26]	16	SDAVM	5.9	NA	85	8.3%
Fox et al. (2017) [39]	10	SDAVF	1	20	80	Radiation burn (1) Pseudomeningocele (1)
Van Dijk et al. (2002) [40]	35	SDAVF	2.7	NA	100	NA
Anson and Spetzler (1995) [41]	24	SDAVF	NA	25	71	NA
Boström et al. (2009) [42]	12	SDAVM	3.9	21.4	80	8% Repeat surgery (1)
Yaşargil et al. (1984) [43]	41	SDAVM	2.9	48.4	31.7	NA
Park et al. (2017) [44]	24	SDAVF, SDAVM	2.7	25	NA	NA
Connolly et al. (1998) [24]	15	SDAVF	8.9	NA	67	7%
Logue (1979) [4]	24	NA	5	20.8	87.5	12.5%
Cogen et al. (1983) [45]	17	SDAVM	5	83	NA	NA
Zozulya et al. (2006) [46]	30	SDAVM	NA	87	NA	NA
Ropper et al. (2012) [47]	11	SDAVF	0.4	0	100	0
Cenzato et al. (2012) [10]	55	SDAVM	3	0	80	0
Kalani et al. (2012) [47]	9	SDAVM	2.4	11	77.8	12.8% Subarachnoid hemorrhage (1) Scrotal swelling (1)

References

1. Bao YH, Ling F. Classification and therapeutic modalities of spinal vascular malformations in 80 patients. Neurosurgery. 1997;40:75–81.
2. Ehresman J, Catapano JS, Baranoski JF, Jadhav AP, Ducruet AF, Albuquerque FC. Treatment of spinal arteriovenous malformation and fistula. Neurosurg Clin N Am. 2022;33:193–206. https://doi.org/10.1016/j.nec.2021.11.005.
3. Akopov SE, Schievink WI. History of spinal cord vascular malformations and their treatment. Seminars in Cerebrovascular Diseases and Stroke, Spinal Cord Vascular Malformations. 2002;2:178–85. https://doi.org/10.1053/scds.2002.128825.
4. Logue V. Angiomas of the spinal cord: review of the pathogenesis, clinical features, and results of surgery. J Neurol Neurosurg Psychiatry. 1979;42:1–11. https://doi.org/10.1136/jnnp.42.1.1.
5. Niimi Y, Sala F, Deletis V, Setton A, de Camargo AB, Berenstein A. Neurophysiologic monitoring and pharmacologic provocative testing for embolization of spinal cord arteriovenous malformations. AJNR Am J Neuroradiol. 2004;25:1131–8.
6. Velat GJ, Chang SW, Abla AA, Albuquerque FC, McDougall CG, Spetzler RF. Microsurgical management of glomus spinal arteriovenous malformations: pial resection technique: clinical article. J Neurosurg Spine. 2012;16:523–31. https://doi.org/10.3171/2012.3.SPINE11982.
7. Spetzler RF, Detwiler PW, Riina HA, Porter RW. Modified classification of spinal cord vascular lesions. J Neurosurg. 2002;96:145–56. https://doi.org/10.3171/spi.2002.96.2.0145.
8. Jellema K, Tijssen CC, van Gijn J. Spinal dural arteriovenous fistulas: a congestive myelopathy that initially mimics a peripheral nerve disorder. Brain. 2006;129:3150–64. https://doi.org/10.1093/brain/awl220.
9. Narvid J, Hett SW, Larsen D, Neuhaus J, Singh TP, McSwain H, Lawton MT, Dowd CF. Spinal dural arteriovenous fistulae: clinical features and long-term results. Neurosurgery. 2008;62:159–67. https://doi.org/10.1227/01.NEU.0000296997.82103.47.
10. Cenzato M, Debernardi A, Stefini R, D'Aliberti G, Piparo M, Talamonti G, Coppini M, Versari P. Spinal dural arteriovenous fistulas: outcome and prognostic factors. Neurosurg Focus. 2012;32(5):E11. https://doi.org/10.3171/2012.2.FOCUS1218.
11. Bakker NA, Uyttenboogaart M, Luijckx GJ, Eshghi OS, Mazuri A, Metzemaekers JDM, Groen RJM, Van Dijk JMC. Recurrence rates after surgical or endovascular treatment of spinal dural arteriovenous fistulas: a meta-analysis. Neurosurgery. 2015;77:137–144; discussion 144. https://doi.org/10.1227/NEU.0000000000000727.
12. Saladino A, Atkinson JLD, Rabinstein AA, Piepgras DG, Marsh WR, Krauss WE, Kaufmann TJ, Lanzino G. Surgical treatment of spinal dural arteriovenous fistulae: a consecutive series of 154 patients. Neurosurgery. 2010;67:1350–1357; discussion 1357-1358. https://doi.org/10.1227/NEU.0b013e3181ef2821.
13. Takai K, Kin T, Oyama H, Iijima A, Shojima M, Nishido H, Saito N. The use of 3D computer graphics in the diagnosis and treatment of spinal vascular malformations. J Neurosurg Spine. 2011;15:654–9. https://doi.org/10.3171/2011.8.SPINE11155.
14. Lane BC, Cohen-Gadol AA. A prospective study of microscope-integrated intraoperative fluorescein videoangiography during arteriovenous malformation surgery: preliminary results. Neurosurg Focus. 2014;36:E15.
15. Ng YP, King NKK, Wan KR, Wang E, Ng I. Uses and limitations of indocyanine green videoangiography for flow analysis in arteriovenous malformation surgery. J Clin Neurosci. 2013;20:224–32. https://doi.org/10.1016/j.jocn.2011.12.038.
16. Bretonnier M, Morandi X, Le Reste P-J. Fluorescein-guided surgery for spinal dural arteriovenous fistulas: a short series. J Clin Neurosci. 2019;70:226–8. https://doi.org/10.1016/j.jocn.2019.08.036.
17. Lane B, Bohnstedt BN, Cohen-Gadol AA. A prospective comparative study of microscope-integrated intraoperative fluorescein and indocyanine videoangiography for clip ligation of complex cerebral aneurysms. J Neurosurg. 2015;122:618–26. https://doi.org/10.3171/2014.10.JNS132766.
18. Yannuzzi LA, Rohrer KT, Tindel LJ, Sobel RS, Costanza MA, Shields W, Zang E. Fluorescein angiography complication survey. Ophthalmology. 1986;93:611–7. https://doi.org/10.1016/S0161-6420(86)33697-2.
19. Bretonnier M, Henaux P-L, Morandi X, Le Reste P-J. Fluorescein-guided resection of brain arteriovenous malformations: a short series. J Clin Neurosci. 2018;52:37–40.
20. Rothrock RJ, Haldeman C, Shah A, Lu VM, Lavi ES, Peterson EC, Levi AD. Challenges in diagnosis and management of previously embolized spinal dural arteriovenous fistulae. World Neurosurg. 2021;154:e710–7. https://doi.org/10.1016/j.wneu.2021.07.122.
21. Fugate JE, Lanzino G, Rabinstein AA. Clinical presentation and prognostic factors of spinal dural arteriovenous fistulas: an overview. Neurosurg Focus. 2012;32:E17.
22. Sure U, Wakat JP, Gatscher S, Becker R, Bien S, Bertalanffy H. Spinal type IV arteriovenous malformations (perimedullary fistulas) in children. Childs Nerv Syst. 2000;16:508–15. https://doi.org/10.1007/s003810000293.
23. Singh B, Behari S, Jaiswal AK, Sahu RN, Mehrotra A, Mohan BM, Phadke RV. Spinal arteriovenous malformations: is surgery indicated? Asian J Neurosurg. 2016;11:134. https://doi.org/10.4103/1793-5482.177663.
24. Connolly ES, Zubay GP, McCormick PC, Stein BM. The posterior approach to a series of glo-

mus (type II) intramedullary spinal cord arteriovenous malformations. Neurosurgery. 1998;42:774–85; discussion 785-786. https://doi.org/10.1097/00006123-199804000-00057.
25. Endo T, Endo H, Sato K, Matsumoto Y, Tominaga T. Surgical and endovascular treatment for spinal arteriovenous malformations. Neurol Med Chir. 2016;56:457. https://doi.org/10.2176/nmc.ra.2015-0327.
26. Wilson DA, Abla AA, Uschold TD, et al. Multimodality treatment of conus medullaris arteriovenous malformations: 2 decades of experience with combined endovascular and microsurgical treatments. Neurosurgery. 2012;71:100–8.
27. Wilson DA, Abla AA, Uschold TD, McDougall CG, Albuquerque FC, Spetzler RF. Multimodality treatment of conus medullaris arteriovenous malformations: 2 decades of experience with combined endovascular and microsurgical treatments. Neurosurgery. 2012;71:100–8. https://doi.org/10.1227/NEU.0b013e318256c042.
28. Elkordy A, Endo T, Sato K, Sonoda Y, Takahashi A, Tominaga T. Exclusively epidural spinal metameric arteriovenous shunts: case report and literature review. Spine J. 2015;15:e15–22. https://doi.org/10.1016/j.spinee.2014.11.022.
29. Gueguen B, Merland JJ, Riche MC, Rey A. Vascular malformations of the spinal cord: intrathecal perimedullary arteriovenous fistulas fed by medullary arteries. Neurology. 1987;37:969–79. https://doi.org/10.1212/wnl.37.6.969.
30. Gross BA, Du R. Spinal pial (type IV) arteriovenous fistulae: a systematic pooled analysis of demographics, hemorrhage risk, and treatment results. Neurosurgery. 2013;73:141–51.
31. Mourier KL, Gobin YP, George B, Lot G, Merland JJ. Intradural perimedullary arteriovenous fistulae: results of surgical and endovascular treatment in a series of 35 cases. Neurosurgery. 1993;32:885–91.; discussion 891. https://doi.org/10.1227/00006123-199306000-00001.
32. Hida K, Iwasaki Y, Ushikoshi S, Fujimoto S, Seki T, Miyasaka K. Corpectomy: a direct approach to perimedullary arteriovenous fistulas of the anterior cervical spinal cord. J Neurosurg. 2002;96(2 Suppl):157–61.
33. Hemphill JC, Smith WS, Halbach VV. Neurologic manifestations of spinal epidural arteriovenous malformation. Neurology. 1998;50:817–9.
34. Clarke MJ, Patrick TA, White JB, Cloft HJ, Krauss WE, Lindell EP, Piepgras DG. Spinal extradural arteriovenous malformations with parenchymal drainage: venous drainage variability and implications in clinical manifestations. Neurosurg Focus. 2009;26:E5. https://doi.org/10.3171/FOC.2009.26.1.E5.
35. Spetzler R, Kondziolka D, Higashida R, Kalani M, (Eds.). Comprehensive management of arteriovenous malformations of the brain and spine. Cambridge: Cambridge University Press; 2015. https://doi.org/10.1017/CBO9781139523943.
36. Rosenblum B, Oldfield EH, Doppman JL, Di Chiro G. Spinal arteriovenous malformations: a comparison of dural arteriovenous fistulas and intradural AVM's in 81 patients. J Neurosurg. 1987;67:795–802. https://doi.org/10.3171/jns.1987.67.6.0795.
37. Ronald AA, Yao B, Winkelman RD, Piraino D, Masaryk TJ, Krishnaney AA. Spinal dural arteriovenous fistula: diagnosis, outcomes, and prognostic factors. World Neurosurg. 2020;144:e306–15. https://doi.org/10.1016/j.wneu.2020.08.126.
38. Fox S, Hnenny L, Ahmed U, Meguro K, Kelly ME. Spinal dural arteriovenous fistula: a case series and review of imaging findings. Spinal Cord Ser Cases. 2017;3:17024. https://doi.org/10.1038/scsandc.2017.24.
39. van Dijk JMC, TerBrugge KG, Willinsky RA, Farb RI, Wallace MC. Multidisciplinary management of spinal dural arteriovenous fistulas. Stroke. 2002;33:1578–83. https://doi.org/10.1161/01.STR.0000018009.83713.06.
40. Anson JA, Spetzler RF. Spinal arteriovenous malformations: surgical treatment. In: Carter LP, Spetzler RF, Hamilton MG, editors. Neurovascular Surgery. New York: McGraw-Hill; 1995. p. 1197–212.
41. Boström A, Krings T, Hans FJ, Schramm J, Thron AK, Gilsbach JM. Spinal glomus-type arteriovenous malformations: microsurgical treatment in 20 cases: clinical article. J Neurosurg Spine. 2009;10:423–9. https://doi.org/10.3171/2009.1.SPINE08355.
42. Yaşargil MG, Symon L, Teddy PJ. Arteriovenous malformations of the spinal cord. Adv Tech Stand Neurosurg. 1984;11:61–102. https://doi.org/10.1007/978-3-7091-7015-1_4.
43. Park JE, Koo H-W, Liu H, Jung SC, Park D, Suh DC. Clinical characteristics and treatment outcomes of spinal arteriovenous malformations. Clin Neuroradiol. 2018;28:39–46. https://doi.org/10.1007/s00062-016-0541-0.
44. Cogen P, Stein BM. Spinal cord arteriovenous malformations with significant intramedullary components. J Neurosurg. 1983;59:471–8. https://doi.org/10.3171/jns.1983.59.3.0471.
45. Zozulya YP, Slin'ko EI, Al-Qashqish II. Spinal arteriovenous malformations: new classification and surgical treatment. Neurosurg Focus. 2006;20:E7. https://doi.org/10.3171/foc.2006.20.5.8.
46. Ropper AE, Gross BA, Du R. Surgical treatment of type I spinal dural arteriovenous fistulas. Neurosurg Focus. 2012;32:E3. https://doi.org/10.3171/2012.1.FOCUS11344.
47. Kalani MYS, Ahmed AS, Martirosyan NL, Cronk K, Moon K, Albuquerque FC, McDougall CG, Spetzler RF, Bristol RE. Surgical and endovascular treatment of pediatric spinal arteriovenous malformations. World Neurosurg. 2012;78:348–54. https://doi.org/10.1016/j.wneu.2011.10.036.

13 Microsurgical Treatment of Perimedullary Fistulae

Daniel C. Walsh

Abstract

Perimedullary arteriovenous fistulae (PMAVF) are a form of spinal intradural vascular malformation wherein there is an arteriovenous shunt irrigated by elements of the intrinsic spinal cord circulation and drained via the coronal venous plexuses without the presence of a nidus. They may present with ischemic radiculomyelopathy or more rarely hemorrhage. Many are amenable to endovascular cure, but where this is not feasible, microsurgical disconnection provides as safe and highly effective alternative providing the angioarchitecture of the shunt is appreciated.

Keywords

Spinal vascular malformation · Perimedullary AVF · Ischemic myelopathy · Fistula Vascular malformation · Arteriovenous Hemorrhage · Spinal cord

D. C. Walsh (✉)
Department of Neurovascular Surgery, King's College Hospital NHS Foundation Trust, London, UK
e-mail: danielwalsh@nhs.net

13.1 Introduction

Perimedullary arteriovenous fistulae (PMAVFs) are a form of spinal intradural vascular malformations wherein there is an arteriovenous shunt irrigated by elements of the intrinsic spinal cord circulation and drained via the coronal venous plexuses without the presence of a nidus. They may easily be confused with dural arteriovenous shunts and other intrinsic spinal cord vascular malformations given their appearance on cross-sectional imaging. The term pial arteriovenous fistula is sometimes applied and, more confusingly, fistulous spinal cord arteriovenous malformation (SCAVM).

13.2 Angioarchitecture and Etymology

PMAVFs can obtain the blood supply from ventral anterior spinal artery and/or dorsal posterior spinal arteries, of which the former is more common. The venous drainage often includes perimedullary veins that extend over many levels with evidence of congestion and venous reflux (Rodesch et al. 2005). Their recognition as a discrete vascular architecture is usually attributed to Rene Djindjian and colleagues in the late 1970s (Djindjian et al. 1977). They subsequently joined the evolving American/British/French classification as type IV lesions [1, 2].

X. Lv (ed.), *Endovascular and Neurovascular Surgery for Spinal Vascular Malformations*,
https://doi.org/10.1007/978-981-97-4661-3_13

Table 13.1 Classification of spinal vascular malformations

Type	Subtype	Designation
I		Spinal dural arteriovenous fistula
	Ia	Single fistula piercing the dural sleeve close to sensory rootlets and arterializing the coronal venous plexus
	Ib	Two or more fistulas arterializing the coronal plexus
II		Intramedullary glomus AVM with AV shunting deep into the pia
III		Metameric AVM
IV		Direct or perimedullary fistulae 1. Single hole fistula with single afferent 2. Single hole fistula draining multiple afferents (ASA and PSA); venous ectasia may be mild or moderate 3. Polyfistulous and/or giant lesions with significant venous ectasia
V		Epidural arteriovenous fistulae

Mourier and Merland further classified perimedullary fistulae in 1993 into three subtypes based on location of the shunt, arterial feeder, venous drainage, flow rate, and caliber of the shunt [3] (Table 13.1).

13.3 Epidemiology and Pathogenesis

Perimedullary fistulae constitute 10–20% of all spinal vascular malformations. It is predominantly known to exist in the thoracolumbar region. Spinal cord PMAVF (ABF type IV) is seen to present earlier in life than those presenting with dural arteriovenous fistula (dAVF) (ABF type I). The common age of presentation is between 30 and 50 years of age (Antonietti et al. 2010). Age at diagnosis for type I PMAVF was found to be later than the detection of type III [4].

Perimedullary arteriovenous fistulae are perhaps the most frequently seen spinal vascular malformation associated with a variety of genetically linked disorders of vasculogenesis, the best characterized being hereditary hemorrhagic telangiectasia (HHT).

13.3.1 Hereditary Hemorrhagic Telangiectasia

HHT is an autosomal dominant inherited condition with a population prevalence estimated at approximately 1 in 5000. Sporadic mutations producing the phenotype are very rare. There are three currently recognized phenotypic subtypes resulting from mutations of the ENG, ACVRL1, MADH4, and SMAD4. Mutations of BMPR9 and RASA1 can produce phenotypically similar illness. Central to the condition is vascular dysplasia resulting from maldevelopment of vascular smooth muscle cells, something implicated in aberrant vasculogenesis and the development of arteriovenous shunts. Central nervous system arteriovenous shunts develop in approximately 10% of cases with only about 1% exhibiting spinal arteriovenous shunts, the architecture of which is typically of PMAVF [5–7].

Eighty-five percent of patients who present with a spinal vascular malformation in association with HHT are under the age of 18 with 40% seen to be under the age of 2 [8].

13.3.2 Capillary Malformation-Arteriovenous Malformation Syndrome

Capillary malformation-arteriovenous malformation syndrome is a more recently described syndrome characterized by multiple capillary malformations of the skin of the face and arm. A proportion of these patients exhibit metameric arteriovenous shunts. There are two subtypes, CM-AVM1 and CM-AVM2, resulting from mutations of the EPHB4 and RASA1 genes, respectively [9–12]. Inheritance is autosomal dominant. Capillary malformations are found in 97% of patients, while arteriovenous malformations and/or AVF occurs in approximately 10% of patients with CM-AVM1 and in about 18% of patients with CM-AVM2. In the series of Revencu et al. 7 of 136 affected individuals exhibited a spinal vascular malformation, most of which as described were likely to represent PMAVFs.

13.3.2.1 Clinical Presentation and Investigation

Symptomatic PMAVFs present with ischemia, hemorrhage, or mass effect. Lower-flow PMAVFs present with a progressive radiculo-myelopathy reminiscent of the picture seen when most spinal dural arteriovenous fistulae (SDAVF). Gait disturbance and sensory symptoms such as patchy sensory loss and radicular pain (Jellema et al. 2003) are early symptoms of an ischemic presentation. Sphincter disturbance is also common. There are typically mixed upper- and lower-motor neuron findings on examination. As with other causes of ischemic myelopathy, the outlook for sphincter recovery is the most guarded with a slightly better outlook for sensory compared with motor symptoms. Our practice is to offer treatment at the earliest opportunity although it remains the case that the diagnosis may not be considered for prolonged periods and that may affect the overall prognosis.

Higher-flow PMAVFs are more likely to present with hemorrhage. Such arteriovenous shunts are more likely to exhibit evidence of vascular wear and tear such as ectasia or aneurysm.

Cross-sectional imaging may be virtually indistinguishable from SDAVF. In our experience with time-resolved contrast MR angiography, while the scan frequently correctly identified the presence of an arteriovenous shunt, it was less reliable in resolving the precise architecture. In a series of intrinsic spinal cord arteriovenous shunts, three proved to be PMAVFs on surgical exploration directed by MRA after catheter angiography has proven technically unsuccessful. However, the criterion standard for the diagnosis of PMAVF remains digital subtraction angiography [13].

13.4 Microsurgical Treatment

Indeed, most perimedullary fistulae are amenable to embolization provided a stable microcatheter position can be maintained at or close to the arteriovenous transition point.

For those that cannot safely be embolized, there will usually be an alternative microsurgical solution. The therapeutic strategy is deceptively simple—disconnection at the transition point as the draining vein or veins are forming. If that point on the pial surface is accessible surgically, point disconnection with low-power diathermy offers a precise and safe means to remedy the problem. The challenge is typically to identify the appropriate place for disconnection and select a safe surgical approach to it.

As described above, most PMAVFs are irrigated by the anterior spinal arterial axis, and the fistulous transition point may lie on the ventral cord surface with the attendant difficulties in access without injuring the cord during manipulation. Careful study of microcatheter angiography together with utilization of 2D flat-panel angio-tomography will facilitate surgical planning, while the use of intraoperative indocyanine green videoangiography and other technologies can facilitate intraoperative visualization. Some authors have advocated for intraoperative digital subtraction angiography with placement of a femoral sheath before prone positioning [14, 15] or access via the popliteal artery [16, 17] while prone. We have found that in most cases, indocyanine green videoangiography will provide the necessary information to guide treatment or on occasion to establish a diagnosis [18, 19].

Below are a series of case examples illustrating some of the operative strategies we have employed in the microsurgical treatment of PMAVFs.

13.4.1 Strategy 1: Point Disconnection on the Dorsal Pial Surface

A 66-year-old woman experienced a progressive loss of sensation in the lower extremities ultimately developing a suspended sensory level at approximately the T12 level. She developed double incontinence and within 2 months of the onset of symptoms was wheelchair dependent. She was extensively investigated for a potential neuroinflammatory causes based on signal change detected in the conus on MRI. The relatively subtle flow voids on the surface of the spinal cord (Fig. 13.1a) were not initially appreciated, but in the absence of any other abnormality, a neurovascular cause was considered.

MR angiography on two occasions did not resolve any arteriovenous shunt but neither could it exclude the diagnosis, so a digital subtraction angiogram was undertaken. Despite a complete interrogation of the spinal cord blood supply, no arteriovenous shunt was identified. Similarly, a spinal CT angiogram did not yield any clue, but the index of clinical suspicion remained high based on the MRA findings. Ultimately, a surgical exploration of the area with the greatest concentration of flow voids, a strategy that had yielded positive results for us in previous cases where no alternative diagnosis could be identified.

The findings at surgery are shown in Fig. 13.1b–e. The direction of blood flow was established by releasing temporary clip occlusion under ICG videoangiography, identifying the arteriovenous transition on the dorsolateral surface of the conus allowing its disconnection with preservation of the intrinsic conus blood supply.

The clinical results were exceptionally rewarding with the patient returning to independent ambulation within a few weeks of the surgery.

13.4.2 Strategy 2: Point Disconnection on the Ventral Pial Surface

When the arteriovenous transition is on the ventral surface, microsurgical access is more challenging, particularly so in the thoracic spinal cord where access anterolaterally is constrained by the thorax.

This 42-year-old male patient presented with a progressive spastic paraparesis worsening for 2 years. The sphincters were not affected, but there was a suspended mid-thoracic sensory level, and MRI demonstrated diffuse thoracic cord edema with dorsal flow voids (Fig. 13.2a).

Time-resolved imaging of contrast kinetics MR angiography (TRICKs-MRA) demonstrated the lesion to be at the level of left-sided T7. Microcatheter digital subtraction angiography was performed at the referring institution with a view to embolization; however, a stable microcatheter position could not be maintained to allow safe injection of a liquid embolic agent. At this point, he was referred to us for an additional opinion on the feasibility of microsurgical treatment. Firstly, another attempt was made at endovascular treatment, however, with the same disappointing result (Fig. 13.2b and c).

A transthoracic approach with corpectomy and the subsequent reconstruction was entertained, but the patient preferred to attempt radiosurgical therapy, which was delivered with the CyberKnife platform. Some susceptibility appeared within the cord on MR, but after 5 years, the PMAVF persisted, while the patient reported fluctuating but overall progressive symptoms. Further radiosurgical treatment was entertained, but a microsurgical attempt was offered from a posterior approach with the benefit of newly introduced microvisualization tools.

A T5–T7 hemilaminectomy and T6 pediculotomy were fashioned to afford dorsolateral thecal exposure. Incision of the dentate ligament and its suspension to rotate the cord gently afforded access for a 45° endoscope and identification of the characteristic vascular anatomy at the arteriovenous transition demonstrated on 2D angiotomography (Fig. 13.2d–g).

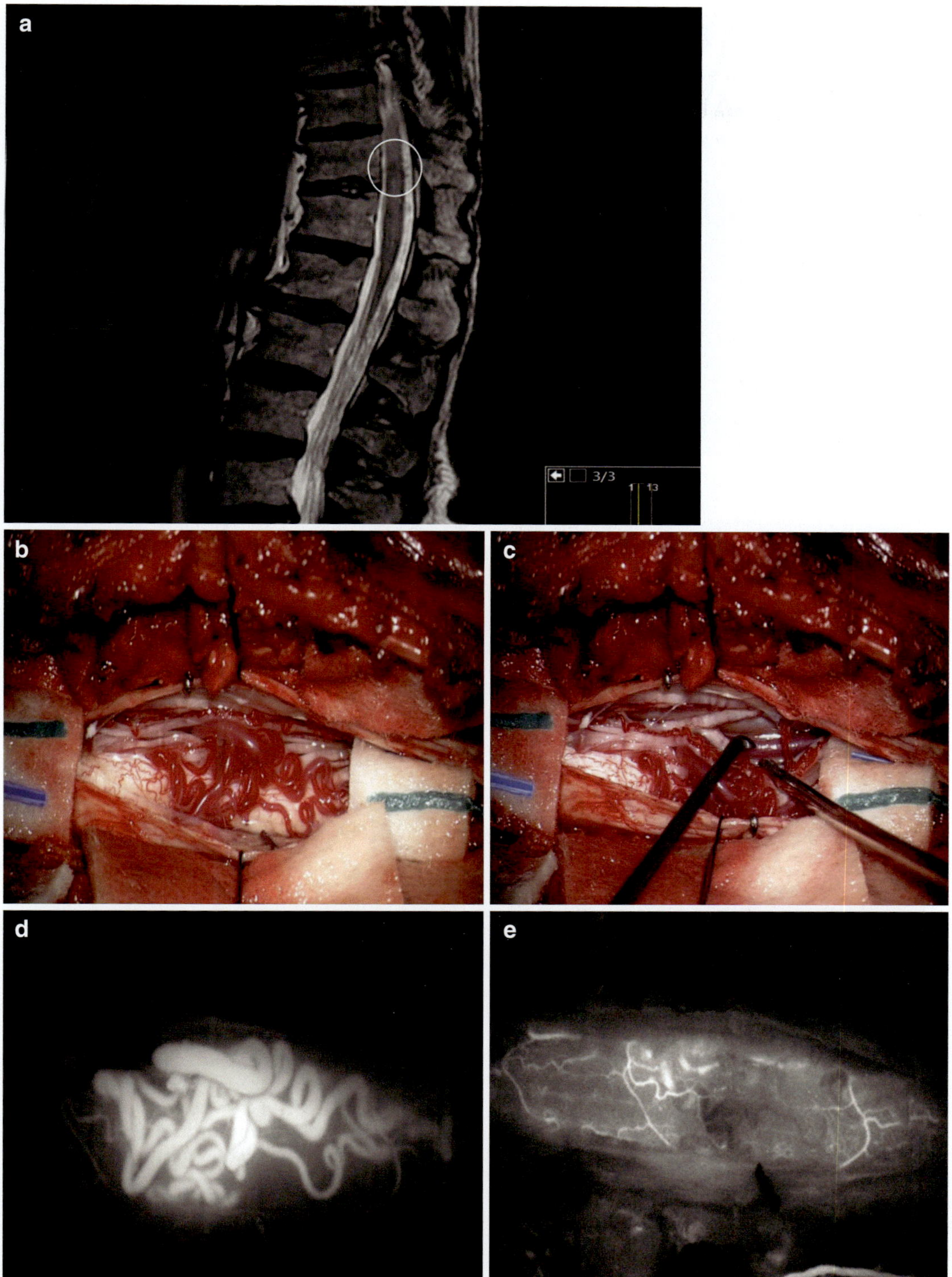

Fig. 13.1 Point disconnection on the dorsal pial surface. (**a**) Sagittal T2 MRI illustrating the expanded conus with central high signal and subtle but prominent flow voids on the cord surface. The area of interest that was ultimately explored is indicated within the circle. (**b**) Clearly arterialized veins are identified on the dorsum of the spinal cord. (**c**) The afferent artery irrigating the shunt is identified entering from caudally. (**d**) The direction of blood flow through the shunt may be demonstrated by releasing temporary clip occlusion of the vessels under ICG videoangiography control. (**e**) The arteriovenous shunt is demonstrably abolished with preservation of the intrinsic arterial vessels on the pial surface

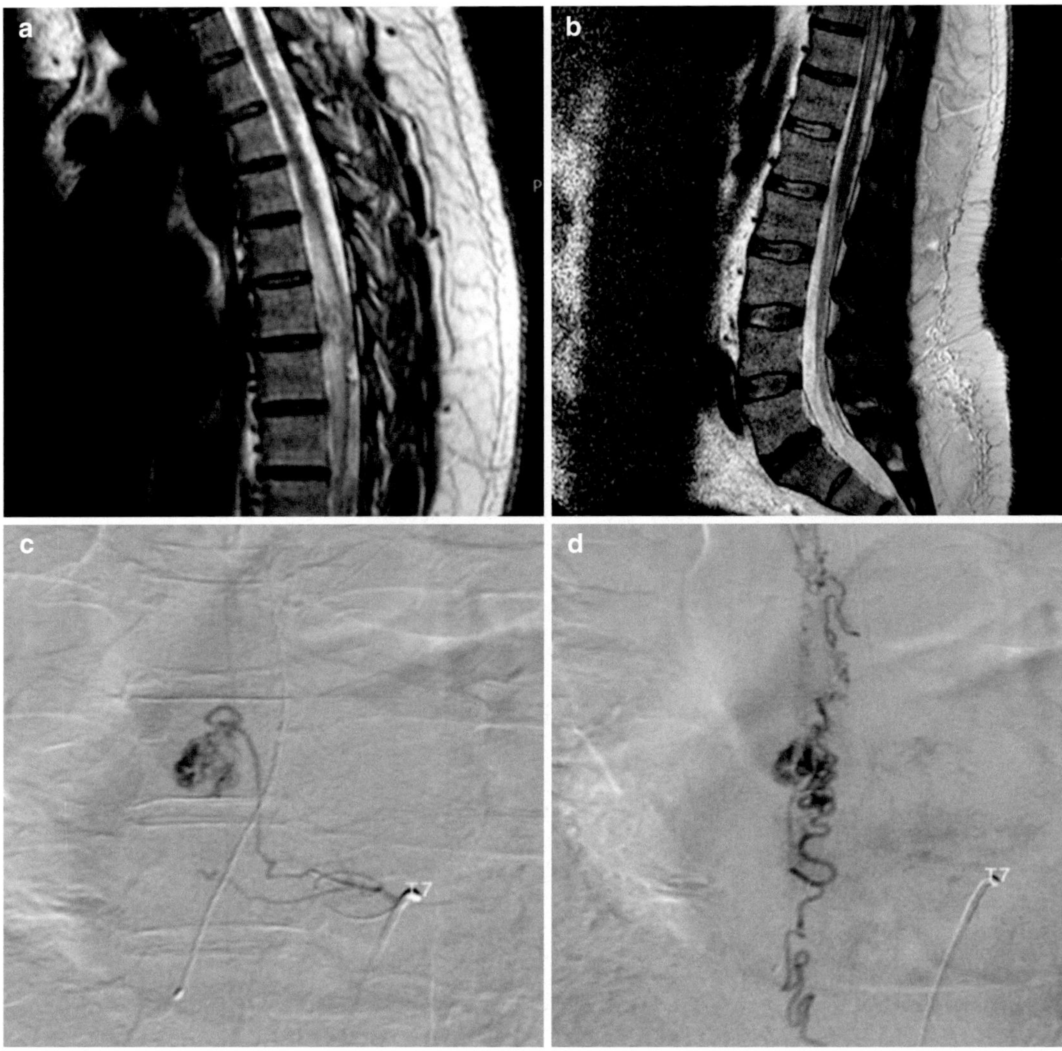

Fig. 13.2 Point disconnection on the ventral pial surface. (**a** and **b**) MRI showing severe thoracic cord swelling with diffuse venous engorgement of the dorsal and coronal venous plexuses. (**c** and **d**) Catheter angiography demonstrating the arteriovenous shunt draining via the ventral coronal venous plexus and located behind the T6 vertebral body. Note the characteristic "Omega" shape formed at the arteriovenous transition point, seen again in panel F on 2D tomography. (**e**) A hemilaminectomy is carried out at the index level, and the pedicle is drilled to afford as much dorsolateral access as possible. The dura is then opened laterally and the dentate ligament section to use as a level in rotating the cord gently away. (**f**) There is a characteristic Omega loop in the vasculature just proximal to the arteriovenous transition shown here on the coronal angiotomogram. Point disconnection precisely at the transition helps to protect the normal intrinsic blood supply and minimize the likelihood of recurrence by ensuring there is no residual venous "escape" that may recruit to the shunt again. (**g**) The QEVO micro-visualization device (Zeiss GmBH) is introduced. Essentially, a 45° endoscope allows identification of the vascular anatomy described above and disconnection with low-powered bipolar diathermy after a period of temporary occlusion under neurophysiological monitoring control

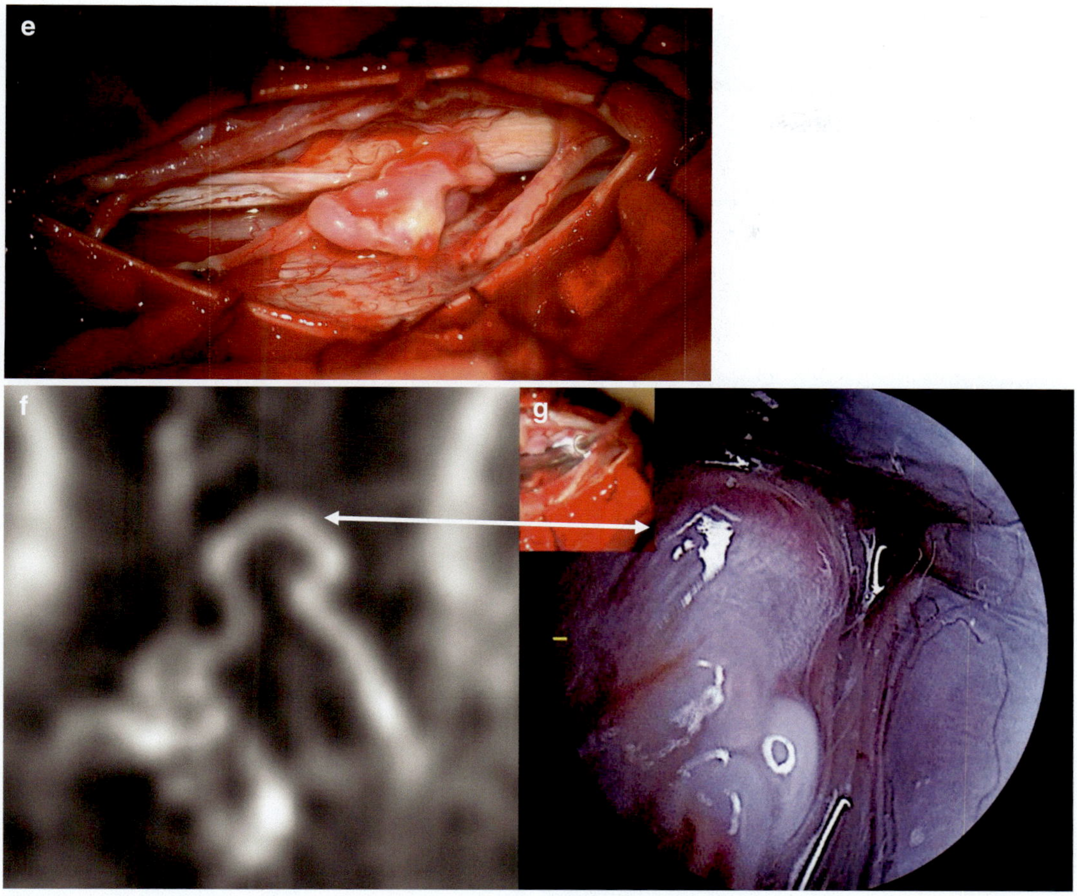

Fig. 13.2 (continued)

The fistulous point was reversibly occluded, while neurophysiological potentials were monitored for more than 10 min without deterioration. Control angiography confirmed complete occlusion of the fistula with subsequent and significant involution of the spinal cord edema present for so many years.

13.4.3 Strategy 3: Retrograde Occlusion from the Venous Side

A 32-year-old woman was running on a treadmill when she developed a sudden pain at around her thoracolumbar junction although this was rapidly superseded by occipito-cervical headache as the pain spread rostrally, and she developed severe nausea. Although not initially appreciated, her first symptom was of a sudden "pop" in her lower back while running on a treadmill rapidly followed by a severe occipito-cervical headache. A CT scan demonstrated cisternal subarachnoid hemorrhage.

CT angiogram and DSA did not reveal any intracranial aneurysm or vascular malformation. She subsequently had an MRI of the whole spine and brain as a part of the follow-up pathway, which revealed the presence abnormal vessels at the L1/L2 level with dilated veins in the spinal canal extending from T12 to the sacral canal caudally. Preoperatively, DSA done showed the fistulous point to be at L2 anterolateral to the termination of the conus (Fig. 13.3a).

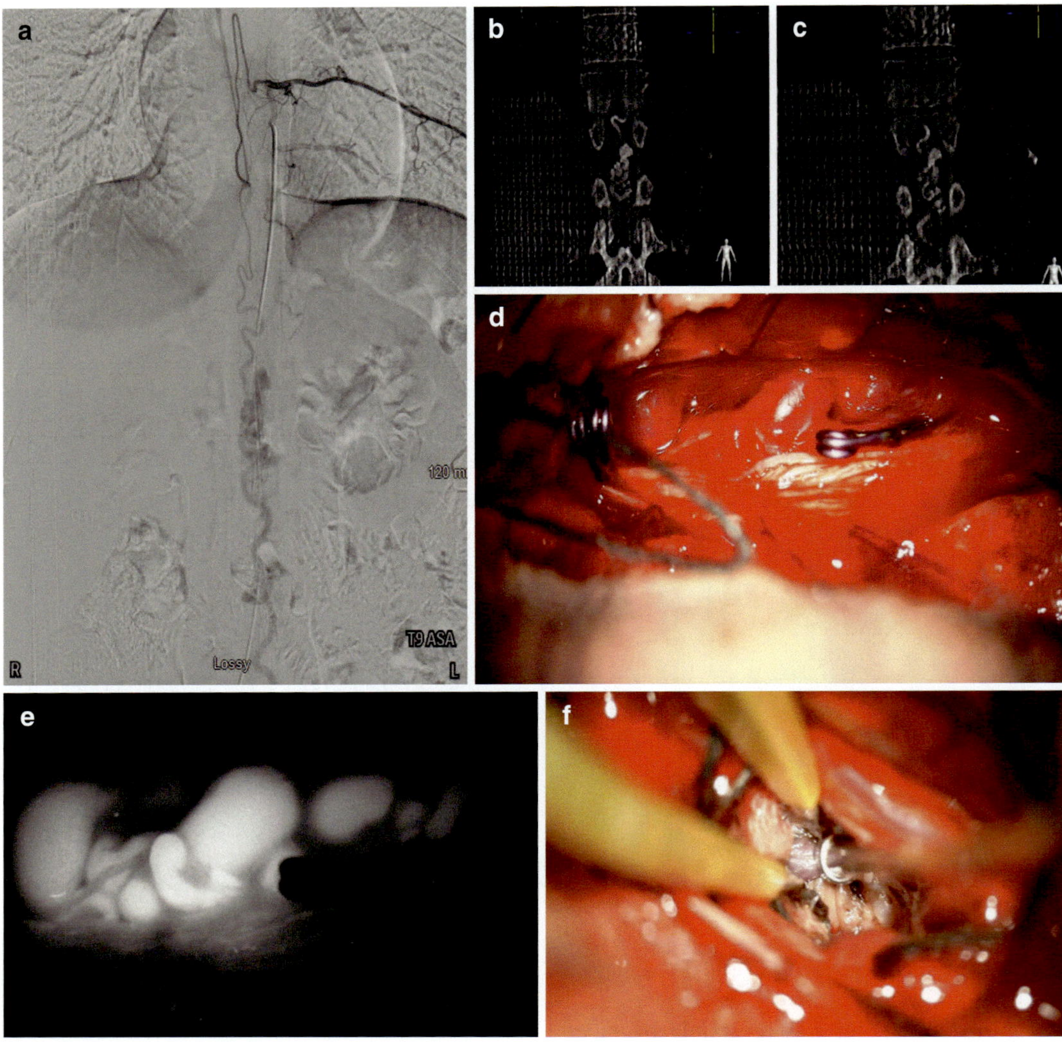

Fig. 13.3 Retrograde diathermy of venous drainage. (**a**) Angiogram illustrating the perimedullary fistula irrigated by the terminating anterior spinal artery and draining caudally within the lumbosacral canal. (**b** and **c**) Coronal angio-tomography illustrating the draining venous complex with ectasia of the veins likely to have been the source of hemorrhage. (**d**) Engorged, friable arterialized veins intimately related to the rootlets of the cauda equina. (**e**) ICG video-angiogram illustrating the arterialization of these veins and showing a distal clip used to collapse a section of the vein before diathermy of the distal outflow proceeding sequentially and rostrally. (**f**) Collapsing the veins to allow access to the transition point at the base of the conus

Endovascular treatment was not favored as the anterior spinal artery terminated in the fistula with little room for reflux of embolic material without potential embarrassment of the *conus basket* vessels.

At operation, very engorged arterialized veins were encountered, which were intimately involved with the cauda equina, sometimes splaying nerve roots. There was evidence of previous arachnoiditis despite not definite history suggestive of previous hemorrhages. Attempts to mobilize these veins to access the point of fistulation produced brisk bleeding. The strategy was then altered to work backward toward the arteriovenous transition point incrementally collapsing the caudal draining veins in the lumbar cistern, with temporary clips and diathermy until the point of fistulation could be secured at the pial surface (Fig. 13.3b–f).

Postoperative angiography demonstrated complete exclusion of the fistula without any evidence of conus ischemia although manipulation of the cauda equina roots did affect bladder function, which was slow to recover.

13.5 Conclusion

As with other types of arteriovenous fistula, PMAVFs are primarily a disease of the venous drainage from the spinal cord. Point disconnection of the arteriovenous transition offers an excellent chance of angiographic cure without embarrassment of the intrinsic arterial supply of the cord. A detailed understanding of the angioarchitecture of the shunt is a prerequisite to planning a suitable microsurgical approach to access this transition point on the pial surface.

References

1. Black P. Spinal vascular malformations: an historical perspective. Neurosurg Focus. 2006;21(6):E11. https://doi.org/10.3171/foc.2006.21.6.2.
2. Heros RC, Debrun GM, Ojemann RG, Lasjaunias PL, Naessens PJ. Direct spinal arteriovenous fistula: a new type of spinal AVM. Case Report. J Neurosurg. 1986;64(1):134–9. https://doi.org/10.3171/jns.1986.64.1.0134.
3. Mourier KL, Gobin YP, George B, Lot G, Merland JJ. Intradural perimedullary arteriovenous fistulae: results of surgical and endovascular treatment in a series of 35 cases. Neurosurgery. 1993;32(6):885–91. https://doi.org/10.1227/00006123-199306000-00001.
4. Gross BA, Du R. Spinal pial (type IV) arteriovenous fistulae: a systematic pooled analysis of demographics, hemorrhage risk, and treatment results. Neurosurgery. 2013;73(1):141–51. https://doi.org/10.1227/01.neu.0000429848.91707.73.
5. McDonald J, Bayrak-Toydemir P, Pyeritz RE. Hereditary hemorrhagic telangiectasia: an overview of diagnosis, management, and pathogenesis. Genet Med. 2011;13(7):607–16. https://doi.org/10.1097/GIM.0B013E3182136D32.
6. Bossler AD, Richards J, George C, Godmilow L, Ganguly A. Novel mutations in ENG and ACVRL1 identified in a series of 200 individuals undergoing clinical genetic testing for hereditary hemorrhagic telangiectasia (HHT): correlation of genotype with phenotype. Hum Mutat. 2006;27(7):667–75. https://doi.org/10.1002/humu.20342.
7. Gallione CJ, Richards JA, Letteboer TG, Rushlow D, Prigoda NL, Leedom TP, Ganguly A, Castells A, Ploos van Amstel JK, Westermann CJ, Pyeritz RE, Marchuk DA. SMAD4 mutations found in unselected HHT patients. J Med Genet. 2006;43(10):793–7. https://doi.org/10.1136/jmg.2006.041517.
8. Brinjikji W, Iyer VN, Yamaki V, et al. Neurovascular manifestations of hereditary hemorrhagic telangiectasia: a consecutive series of 376 patients during 15 years. Am J Neuroradiol. 2016;37(8):1479–86. https://doi.org/10.3174/ajnr.a4762.
9. Wooderchak-Donahue WL, Akay G, Whitehead K, et al. Phenotype of CM-AVM2 caused by variants in EPHB4: how much overlap with hereditary hemorrhagic telangiectasia (HHT)? Genet Med. 2019;21(9):2007–14. https://doi.org/10.1038/s41436-019-0443-z.
10. Amyere M, Revencu N, Helaers R, et al. Germline loss-of-function mutations in EPHB4 cause a second form of capillary malformation-arteriovenous malformation (CM-AVM2) deregulating RAS-MAPK signaling. Circulation. 2017;136:1037–48.
11. Thiex R, Mulliken JB, Revencu N, et al. A novel association between RASA1 mutations and spinal arteriovenous anomalies. Am J Neuroradiol. 2010;31(4):775–9. https://doi.org/10.3174/ajnr.A1907.
12. Revencu N, Boon LM, Mendola A, et al. RASA1 mutations and associated phenotypes in 68 families with capillary malformation-arteriovenous malformation. Hum Mutat. 2013;34(12):1632–41. https://doi.org/10.1002/HUMU.22431.
13. Amarouche M, Hart JL, Siddiqui A, Hampton T, Walsh DC. Time-resolved contrast-enhanced MR angiography of spinal vascular malformations. Am J Neuroradiol. 2015;36(2):417–22. https://doi.org/10.3174/AJNR.A4164.
14. Schievink WI, Vishteh AG, Mcdougall CG, Spetzler RF. Intraoperative spinal angiography. J Neurosurg. 1999;90(1 Suppl):48–51. https://doi.org/10.3171/SPI.1999.90.1.0048.
15. Orru E, Sorte DE, Gregg L, et al. Intraoperative spinal digital subtraction angiography: indications, technique, safety, and clinical impact. J Neurointerv Surg. 2017;9(6):601–7. https://doi.org/10.1136/NEURINTSURG-2016-012467.
16. Villelli NW, Lewis DM, Leipzig TJ, DeNardo AJ, Payner TD, Kulwin CG. Intraoperative angiography via the popliteal artery: a useful technique for patients in the prone position. J Neurosurg Spine.

2018;29(3):322–6. https://doi.org/10.3171/2018.1.SPINE171257.
17. Maeda Y, Mitsuhara T, Kume S, et al. Assessment of intraoperative spinal angiography via the popliteal artery for spinal vascular diseases. World Neurosurg. 2023;169:1–8. https://doi.org/10.1016/J.WNEU.2022.10.040.
18. Hettige S, Walsh D. Indocyanine green video-angiography as an aid to surgical treatment of spinal dural arteriovenous fistulae. Acta Neurochir. 2010;152(3):533. https://doi.org/10.1007/s00701-009-0445-8.
19. Walsh DC, Zebian B, Tolias CM, Gullan RW. Intraoperative indocyanine green video-angiography as an aid to the microsurgical treatment of spinal vascular malformations. Br J Neurosurg. 2013;28(2):259–66. https://doi.org/10.3109/02688697.2013.829556.

14 Surgical Management of Spinal Cord AVMs

David Felzensztein, Eilat Sapirstein, Eyal Hendler, and Eyal Itshayek

Abstract

Surgical management of spinal vascular lesions is challenging owing to the location of the lesion (i.e., intramedullary), blood supply (intrinsic spinal cord vessels, direct aortic tributaries), preoperative diagnostic accuracy, and intraoperative identification of the lesion.

The clinical presentation of spinal cord AVMs is characterized by myelopathy due to different pathological mechanisms. Reduced blood supply, increased venous pressure, and hemorrhage have all been described as culprits for neurological manifestations. Second-hit events, such as hemorrhage, are as high as 10% per year with detrimental consequences, so early and definitive treatment of these lesions is paramount for optimal clinical outcomes.

Unlike brain AVMs, partial treatment of spinal cord lesions is safe and allows preservation of spinal feeding arteries while reducing the risk of rebleeding and improving long-term outcomes.

Surgical resection of spinal AVMs depends on favorable angioarchitecture, allowing a safe resection without risking the spinal cord blood supply.

Several classifications have been proposed to aid in the diagnostic and therapeutic management of these lesions. Most recently, the Toronto classification has been proposed with guidance on treatment modality and occlusion success rate.

This chapter describes spinal cord vascular lesions' diagnostic course and surgical management.

Keywords

Spinal cord · Vascular malformation
Vascular lesions · Surgical management
Indocyanine green

14.1 Introduction

Vascular spine lesions are classified according to their location in relationship to the spinal cord [1]. These uncommon lesions represent a heterogeneous group of diseases, with an annual incidence of 5–10 per million. Among these lesions, DAVFs are the most common ranging from 60 to 80%, with a male-to-female ratio of 5:1 [2]. DAVFs are diagnosed between the sixth and eighth decades of life, mostly in the thoracic and lumbar regions [3]. Spinal AVMs appear in the third decade of life and occasionally are associated with genetic syndromes [4].

D. Felzensztein · E. Sapirstein · E. Hendler ·
E. Itshayek (✉)
Department of Neurosurgery, Rabin Medical Center, Petah Tikva, Israel
e-mail: eyalhe1@clalit.org.il

X. Lv (ed.), *Endovascular and Neurovascular Surgery for Spinal Vascular Malformations*,
https://doi.org/10.1007/978-981-97-4661-3_14

Table 14.1 Toronto classification of arteriovenous malformations of the spine

Vascular lesions	Topography of the shunt
Spinal cord AVM	Intradural intramedullary
Pial AVF	Intradural pial
Microfistula	
Macrofistula	
Dural AVF	Dural
Epidural AVF	Epidural
Paraspinal AVF	Paraspinal space
SAMS	Multiple

AVF arteriovenous fistula, *AVM* arteriovenous malformation, *SAMS* spinal arteriovenous metameric syndrome

Several classification systems have been proposed to describe these lesions [2, 4–6]. Most recently, the Toronto classification has been proposed based on the anatomical relationship with the spinal cord and surrounding structures [7] (Table 14.1). Both microsurgical techniques and endovascular treatments are available, aiming to arrest and prevent further neurological deficits. The treatment approach is decided based on angiographic characteristics and the lesion's anatomical location [8]. Surgical management of vascular spine lesions has remained an important treatment tool in the armamentarium and should be available for practicing spinal surgeons.

14.2 Patient Assessment

Clinical presentation of arteriovenous malformations of the spine varies depending on their type and the local and regional hemodynamic effects [9]. Therefore, a detailed history and physical examination are necessary to expedite diagnosis and offer early treatment [10]. The clinical features include radicular symptoms, back pain, limb weakness, paresthesia and proprioceptive disturbances, autonomic dysfunction, bowel and bladder dysregulation, and most severely Foix-Alajouanine syndrome [10]. The presenting symptoms and clinical course depend on the vascular pathology and flow intensity [9]. For instance, high-output cardiac failure may occur in rare cases of pediatric patients with high-flow fistulas [11]. Venous congestion is proposed as a pathophysiological mechanism for chronic and subacute clinical presentations. It is caused by reflux of spinal draining veins with subsequent venous congestion. Due to anatomical venous outflow, the clinical presentation is typically caudal to cranial [12]. Hemorrhage is another culprit for clinical deterioration. Due to different mechanisms, arteriovenous shunt and AVMS can cause bleeding at any point in the spinal canal. Up to 50% of intradural AVMs present with spontaneous rupture with a yearly rupture rate of 4% [13–15]. Rebleeding risk increases to 10% during the first month and up to 40% within the first year. The mortality rate from each bleeding reaches 20% [13–16]. Bleeding is associated with a ruptured aneurysm in 29%, mainly at the cervical level. In other cases, the bleeding occurs at the nidal site due to increased intranidal pressure [11]. Finally, local compression may occur due to venous tortuosities, aneurysms, and rarely spinal artery aneurysms [17].

The Aminoff and Logue disability scale score is used to classify the clinical severity of spinal malformations type I [18] (Table 14.2).

Table 14.2 Aminoff and Logue disability scale score (Gokhale, Sankalp & Khan, Shariq & McDonagh, David & Britz, Gavin. (2014). Comparison of surgical and endovascular approach in management of spinal dural arteriovenous fistulas: a single center experience of 27 patients. Surgical neurology international. 5. 7. 10.4103/2152-7806.125628) [19]

Classification of gait disturbance
Grade 1: Leg weakness or abnormal gait, no restricted activity
Grade 2: Grade 1 with restricted activity
Grade 3: Requires cane or similar support for walking
Grade 4: Requires walker or crutches for walking
Grade 5: Update to stand, confined to bed or wheelchair
Classification of micturition
Grade 1: Hesitancy, urgency, or frequency
Grade 2: Occasional urinary incontinence or retention
Grade 3: Total urinary incontinence or retention

14.3 Imaging Modalities

Clinical suspicion is confirmed with imaging studies. MRI and MRA are indispensable in the diagnosis of clinical myelopathy as well as vascular assessment. Anatomical features are well depicted, and the relationship of the lesion to the spinal cord is established [20]. MRI can localize many fistulous connections and differentiate between intramedullary and extramedullary components (Figs. 14.1 and 14.2) [21]. Once a vascular pathology has been suggested in the MRI, it is necessary to perform a catheter-based digital subtraction angiography (DSA) [21]. It is used for lesion characterization, localization, and flow assessment. Spinal cord vasculature is established and differentiated from the pathological angioarchitecture.

Regarding nidal malformations, bilateral injections are performed to assess better the feeders, flow-related aneurysms, and en passage vessels (Fig. 14.3). Treatment planning, either surgical or endovascular, can then take place. Preoperative marking is also performed to assist in the surgical localization of the AVS [21].

Another promising tool for preoperative surgical assessment is diffusion tensor imaging (DTI) [22]. Its use in the spine is technically complex owing to its small cross-sectional size and susceptibility-induced field inhomogeneity [22]. However, new techniques are evolving to provide improved accuracy and anatomical consistency even in the event of metallic implants [22]. This promising technology will assist in studying long fiber tracts and their relationship with the AVS and assist in safer resections.

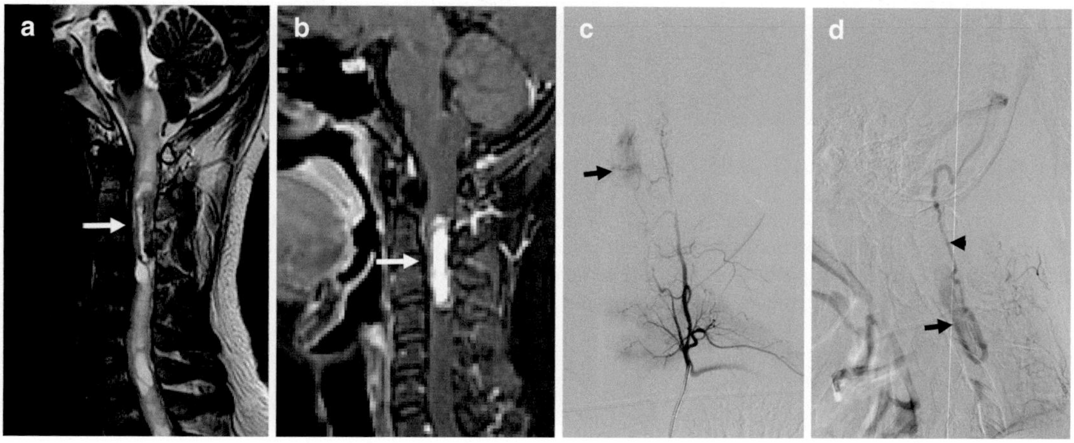

Fig. 14.1 A 24-year-old male patient presented with progressive right upper limb weakness for 1 year. Cervical MRI (**a**) and contrast-enhanced MRI (**b**), sagittal views, showed a C3–C5 level intramedullary hemangioblastoma (arrows). The left thyrocervical trunk angiography, anteroposterior view (**c**) and lateral view (**d**), showed obvious tumor staining (arrows) and draining to intracranial vein (arrowhead)

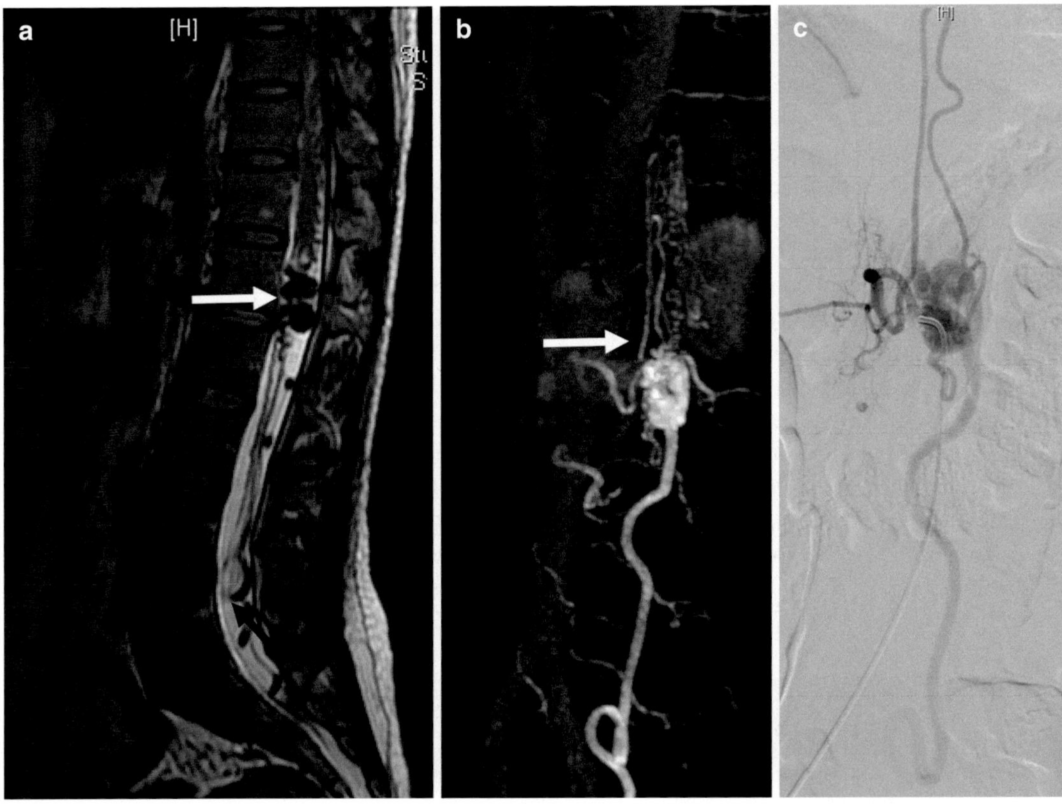

Fig. 14.2 A 36-year-old female patient presented with subarachnoid hemorrhage. (**a**) The lumbar spine MRI, sagittal view, showed multiple vascular flow voids on the surface of the L1 level spinal cord. (**b**) Magnetic resonance angiography suggests spinal vascular malformation at L1 level. (**c**) The right L1 segmental artery angiography, anteroposterior view, showed an L1 level perimedullary arteriovenous fistula supplied by the L1 radiculomedullary artery and anterior spinal artery. The downward vein drainage was thickened and had aneurysmal dilation at the proximal end

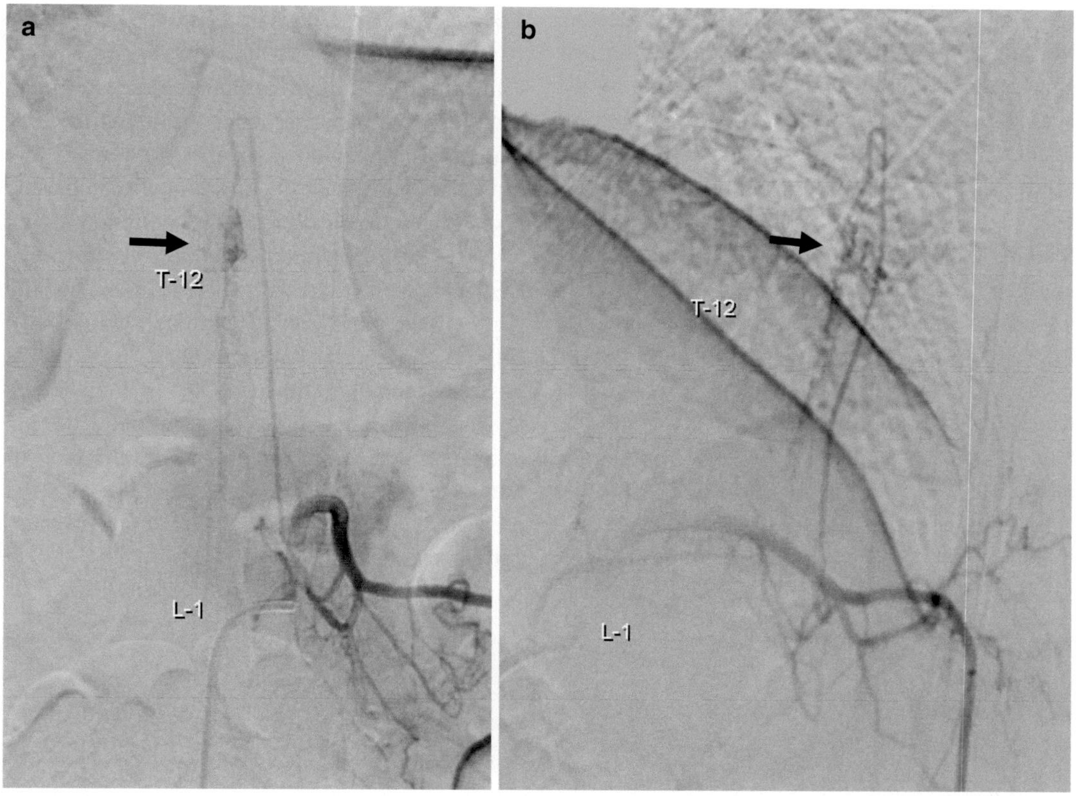

Fig. 14.3 A 29-year-old female patient presented with a sudden onset of paralysis of both lower limbs and difficulty urinating for 10 days. Thoracolumbar CTA examination revealed a high-density lesion in the spinal cord with bleeding. The left L1 segmental artery angiography, anteroposterior view (**a**) and lateral view (**b**), showed a T12 level intramedullary arteriovenous malformation supplied by the L1 radiculomedullary artery and anterior spinal artery and drained downward to the veins

14.4 Treatment Approach and Surgical Technique

Surgery aims to disrupt the vascular fistulas, whether AVM or AVF, and resect enough of the lesion to alleviate venous hypertension while preserving neurological function. Localization of the lesion depends on preoperative imaging and is aided by endovascular markings [23]. Once identified, exposure must permit vascular control and neural protection [24]. In some cases, such as DAVF, identification of the fistula arising from the radicular artery and resecting part of the draining vein is enough for adequate treatment [25]. However, in AVMs, more extensive exposure that allows the identification of the lesions' angioarchitecture is necessary [26].

The surgical approach is then chosen depending on the type and location of the lesions. Whether minimal access approaches or motion-preserving techniques are used, one must consider optimal lesion exposure.

Once the vascular lesion has been located and adequate exposure has been achieved, the vascular shunt is disconnected. DAVS usually have a single radicular feeder that can be coagulated and sectioned safely. In case of proximity to the Adamkiewicz, care must be taken not to disrupt its supply to the spinal cord. The complete draining vein resection was performed in previous years with neurological consequences [27]. More recent studies have shown that limited venous resection is enough to prevent revascularization of the fistula [25]. Lesions located intramedullary are approached via the shortest route to the lesion. Midline myelotomy is a safe corridor with low surgical morbidity [28]. Prior mapping of the actual midline is paramount to avoid neurological insult. If the lesion is superficial and represented on the surface, it is safe to approach the pathology via this route. Sharp subpial resection of the feeding vessel is performed under microscopic augmentation, and continuous monitoring is observed. Minimal retraction and retraction breaks are essential to prevent retraction-related injury. The pial resection technique is another technique utilized for the resection of AVMs. The feeding arteries and draining veins are coagulated and divided along the surface of the spinal cord. This partial devascularization appears sufficient to reduce venous hypertension [26].

14.4.1 Lesion-Specific Consideration

Care must be used when surgically addressing each different vascular shunt. Although the ultimate goal of fistulous disconnection remains the same, specific lesion considerations must be taken. In the case of the most common lesion (type I malformation or DAVF), preoperative DSA assessment can demonstrate branches and feeders that must not be sacrificed (Fig. 14.4). Either the anterior radicular artery (PSA) or the posterior radicular artery (ASA) can branch from the fistulous radicular artery. Ligation of the fistula must take into account the preservation of these vessels. The Adamkiewicz artery must be identified in the preoperative DSA to avoid inadvertent sacrifice.

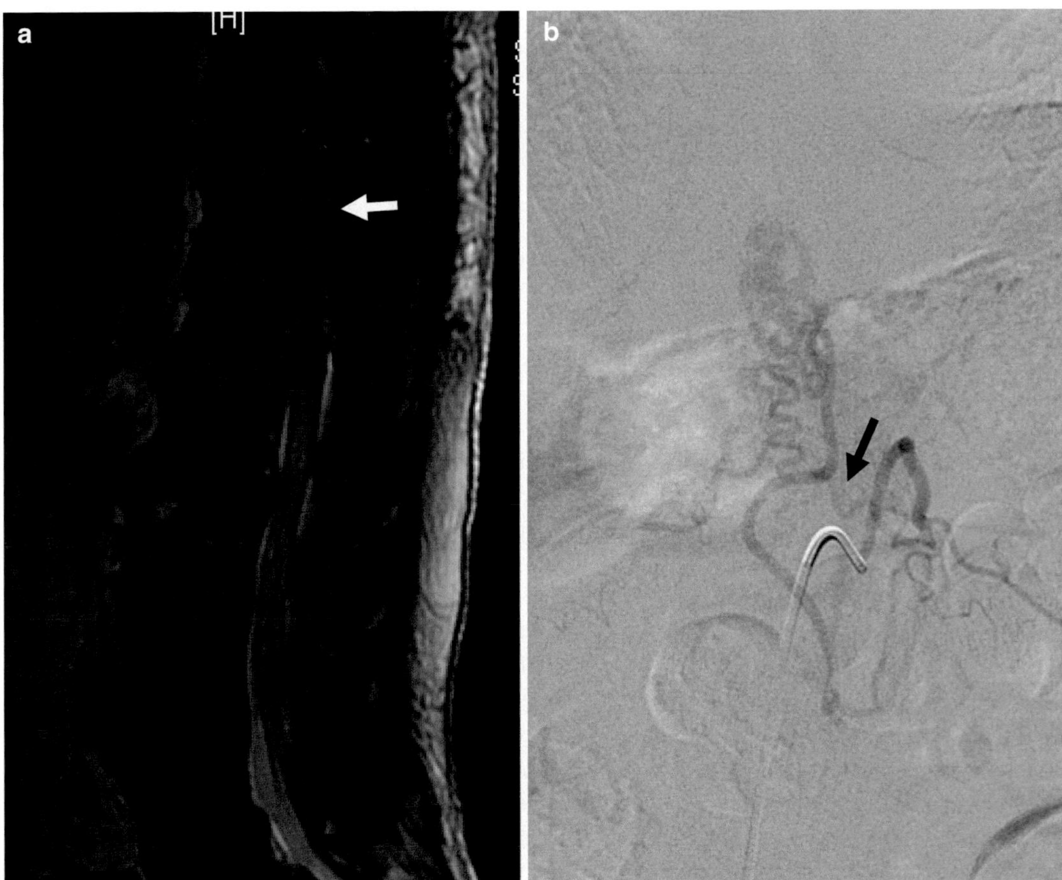

Fig. 14.4 A 51-year-old male patient presented with numbness in the right lower limb for 1 month. (**a**) Thoracolumbar MRI examination showed multiple vascular flow voids on the surface of the spinal cord. (**b**) The left thoracic segmental artery angiography, anteroposterior view, showed a dural arteriovenous fistula supplied by the radiculomeningeal artery and drained downward to the veins on the surface of the spinal cord

In a recent study [29], resection of the proximal end of the draining vein was enough to prevent a recurrence, thus avoiding venous stripping along the entire lesion.

Spinal extradural arteriovenous fistulas (AVFs) are divided into type A (with retrograde parenchymal drainage) and type B (pure extramedullary). An endovascular approach is advised for type A, with an extradural draining vein [30]. When embolization cannot be performed safely, a surgical approach to the fistula is recommended. The treatment consists of obliteration of the intradural drainer. Type B lesions are effectively treated via the endovascular route [30].

The approach to intramedullary arteriovenous malformations (AVMs) (glomus type) is similar to intracranial malformations (Fig. 14.3). First-line treatment remains endovascular owing to the increased surgical risk. A surgical approach, either in combination or alone, is considered when there is a significant risk to the intrinsic spinal arteries or is deemed too hazardous. Rebleeding risk decreased to 8% with either partial or complete lesion treatment [31].

Conus medullaris AVMs are complicated due to the arcade of vessels formed by communications of the PSA and ASA. The afferents are usually small, multiple, and difficult to catheterize. Surgical resection is advised over embolization [32].

Cobb syndrome and the complete form of the spinal arteriovenous metameric syndrome (SAMS) include multiple malformations that derive from the same metameric segment [7]. These lesions can be localized in any derivative of the metamer, from the skin to the intramedullary segment. There is no established optimal treatment for these lesions [33]. Treatment is aimed at reducing the progression of neurological deficits. Most series report combined surgical and endovascular approaches [7, 33].

Perimedullary shunts, otherwise classified as type IV malformations, were first described by Djindjian et al. [34] (Fig. 14.2). These lesions can be subdivided into type IVa, type IVb, and type IVc depending on the number and diameter of feeding arteries and draining veins, with overall bleeding risk of 2.5% [35].

14.4.2 Surgical Aids

Intraoperative monitoring has been shown to improve neurological outcomes in resecting the intramedullary lesion [36]. Both continuous monitoring and mapping have been used [37]. IONM can be helpful in vascular surgery before definitive vessel ligation [38].

Intraoperative micro-ultrasound is another adjunct tool that can assist in the microsurgery of spinal AVS [39].

Combined surgical and intraoperative endovascular modalities are used in specific centers [40]. This approach allows real-time analysis of the spinal vasculature and can help determine the extent of resection and en passage of arteries. However, the technical difficulty of this approach precludes its widespread use.

Recently ICG (indocyanine green) angiography has been used with comparable results to catheter-based studies. FL 800 filter is used in the microscope, and real-time manipulation of the vessels can be performed safely [41]—identification of residual and early-filling pedicles that are then addressed. ICG has been extensively used in resecting brain vascular lesions with favorable outcomes [42].

14.5 Case Illustration

14.5.1 Case Presentation

A 68-year-old male patient with a history of two recent surgeries performed under spinal anesthesia presented to the emergency department with spastic paraparesis, urinary urgency, and lower limb dysesthesia.

The patient had symmetric lower limb weakness 3/5, spasticity, hyperreflexia, and positive Babinski sign on examination.

MRI was performed, evidencing spinal cord edema suggestive of an arteriovenous shunt with engorged epidural vessels.

Diagnostic angiography was performed. A DAVF originating from the right T6 radicular artery and engorged perimedullary veins are shown. The Adamkiewicz artery originated from

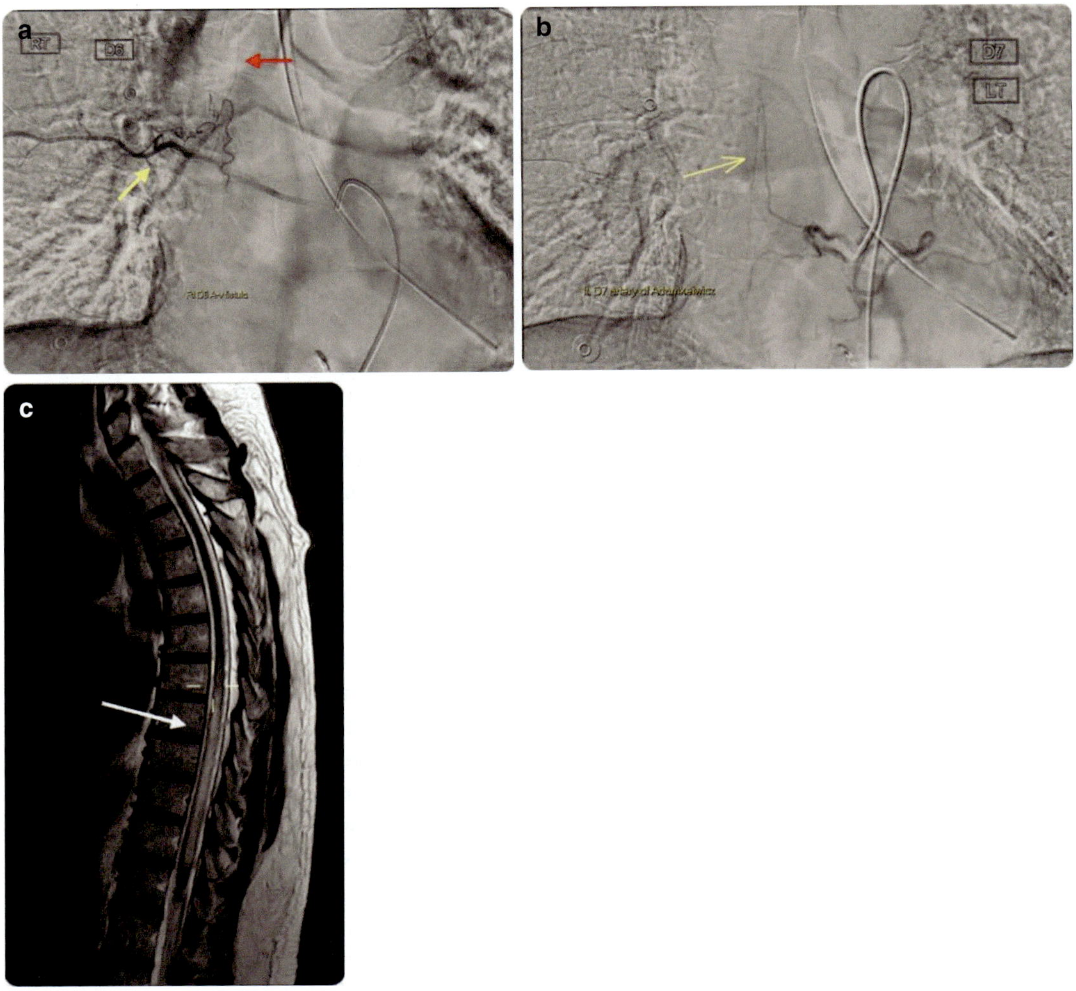

Fig. 14.5 Right T6 radicular artery feeder—dural arteriovenous fistula. (**a**) Angiographic representation of the fistula arising from the right T6 radicular artery (yellow arrow). The right PSA branches at this level (red arrow). (**b**) The Adamkiewicz artery from the left T7 radicular artery (yellow arrow). (**c**) T2WI of the thoracic spine showing spinal cord edema and engorged perimedullary vein (white arrow)

the left T7 radicular artery (Fig. 14.5). Supply to the right PSA distal to the fistula precludes endovascular treatment due to the high risk of iatrogenic closure.

14.5.2 Surgical Approach

Standard T5 and T6 laminectomy is performed. Midline durotomy and retraction sutures are put in place. The central arterialized draining vein is identified and followed cranially until the fistula is located just below the T6 pedicle. Fistulous vessels are identified with the use of ICG. Once the fistula is isolated, coagulation and transaction of the fistula are performed proximal to the exit of the right-sided PSA. Visual confirmation with ICG and reduced engorgement of the arterialized veins are seen. Standard closure follows (Fig. 14.6).

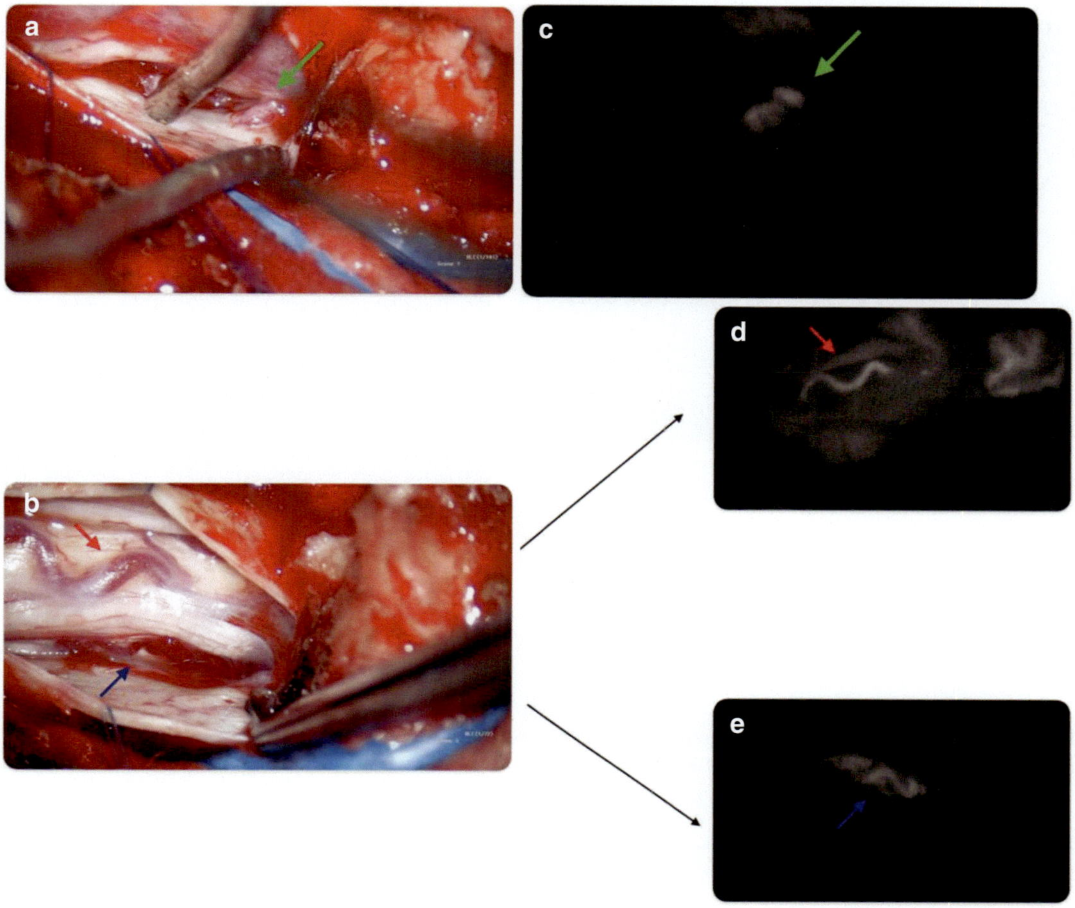

Fig. 14.6 Right T6 radicular artery feeder—dural arteriovenous fistula. (**a**) Surgical field view of the fistula (green arrow) and engorged perimedullary veins. (**b**) Arterialization of the posterior perimedullary vein (red arrow) and dilatation of the anterior perimedullary veins (blue arrow). Confirmation of the fistula is demonstrated with ICG (corresponding colored arrows **c**, **d**, **e**)

Gradual clinical recovery is seen during the following months with residual limb weakness. Follow-up angiography and MRI at 3 years show no residual cord edema, and no remaining fistula is observed (Fig. 14.7).

Disclosures and Acknowledgments No disclosures.

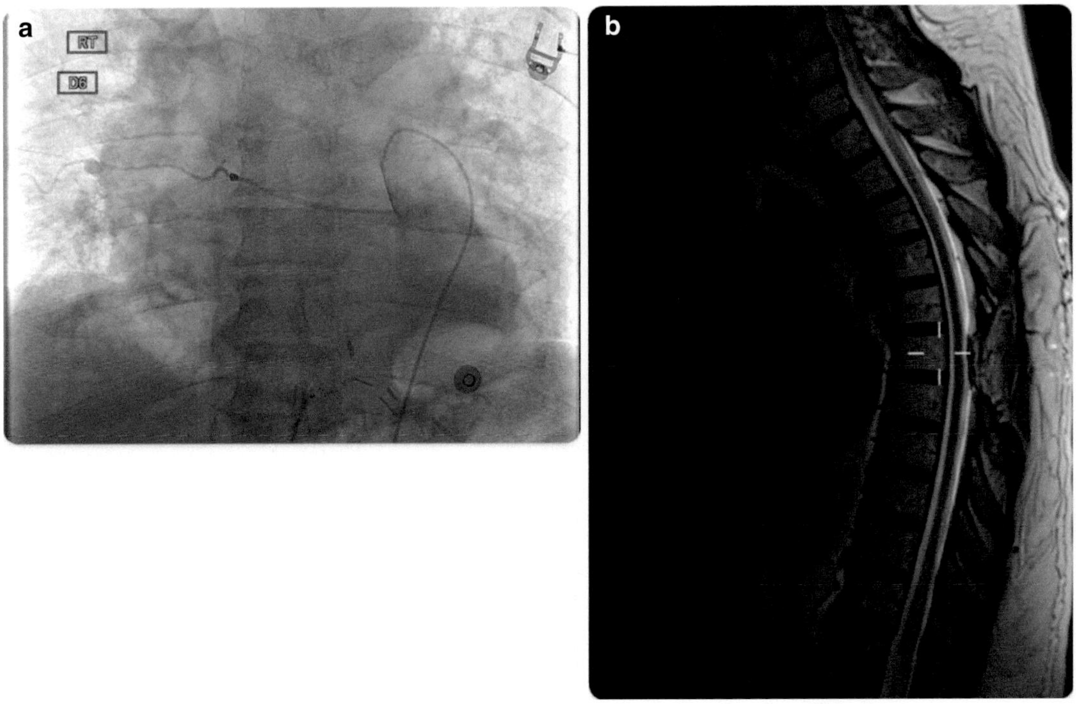

Fig. 14.7 Three-year follow-up angiography showing no residual fistula. (**a**) T2WI with complete resolution of the spinal cord edema. Some cord atrophy is observed on panel **b**

References

1. Rubin MN, Rabinstein AA. Vascular diseases of the spinal cord. Neurol Clin. 2013;31:153–81.
2. Spetzler RF, Detwiler PW, Riina HA, Porter RW. Modified classification of spinal cord vascular lesions. J Neurosurg. 2002;96:145–56.
3. Kiyosue H, Matsumaru Y, Niimi Y, Takai K, Ishiguro T, Hiramatsu M, et al. JSNET spinal AV shunts study group. Angiographic and clinical characteristics of thoracolumbar spinal epidural and dural arteriovenous fistulas. Stroke. 2017;48:3215–22. https://doi.org/10.1161/STROKEAHA.117.019131.
4. Rodesch G, Hurth M, Alvarez H, Tadie M, Lasjaunias P. Classification of spinal cord arteriovenous shunts: proposal for a reappraisal–the Bicetre experience with 155 consecutive patients treated between 1981 and 1999. Neurosurgery. 2002;51:374–9; discussion 379–80.
5. Abecassis IJ, Osbun JW, Kim L. Classification and pathophysiology of spinal vascular malformations. Handb Clin Neurol Elsevier. 2017;143:135–43.
6. Geibprasert S, Pereira V, Krings T, Jiarakongmun P, Toulgoat F, Pongpech S, Lasjaunias P. Dural arteriovenous shunts: a new classification of craniospinal epidural venous anatomical bases and clinical correlations. Stroke. 2008;39:2783–94.
7. Lenck S, Nicholson P, Tymianski R, Hilditch C, Nouet A, Patel K, Krings T, Tymianski M, Radovanovic I, Mendes PV. Spinal and Paraspinal arteriovenous lesions. Stroke. 2019;50(8):2259–69. https://doi.org/10.1161/STROKEAHA.118.012783.
8. Endo T, Endo H, Sato K, Matsumoto Y, Tominaga T. Surgical and endovascular treatment for spinal arteriovenous malformations. Neurol Med Chir (Tokyo). 2016;56(8):457–64. https://doi.org/10.2176/nmc.ra.2015-0327.
9. Söderman M, Mauti M, Löfgren J, et al. Clinical presentation of spinal arteriovenous malformations and aneurysms. Neuroradiology. 2013;55(8):925–33.
10. Kreppel D, Nacey N. Spinal arteriovenous malformations. J Clin Neurosci. 2015;22(1):19–25.
11. Müller M, Rohde V, Vajkoczy P. Spinal arteriovenous malformations: experience with surgical treatment in 60 patients. Neurosurgery. 2012;70(4):874–84.
12. Hoh BL, Chapman PH, Loeffler JS, Carter BS, Ogilvy CS. Results of multimodality treatment for 141 patients with brain arteriovenous malformations and seizures: factors associated with seizure outcomes. Neurosurgery. 2012;70(3):531–8.

13. Amin-Hanjani S, Barker FG, Charbel FT, Connolly ES, Morcos JJ, Thompson BG. Treatment of spinal arteriovenous malformations: a multicenter study of 39 patients. Neurosurgery. 2014;74(1):51–60.
14. Fifi JT, Meyers PM, Lavine SD, et al. Complications of modern diagnostic cerebral angiography in an academic medical center. J Vasc Interv Radiol. 2014;25(5):825–31.
15. Walcott BP, Smith ER, Scott RM, Orbach DB. Spinal arteriovenous malformations in children. J Neurosurg Pediatr. 2014;14(1):1–12.
16. Winkler EA, Rutledge WC, Ko NU. The future of arteriovenous malformation management: interventional neurology. Curr Opin Neurol. 2014;27(1):91–7.
17. Pivovarnik JM, Chen S. Spinal cord compression due to spinal artery aneurysm in an otherwise healthy patient: a case report and literature review. Cureus. 2019;11(1):e3853.
18. Aminoff MJ, Logue V. The prognosis of patients with spinal cord malformations. Brain. 1974;97(1):211–24.
19. Gokhale S, Khan S, McDonagh D, Britz G. Comparison of surgical and endovascular approach in management of spinal dural arteriovenous fistulas: a single center experience of 27 patients. Surg Neurol Int. 2014;5:7. https://doi.org/10.4103/2152-7806.125628.
20. Miyamoto T, Iwasaki Y. Diagnostic imaging for spinal vascular malformations. Neurol Med Chir. 2014;54(12):947–56.
21. Vilela P, Goulão A, Gomes L. Spinal arteriovenous shunts: imaging and intervention. Eur J Radiol. 2013;82(2):221–32. https://doi.org/10.1016/j.ejrad.2012.08.023.
22. Hua X, Zhao T, Sun H, Li Z, Chen X. Application of diffusion tensor imaging in the surgical treatment of spinal vascular malformations. J Clin Neurosci. 2015;22(11):1741–6.
23. Zaidi HA, Montoure A, El Tecle NE, et al. Spinal arteriovenous fistulas and malformations: a review of imaging and treatment options. Neurosurg Focus. 2019;46(4):E4. https://doi.org/10.3171/2019.1.FOCUS18641.
24. Gupta A, Bansal S, Satyarthee GD, Kumar A, Sharma BS. Surgical treatment of spinal arteriovenous malformations: an institutional experience. Asian J Neurosurg. 2017;12(3):435–43. https://doi.org/10.4103/1793-5482.175620.
25. Diaz OM, Alturki AY, Arnaout OM, et al. Treatment strategies for spinal dural arteriovenous fistulas: a comprehensive review. Neurosurg Focus. 2019;46(4):E3. https://doi.org/10.3171/2019.1.FOCUS18615.
26. Lawton MT, Porter RW, Heiserman JE, Jacobowitz R, Sonntag VK, Dickman CA. Surgical management of spinal arteriovenous lesions: clinical article. J Neurosurg Spine. 2017;26(4):497–511. https://doi.org/10.3171/2016.8.SPINE16549.
27. Schick U, Hassler W, Hennes C, et al. Spinal dural arteriovenous fistulae: surgical and endovascular treatment. Neurosurgery. 2019;85(2):E270–8. https://doi.org/10.1093/neuros/nyy579.
28. Samadian M, Izadpanahi A, Safari A, et al. Spinal intramedullary cavernous hemangiomas: surgical strategies and outcomes. J Neurol Surg A Cent Eur Neurosurg. 2018;79(5):395–404. https://doi.org/10.1055/s-0038-1636915.
29. Hu P, Chen J, Gu Y, Xu B, Xu K, Fang Y, et al. Resection of proximal end of the draining vein alone for the treatment of spinal dural arteriovenous fistula. Acta Neurochir. 2021;163(4):1009–16. https://doi.org/10.1007/s00701-021-04810-z.
30. Katsaridis V, Papagiannaki C, Aimar E. Endovascular treatment of spinal cord arteriovenous fistulae. J Neurol Neurosurg Psychiatry. 2008;79(2):125–9. https://doi.org/10.1136/jnnp.2006.108175.
31. Liu P, Yang X, Wang Y, Cai L, He X, Zhu Y. Surgical treatment of conus medullaris arteriovenous malformations: a retrospective study of 20 patients. J Neurosurg Spine. 2013;18(3):236–43.
32. Kim BS, Kim HJ, Kim JT, Kim KH, Moon KS. Clinical outcomes of surgical and endovascular treatment for spinal arteriovenous malformations. Neurosurgery. 2019;85(4):E709–17.
33. Consoli A, Coskun O, Di Maria F, Gratieux J, Condette-Auliac S, Smadja S, Boulin A, Rodesch G. Spinal cord arteriovenous shunts: from classification to therapeutic management. Rev Neurol. 2021;177:469–76.
34. Djindjian R, Merland JJ, Cophignon J, Rey A. Shunts artério-veineux péri-médullaires intradurals. Journal de radiologie, d'électrologie, et de médicine nucléaire. 1976;57(10):687–704.
35. Yamada SM, Spetzler RF, Haid RW, Zabramski JM. Perimedullary arteriovenous fistulas: a review. Neurosurg Focus. 2003;14(6):e7.
36. Dong C, Zhang T, Qiu Y, Hao S. The role of intraoperative neurophysiological monitoring in the resection of intramedullary lesions. Neurol Sci. 2021;42(2):491–8. https://doi.org/10.1007/s10072-020-04814-1.
37. Jiang B, Liu X, Liu Z, Feng X. Intraoperative neurophysiological monitoring for spinal cord tumor surgery: a systematic review and meta-analysis. World Neurosurg. 2021;150:429–439.e2. https://doi.org/10.1016/j.wneu.2021.05.038.
38. Cheng L, Li X, Wang Y, Yang M, Jia X. The clinical application of intraoperative neurophysiological monitoring in intracranial aneurysm surgery. World Neurosurg. 2018;111:e428–35. https://doi.org/10.1016/j.wneu.2017.12.050.
39. Raza SM, Donaldson AM, Lieber B, Wang WH. Intraoperative micro-ultrasound in spinal surgery. J Clin Neurosci. 2018;53:186–91. https://doi.org/10.1016/j.jocn.2018.05.051.
40. Alfano JM, Cmelak AJ, Ding D, Mehra S. Combined surgical and endovascular approach for resection of spinal arteriovenous malformations: a case series and

technical report. World Neurosurg. 2020;138:468–77. https://doi.org/10
41. Pirris SM, Abla AA, Yu C, Chang SD, Theodosopoulos PV. Indocyanine green fluorescence angiography for intracranial dural arteriovenous fistulae: surgical technique and nuances. J Neurosurg. 2019;132(4):1114–20. https://doi.org/10.3171/2018.11.JNS182686.
42. Chang JW, Park YG, Lee DH, Kim DH, Chung SS. Indocyanine green angiography in the surgical treatment of brain arteriovenous malformation: a single institutional experience with 68 patients. J Cerebrovasc Endovasc Neurosurg. 2020;22(1):6–14. https://doi.org/10.7461/jcen.2020.22.1.6.

Spinal Aneurysm

15

Shuroq Alshehri, Mustafa Ismail, Hajer Al Naqbi, Hosam Al-Jehani, Faisal Mishaal Alabbas, Zaid Aljuboori, and Samer S. Hoz

Abstract

Spinal aneurysms (SAs) are a very rare pathology to be encountered as compared to intracranial aneurysms. The first ever described spinal aneurysm was in 1930. Djindjian and his colleagues found that the incidence rate is less than 1 in every 3000 cases who had a spinal angiogram. Given its rarity, there is no unified system to classify spinal aneurysms. Nearly 55% of all presented SAs were isolated once.

Unlike intracranial aneurysms, spinal aneurysms are usually lacking a surgical neck. Histopathology was described as dissecting aneurysms, and the incidence of a fusiform aneurysm in the spine was found to be more common. However, saccular aneurysms were also reported.

Most cases present with ruptured spinal aneurysms, usually smaller than intracranially (<3 mm in diameter) and located at the cervical level. Also, the mean diameter of aneurysms was 9 mm (range 3–27 mm).

The clinical presentation usually varies, but the sudden onset of low back pain is the most common. Presenting with or without hemorrhage in the subarachnoid space was irrelevant to its size or predictive of the outcome or mortality as in those with cranial origin.

An earlier review in 1957 by Henson and Crof described cervical aneurysms as unlikely to present in a living patient.

The management of spinal aneurysms includes conservative or surgical or endovascular options. The choice of treatment pathway should be individualized according to the case as it varies with the location of the aneurysm, rupture status, related angiographic findings, clinical status of the patient, and time frame from presentation in cases with a significant deficit. We will explore the treatment principles with case examples in this chapter.

Keywords

Spinal aneurysm · Surgery · Embolization Treatment

S. Alshehri · H. Al-Jehani · F. M. Alabbas
Department of Neurosurgery, Imam Abdulrahman Bin Faisal University, Dammam, Saudi Arabia

M. Ismail
Department of Neurosurgery, Neurosurgery Teaching Hospital, Baghdad, Iraq

H. Al Naqbi
Department of Neurosurgery, Rashid Hospital, Dubai, UAE
e-mail: hmalnaqbi@dha.gov.ae

Z. Aljuboori
Department of Neurosurgery, Geisinger Commonwealth School of Medicine, Geisinger, PA, USA
e-mail: Zaljuboori1@geisinger.edu

S. S. Hoz (✉)
Department of Neurosurgery, University of Cincinnati College of Medicine, Cincinnati, OH, USA

X. Lv (ed.), *Endovascular and Neurovascular Surgery for Spinal Vascular Malformations*,
https://doi.org/10.1007/978-981-97-4661-3_15

15.1 Introduction

Compared to intracranial aneurysms, spinal aneurysms are a very rare pathology to be encountered. The first ever described spontaneous spinal subarachnoid hemorrhage was by Balk in 1900. Djindjian and his colleagues found the incidence rate is less than 1 in every 3000 cases who had a spinal angiogram. Given its rarity, there is no unified system to classify spinal aneurysms, but in literature, it was classified as an AVM-related aneurysm (AVM-SA) and isolated aneurysms (iSA), and AVM-related aneurysms are more common [1–3].

Spinal arteriovenous malformation accounts for 5–9% of all central nervous system arteriovenous malformations (AVMs), and only 3–4% are located intradurally. Aneurysms with arteriovenous malformation association (SA-AVM) were found in 44.7% of all patients. Mainly "glomus"-type AVM is the most commonly associated with aneurysms [4, 5].

Current data is an ambiguous predominance in gender and ethnicity. However, in one systemic review of the literature, the group of AVM-associated aneurysms tends to occur more in younger age groups compared to solitary ones. In one retrospective review, they encountered 7 out of 11 patients who were females (63.3%) with a median age of 60. Another systemic review that was published in 2013 disclosed a median age of presentation as 38 years where less than 10% of them were below the age of 10. The mean age of presentation of iSA is 49 ± 17.8 years and SA-AVM is 23 ± 16.9 [3, 6].

15.2 Pathophysiology

Unlike intracranial aneurysms, spinal aneurysms are usually lacking a surgical neck. Histopathologically, they were described as dissecting aneurysms, and incidents of fusiform aneurysms in the spine were found to be more common. However, saccular aneurysms were also reported.

The natural history of spinal aneurysms is still not clear, but a couple of theories were suggested. Any given pathology that causes high flow within spinal vascular circulation may increase the hemodynamic stress on the vascular wall, which is a direct contributing factor in the formation of spinal aneurysms. Thus, spinal aneurysms were found to be associated with arteriovenous malformations, arteriovenous fistula, and coarctation of the aorta and were rarely discovered in isolation. In 1980, Caroscio data included 30 patients with spinal artery aneurysms: 15 were with AVMs, 12 had coarctation of the aorta, and 3 cases were isolated. In addition, it was linked to several comorbidities such as connective tissue disease, infectious or inflammatory vasculopathy, bilateral vertebral artery occlusion, and patient post-renal transplant. However, the data on isolated spinal aneurysms still are inadequate.

Most cases are present with ruptured spinal aneurysms, and they usually come smaller in size in comparison with those intracranially (<3 mm in diameter). Also, the average diameter is 10.5 mm. A study published in 2018 found only 8 out of 91 patients who presented with AVM had an aneurysm, in which 4 of them were located at the cervical level. Also, the mean diameter of aneurysms was 9 mm (range 3–27 mm). The percentage of presentation with the ruptured aneurysm is not yet clear. But it was found a higher rate of hemorrhage in cases where the spinal arteriovenous malformation (AVM) was associated with an aneurysm compared to those AVM without. The incidence of ruptured spinal aneurysms is 92%, and ruptured spinal aneurysms associated with AVMs are 79%. An intranidal aneurysm is more likely to bleed than those located along the feeding artery. All patients who presented with or without hemorrhage in the subarachnoid space did not have relevance to its size or predictive of the outcome or mortality as in those with cranial origin [6–9].

15.3 Classification of Spinal Aneurysms

One of the proposed classifications of spinal aneurysms is to divide them into two groups. **Type I** is spinal aneurysms (SAs) associated with

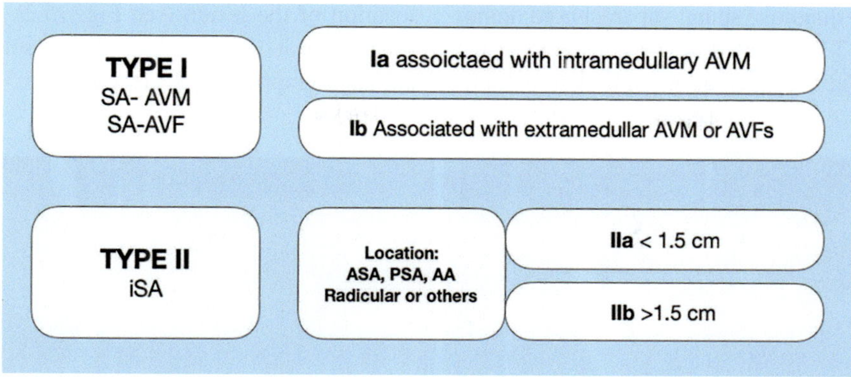

Fig. 15.1 Classification of spinal aneurysm (*SA-AVM* spinal aneurysms associated with arteriovenous malformation, *SA-AVF* spinal aneurysms associated with arteriovenous fistula, *iSA* isolated spinal aneurysm, *ASA* anterior spinal artery, *PSA* posterior spinal artery, *AA* artery of Adamkiewicz) [6]

arteriovenous malformations (AVMs) or dural arteriovenous fistulas (AVFs). Furthermore, it can be divided into **type Ia** spinal aneurysms associated with intramedullary AVM (along the feeding artery or in the nidus) and **type Ib** spinal aneurysms associated with extramedullary AVM or AVFs. **Type II** is an isolated spinal aneurysm (iSA), and it can be subclassified based on the lesion or the aneurysm size and location of the anterior spinal artery (ASA), posterior spinal artery (PSA), artery of Adamkiewicz (AA), and radicular or radiculopial lateral spinal artery: **type IIa** < 1.5 cm in diameter and **type IIb** > 1.5 cm [6] (see Fig. 15.1).

15.4 Presentation

The clinical presentation usually varies, but the sudden onset of low back pain is the most common presentation. Also, lower limb weakness, sphincter abnormalities, and paresthesia were reported [6, 10, 11].

A cervical aneurysm is more commonly linked to devastating morbidity and mortality. An earlier review in 1957 by Henson and Crof described cervical aneurysm as unlikely to be present in a living patient. High clinical suspicion of cervical SA should be raised whenever subarachnoid and intraventricular hemorrhage is seen in the posterior fossa with a history of sudden neck pain and nuchal rigidity with a negative CTA of the brain [11, 12].

Intradural and extramedullary located aneurysms were the most common locations, and both can cause subarachnoid hemorrhage. Aneurysmal subarachnoid hemorrhage is considered an unfortunate and even fatal presentation in most intracranial origin cases; it was reported less than 1% of presented cases had a spinal origin of SAH. However, the presentation of SAH wasn't linked to the outcome like intracranial presentations [13].

Radiologically, CT of the spine can be done initially as a screening tool to rule out other spinal pathologies; 9 out of 10 patients who have positive CT for SA had a spinal subarachnoid hemorrhage or subdural hematoma or even both. In the same series, 0 patients presented with hematomyelia. However, an MRI of the spine can give a clear idea of any signal changes within the cord and can show the presence of vascular pathologies, swelling of the spinal cord, and dilated veins [14–16].

15.5 Investigation

CTA and MRA also are great modalities as noninvasive imaging of the spine to determine the size as well as the orientation of the aneurysm; three out of four patients had evidence of spinal aneurysm. MRI T1 and FLAIR signal sequences can help to diagnose spinal subarachnoid hemorrhage, and T2-weighted image is used to visualize flow void in case of an AVM to determine the location of the lesion (see Fig. 15.2). The most sensitive tool or the gold standard is selective spinal angiography or DSA (see Fig. 15.3).

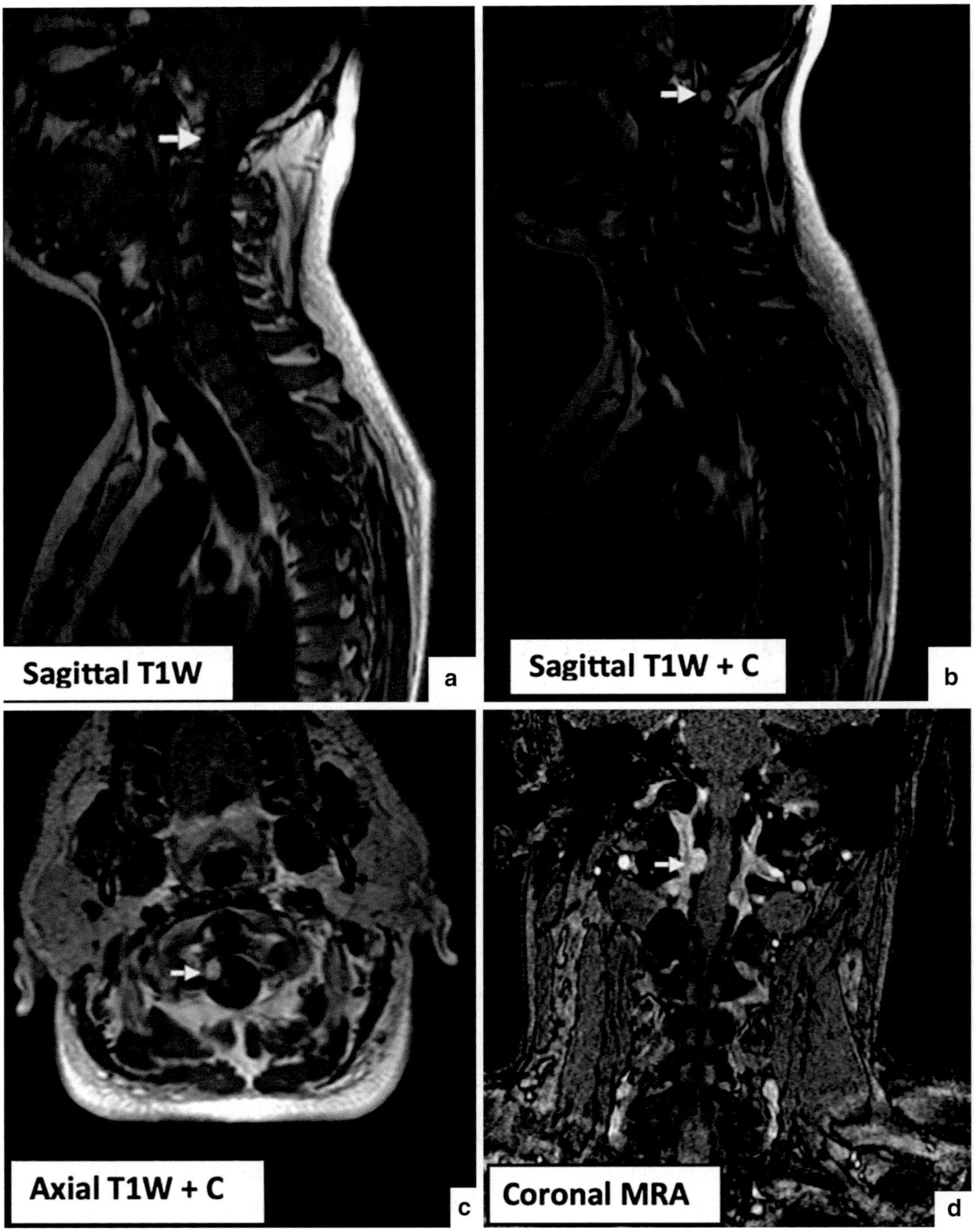

Fig. 15.2 MR images (**a–d**) of the cervical spine of a 30-year-old patient demonstrated small saccular aneurysm with wide neck (arrows) arising from medial side of the right V3 segment of the vertebral artery at C1 and C2 level which indentation the spinal cord and causing spinal canal stenosis. (Courtesy of Dr. Xian Li, School of Clinical Medicine of Tsinghua University, China)

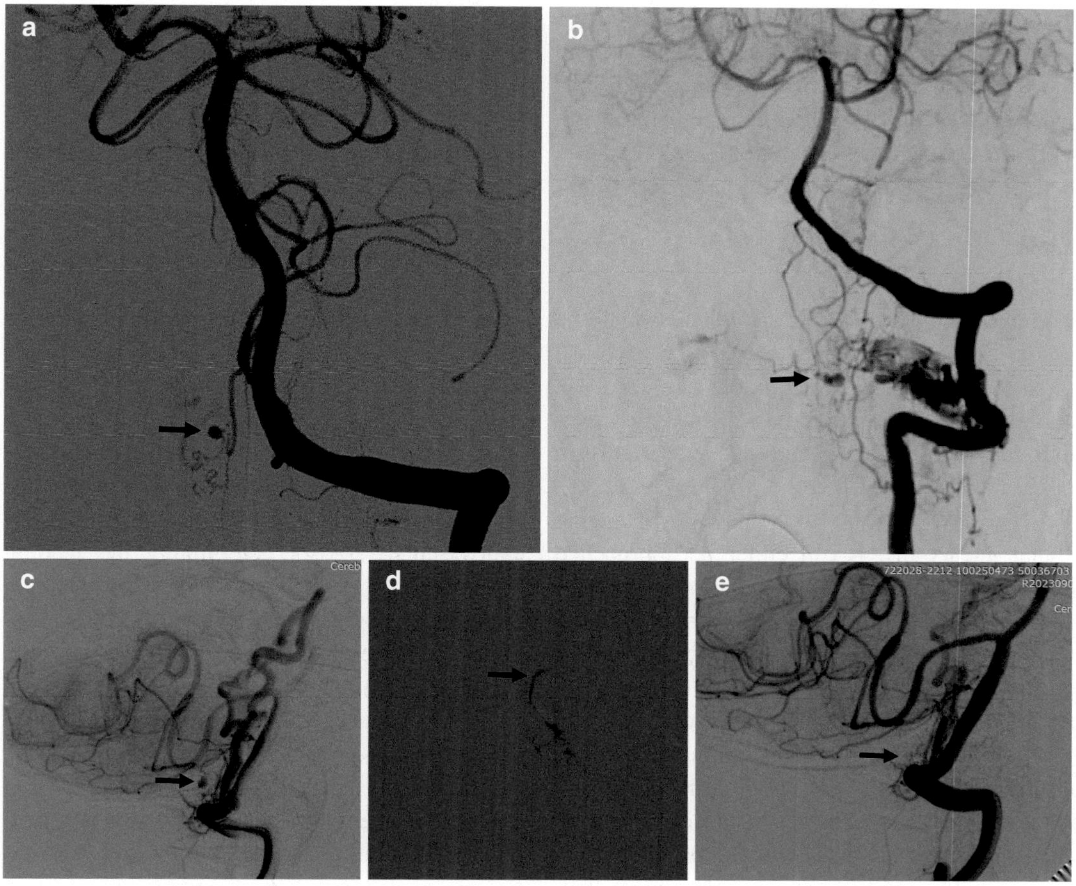

Fig. 15.3 (**a**) A 64-year-old male patient presented with subarachnoid hemorrhage. The left vertebral artery angiography showed an anterior spinal artery aneurysm with a small arteriovenous malformation at the distal end (type Ia). (**b**) A 73-year-old female patient presented with subarachnoid hemorrhage. The conventional angiography showed an anterior spinal artery aneurysm with extramedullary dural arteriovenous fistula (type Ib). (**c** and **d**) A 53-year-old male patient presented with subarachnoid hemorrhage. The conventional angiography showed a left C1 radicular artery aneurysm with an extramedullary dural arteriovenous fistula (type Ib) (arrow in panel **c**). The aneurysm was embolized with Onyx-18 (arrow in panel **d**). The control angiogram showing the disappearance of the aneurysm and the partial occlusion of the dural fistula (arrow in panel **e**). (Courtesy of Dr. Xian Li, School of Clinical Medicine of Tsinghua University, China)

Aneurysms, located in the anterior spinal artery, are more commonly encountered rather than posterior spinal aneurysms. They can originate from different segments, such as radicular and radiculomedullary junction, and from a sulcal-commissural artery leading to the formation of intramedullary arteriovenous malformation. Geibprasert and his colleagues studied 32 cases of spinal aneurysms and found nearly 60% originated from anterior spinal artery aneurysms [16–18].

In a retrospective study, 9 out of the 11 cases had a radiculopial artery aneurysm, 3 patients had radiculomedullary aneurysms, and 2 patients had multiple sclerosis aneurysms. Radiculomedullary artery aneurysms were associated with subdural hemorrhage, and radiculopial artery aneurysms were associated with subarachnoid hemorrhage. Anatomically, radiculomedullary artery courses along the dural sleeve, and any bleeding can lead to the splitting off of the dural layers leading to the SDH. In addition, the radiculopial artery aneurysms are located intradurally, and their course is wrapped around the spinal cord. Spinal angiography or DSA provides critical information to help guide the management and predict the outcome [3].

15.6 Management

The management of spinal aneurysms should be tailored for every case, depending on the clinical picture, neurological presentation, size, location, and relation to the parent vessel, feeding artery, draining veins, aneurysm type, and aneurysm orientation.

There are different approaches to managing spinal aneurysms. It can either be approached conservatively or by endovascular procedure, surgical procedure, or a combination of both. Conservative management and watchful waiting are not at all uncommon approach to the spinal aneurysm, especially in isolated type.

Observation is recommended in cases with multiple aneurysms and cases with underlying connective tissue disease, vasculitis, infection, and post-transplant since those conditions can present with pseudoaneurysms. On top of that, patients are most likely to have serious comorbidities, which can correlate to overall poor outcomes. Longatti and his colleagues suggested a conservative approach is best for small aneurysms with distal blood flow and in the absence of spinal cord compression. However, during the observation, patient's blood pressure should be tightly controlled and should be followed by DSA from time to time to look for any morphological changes in the aneurysm. Watchful waiting provided an observation in which 50% of the cases can have regression or obliteration of the aneurysm for an obscure cause. Despite a lot of neurosurgeons advocating for observation, this decision has to be tailored for every single case since some cases in the literature reported patient demise with suspicion of rebleeding as the cause of death [2, 19–21]. The risk of rebleeding after a conservative approach is still unclear, but in a couple of cases in the literature, patients died while they are in observation and the presumption was due to rebleeding.

According to Lasjaunias et al., the indications to treat spinal cord AVM include all patients with symptomatic lesions that can be cured. If cure of the lesion is not possible, structures that represent the anatomical risk factors, such as associated aneurysms, should be treated [13].

The utilization of endovascular treatment should be practiced whenever possible due to its less invasive approach and a perfect choice for elderly patients or those who have serious morbidities.

In cases of AVM, morphological features (saccular vs. fusiform) as well as the extent of nidus play a crucial point before approaching any AVM endovascularly. Also, determining the feeding artery in an AVM is a crucial step in the management to avoid further neurological defects secondary to ischemia or decrease blood flow to the spinal cord.

Endovascular embolization for spinal aneurysms by Onyx or glue as well as coils can be used to treat cases of arteriovenous malformation and anterior-venous fistula in order to decrease blood flow within the lesion. However, treating vascular malformation with embolization can be obliterated in stages or complete obliteration or used in synergy with surgical intervention. For an aneurysm associated with AVF, the main target of obliteration by any means is the fistulous part where the feeding artery meets the draining vein and thus decreases the hemodynamic stress in which the flow decreased within the aneurysm. When an artery is occluded or sacrificed, there has to be a clear visualization of blood flow coming from the contralateral side to avoid a considerable risk of spinal cord infarction in order to avoid further deterioration of the neurological status. Natsumi et al. suggested embolization as an optimal approach for spinal glomus AVM [21] (see Fig. 15.4).

The surgical approach can be challenging depending on the presentation. In case the patient presents with acute neurological deterioration secondary to cord compression, surgical decompression is urgently recommended to ensure a

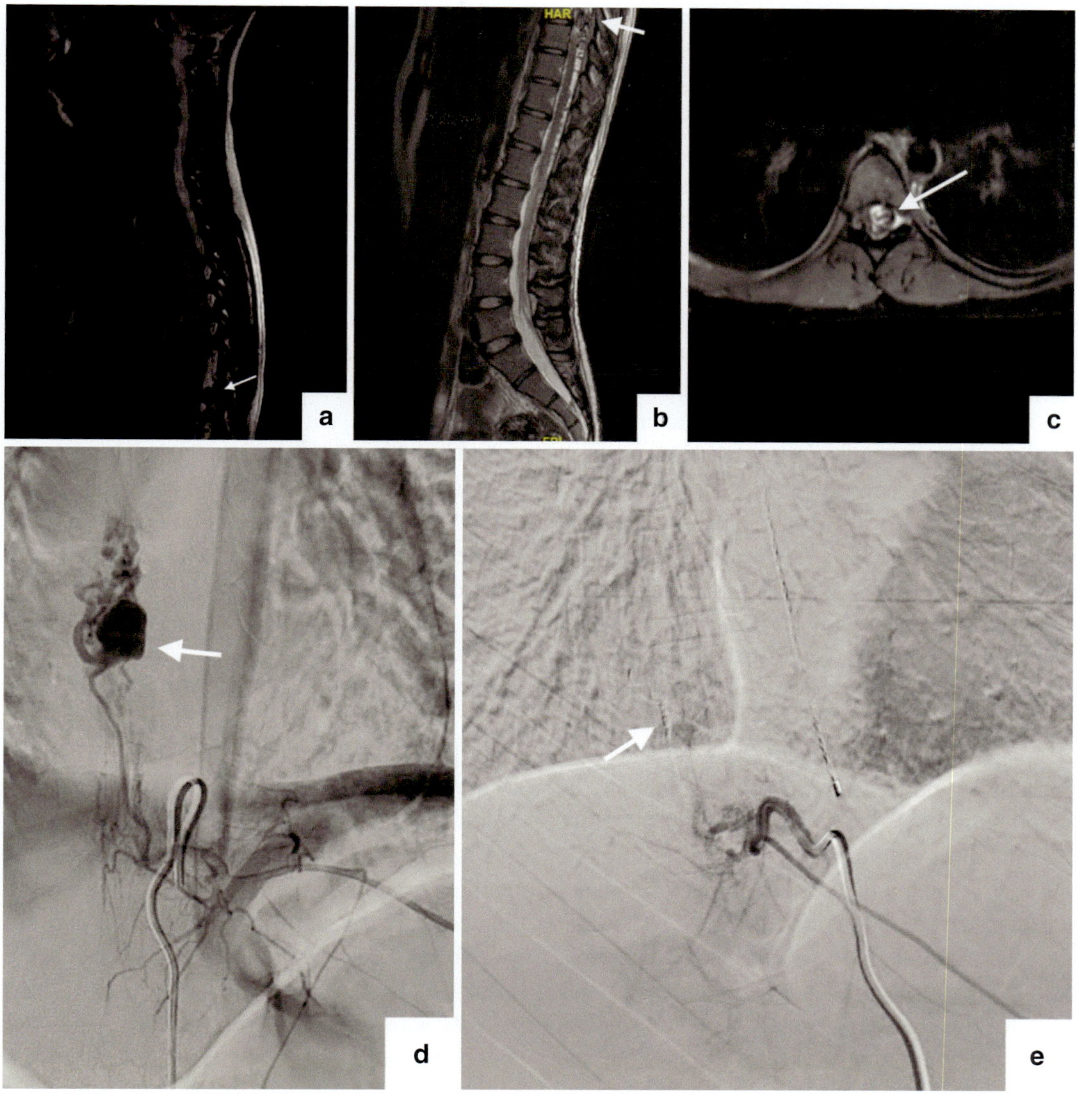

Fig. 15.4 A 17-year-old female who presented with left lower limb spasticity for 4 months. MRI of the spine (**a**–**c**) showed a flow void extending from T5 to T11, suggestive of an AVM with associated aneurysm. In conventional angiography (**d**), a left T8 arteriovenous fistula supplied by anterior spinal artery and draining intradurally. Also, another feeder seen at the level of T11 on the left side, which has large fistula and peri-nidal aneurysm. No other feeders identified. A selective left T11 spinal artery embolization (**d**) was done using a microcatheter that was introduced through the marginal artery toward the anterior spinal artery, as getting close to the peri-nidal aneurysm, coils then were deployed and the final run (**e**) demonstrated a successful embolization of the perimedullary AVM through T11 feeder. A second stage is needed to embolize the left T8 aVF. (Courtesy of Dr. Faisal Alabbas and Dr. Abdulrahman Alabdulwahab, Imam Abdulrahman Bin Faisal University, Saudi Arabia)

better neurological outcome. On the other hand, surgery is recommended as well in cases where the saccular or surgical neck is present with easy accessibility with the posterior approach. Clipping aneurysms can be used when they have a clear surgical neck; however, most spinal aneurysms are fusiform in shape, which makes this option unsuitable for most patients. Wrapping of aneurysms with muscle, gauze, or muslin can be used in cases of the fusiform type where it is located at the long axis of the anterior and posterior spinal aneurysms where the risk of infarction is higher in case of injury. In cases where surgical management is indicated and it was delayed for any reason, a repeated angiography is mandatory because of the high probability of spontaneous regression. For lesions that are located ventrally at the cervical and upper thoracic levels, the anterior approach with corpectomy can be used with better exposure can be obtained by partial removal of the manubrium of the sternum or part of the clavicle, after surgical resection or clipping cervical reconstruction using expandable cages and plating can be used. For lesions that occupied the neural foramina in the thoracic area, a posterolateral thoracotomy may provide an accessible window. Ventrally located thoracic and lumbar aneurysms are very challenging because of the limitation of the exposure, but usually, they are surgically treated by posterior or posterolateral approach by partial facetectomy or ipsilateral pedicle removal to facilitate wider exposure [18, 22, 23].

However, the surgical option is maintaining adequate blood perfusion to the spinal cord throughout the surgery, which is essential, by keeping the MAP above 90 mmHg. Additionally, neuromonitoring during surgery is useful; while spinal cord manipulation is attempted, somatosensory evoked potentials (SSEPs) and motor evoked potentials (MEPs) can be used. Steroid administration such as methylprednisolone may have a protective property in preventing neural death and improving collateral circulation, and some other agents aid in the prevention of reperfusion injury, which can play a key role in delayed spinal cord injury. Examples of those are local vasodilators (papaverine), vasopressors (epinephrine, norepinephrine, and phenylephrine), agents that can cause reduction of neuronal excitotoxicity (steroids, riluzole, MgSo4, basic fibroblast growth factor, and dehydroepiandrosterone (DHEA)), and agent causing prevention of ischemia and causing reperfusion such as statins [24].

Some authors proposed surgical treatment for cases with poor neurological status on presentation (ASIA scores A and B), evidence of spinal infraction, and size progression as well as thrombosed spinal aneurysms. In addition to aneurysms located in the posterior spinal artery (PSA), it is easily accessed surgically. It should be taken into consideration that PSA has abundant anastomosis to supply the spinal cord and sacrificing one vessel is unlikely to cause a spinal infarction, and its smaller diameter compared to ASA makes the surgical option more reasonable than endovascular management. However, dealing with ASA aneurysms is more complex since they carry a very serious neurological sequela if any complications happened especially in a neurologically intact patient. In cases where they have an aneurysm associated with AVM, both endovascular and surgical management can be done.

The spinal aneurysm risk of rebleeding after conservative vs. endovascular and surgical management is still unclear due to underreporting in the literature.

15.7 Prognosis and Outcome

Overall, isolated and AVM-associated spinal aneurysms have good or fair neurological outcomes. But aggressive management of cervical aneurysms should be provided since it carries significant morbidity and mortality compared to thoracolumbar aneurysms (33% vs. 0% mortality). Some suggested presenting symptoms at the onset usually correlate with the outcome, and patients who presented with headache and N/V and back pain will show some to significant improvement compared to patients who presented with spinal cord compression secondary to subarachnoid hemorrhage or subdural hematoma (100% vs. 40% improvement). However, the worst of them all are those patients who presented with hematomyelia; only 14% of patients can present with intramedullary bleeding or hematomyelia.

In a retrospective study of 11 patients with a radiculomedullary artery or radiculopial artery, 87.5% of patients were functionally independent with a mean clinical follow-up of 20 months. During follow-up, four patients (36.4%) who had an MRI of the spine had persistent abnormal signal changes in the spinal cord, and two patients had adhesive arachnoiditis (18.2%). In another series, Rosenblum et al. reported good functional status in 88% of those with aneurysms associated with AVFs and 49% with intramedullary AVMs and 71% of patients with both isolated spinal aneurysms and spinal aneurysms associated with AVMs [6, 25, 26].

As soon as the proper intervention is carried out, the patient should be referred to extensive rehabilitation since most of the patients showed great neurological improvement after discharge. The outcomes for spinal aneurysm cases varied based on the age and duration of symptoms. The good outcome represents 44–45% for young patients with chronic presentation, while it is 40–63% for older patients [6].

15.8 Conclusion

The spinal artery aneurysm's natural history and management are still not clear due to its rare presentation. Sudden onset of back pain with lower limb weakness, headache, nausea, or vomiting might be an indication of a ruptured spinal aneurysm. Once an aneurysm is diagnosed, the management should be tailored accordingly. Finally, more data is needed to determine or help establish guidelines to approach spinal aneurysms.

References

1. Djindjian R, Dumesnil M, Faure C, Lefebvre J, Leveque B. Etude angiographique d'un angiome intrarachidien. Rev Neurol. 1962;106:278–85.
2. Henson RA, Croft PB. Spontaneous spinal subarachnoid haemorrhage. QJM. 1956;25(1):53–66.
3. Renieri L, Raz E, Lanzino G, Krings T, Shapiro M, Shirani P, Brinjikji W. Spinal artery aneurysms: clinical presentation, radiological findings, and outcome. J Neurointerv Surg. 2018;10(7):644–8.
4. Varshneya K, Pendharkar AV, Azad TD, Ratliff JK, Veeravagu A. A descriptive analysis of spinal cord arteriovenous malformations: clinical features, outcomes, and trends in management. World Neurosurg. 2019;131:e579–85.
5. Kim LJ, Spetzler RF. Classification and surgical management of spinal arteriovenous lesions: arteriovenous fistulae and arteriovenous malformations. Neurosurgery. 2006;59(suppl_5):S3–195.
6. Madhugiri VS, Ambekar S, Kumar VR, Sasidharan GM, Nanda A. Spinal aneurysms: clinicoradiological features and management paradigms: a systematic review. J Neurosurg. 2013;19(1):34–48.
7. Massand MG, Wallace RC, Gonzalez LF, Zabramski JM, Spetzler RF. Subarachnoid hemorrhage due to isolated spinal artery aneurysm in four patients. AJNR Am J Neuroradiol. 2005;26(9):2415–2419.
8. Caroscio JT, Brannan T, Budabin M, Huang YP, Yahr MD. Subarachnoid hemorrhage is secondary to spinal arteriovenous malformation and aneurysm: report of a case and review of the literature. Arch Neurol. 1980;37(2):101–3.
9. Jung SC, Song Y, Cho SH, Kim J, Noh SY, Lee SH, Suh DC, et al. Endovascular management of aneurysms associated with spinal arteriovenous malformations. J NeuroInterv Surg. 2018;10(2):198–203.
10. Moore DW, Hunt WE, Zimmerman EJ. Ruptured anterior spinal artery aneurysm: repair via a posterior approach. Neurosurgery. 1982;10(5):626–30.
11. Wisoff HS, Jacobs GB, Rubin RC, Hubbard JH, Wille RL. Arteriovenous malformations of the spinal cord. J Neurosci Nurs. 1979;11(1):16–20.
12. Di Chiro G. Development of spinal cord angiography. Acta Radiol Diagn. 1972;13(P2):767–70.
13. Lasjaunias P, Berenstein A, ter Brugge KG. Surgical neuroangiography. 2, clinical and endovascular treatment aspects in adults: 2. Cerebral arteriovenous shunts, spinal arteriovenous shunts, spinal vascular tumours, technical aspects of endovascular neurosurgery: 155 tables. Springer; 2004.
14. Rengachary SS, Duke DA, Tsai FY, Kragel PJ. Spinal arterial aneurysm: case report. Neurosurgery. 1993;33(1):125–9.
15. Kim HJ, Choi IS. Dissecting aneurysm of the posterior spinal artery: case report and review of the literature. Neurosurgery. 2012;71(3):E749–56.
16. Koc O, Ozbek O, Paksoy Y, Kocaogullari Y. Anterior spinal artery aneurysm presenting with spinal cord compression: MRI and MRI angiographic findings. J Neurol Neurosurg Psychiatry. 2010;81(7):771–2.
17. Yonas H, Patre S, White RJ. Anterior spinal artery aneurysm: case report. J Neurosurg. 1980;53(4):570–3.
18. Geibprasert S, Krings T, Apitzsch J, Reinges MHT, Nolte KW, Hans FJ. Subarachnoid hemorrhage following posterior spinal artery aneurysm: a case report and review of the literature. Interv Neuroradiol. 2010;16(2):183–90.
19. Koçak A, Ateş Ö, Çayli SR, Saraç K. Isolated posterior spinal artery aneurysm. Br J Neurosurg. 2006;20(4):241–4.
20. Berlis A, Scheufler KM, Schmahl C, Rauer S, Götz F, Schumacher M. Solitary spinal artery aneurysms as a rare source of spinal subarachnoid hemorrhage: potential etiology and treatment strategy. Am J Neuroradiol. 2005;26(2):405–10.

21. Baba N, Horiuchi R, Yagi T, Kanemaru K, Yoshioka H, Kinouchi H. Spinal glomus AVM presenting solely with groin pain: illustrative case. J Neurosurg. 2022;3(24):CASE22105.
22. Garcia CA, Dulcey S, Dulcey J. Ruptured aneurysm of the spinal artery of Adamkiewicz during pregnancy. Neurology. 1979;29(3):394.
23. Friedrich H, Hänsel-Friedrich G, Zeumer H. Intramedullary vascular lesions in the high cervical region: transoral and dorsal surgical approach. Two case reports. Neurosurg Rev. 1990;13:65–71.
24. Kemp CM, Feng Z, Aftab M, Reece TB. Preventing spinal cord injury following thoracoabdominal aortic aneurysm repair: the battle to eliminate paraplegia. JTCVS Techniq. 2021;8:11–5.
25. Hill TC, Tanweer O, Thomas C, Engler J, Shapiro M, Becske T, Huang PP. Posterior spinal artery aneurysm presenting with leukocytoclastic vasculitis. J Cerebrovasc Endovasc Neurosurg. 2016;18(1):42–7.
26. Rosenblum B, Oldfield EH, Doppman JL, Di Chiro G. Spinal arteriovenous malformations: a comparison of dural arteriovenous fistulas and intradural AVM's in 81 patients. J Neurosurg. 1987;67(6):795–802.

Surgical Treatment of Spinal Arteriovenous Malformations

16

Guangyu Wang

Abstract

Spinal vascular malformation in children is a rare disease in clinic. At present, there are many disputes about its etiology, clinical features, examination methods, and surgical treatment strategies. With our in-depth understanding of this disease, its pathophysiological process and anatomical classification become more and more clear, which plays a very important role in the diagnosis and treatment of the disease. By studying the literature reports published by scholars in recent years, combined with the summary of their own clinical work, the author clarifies the disease.

Keywords

Surgery · Treatment · Spinal · Arteriovenous malformation

16.1 Background

Spinal vascular malformation in children is a rare lesion, and the lesion has many manifestations. With the in-depth understanding of the disease, its naming and classification are also constantly improving. According to the naming and classification of these diseases, it can help us to better understand its pathophysiological process, so as to formulate a more reasonable treatment plan.

Spinal arteriovenous malformations were first described by Gaupp in 1888. The initial classification was mainly based on pathological features and later adopted anatomical structure criteria. With the deepening of the understanding of these lesions, a lot of improvements and supplements to the classification of these diseases have been put forward. In 2002, Chowdhry and other scholars proposed a classification system based on vascular structure and pathophysiological characteristics of spinal cord vascular malformations.

Spinal vascular malformations may be attributed to tumor lesions (hemangioblastoma and cavernous hemangioma), arteriovenous fistula (AVF), and arteriovenous malformations (AVM). Unrelated to arteriovenous malformations, spinal cord aneurysms caused by blood flow changes and arterial dissection are rare and have not been reported in children.

Spinal arteriovenous fistula is more common in adults and usually occurs in progressive myelopathy [1]. They are divided into epidural, intradural dorsal, and intradural ventral arteriovenous fistulas. Spinal epidural arteriovenous fistula is not common. They are characterized by direct communication between nerve root artery branches and epidural venous plexus (Figs. 16.1, 16.2, and 16.3). The clinical symptoms are mainly related to venous dilatation and space-

G. Wang (✉)
Department of Neurosurgery, Qilu Children's Hospital, Shandong University, Jinan, China

X. Lv (ed.), *Endovascular and Neurovascular Surgery for Spinal Vascular Malformations*,
https://doi.org/10.1007/978-981-97-4661-3_16

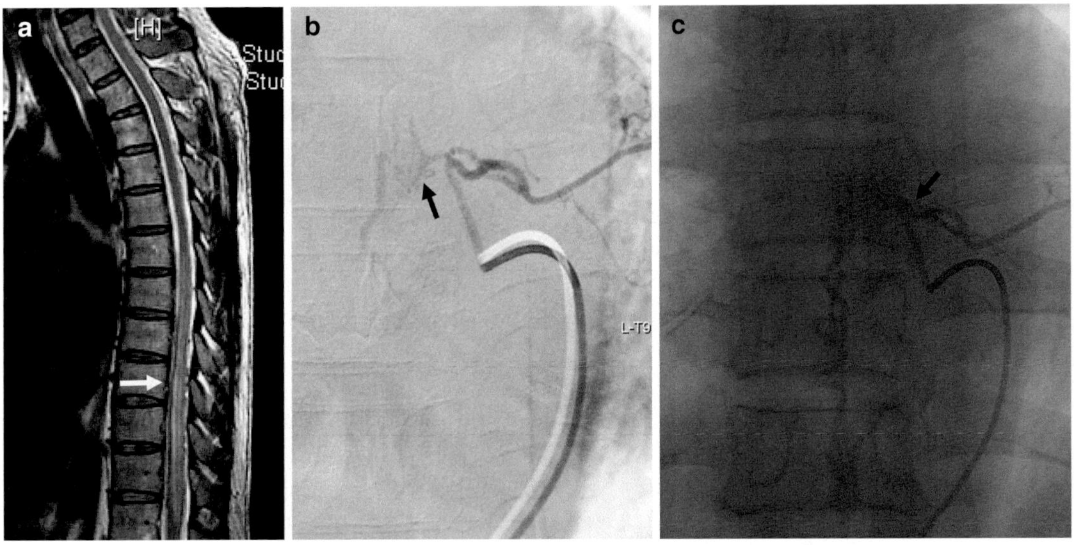

Fig. 16.1 A 47-year-old male patient presented with numbness and pain in both lower limbs for 3 months. (**a**) Thoracolumbar magnetic resonance imaging, sagittal review, revealed spinal cord edema in the thoracolumbar region with multiple flow void signals on the surface of the spinal cord (arrow). (**b**) Left T9 segmental artery angiography revealed a left T9 dural arteriovenous fistula (arrow). (**c**) The non-subtractive image showed that the fistula was located in the intervertebral foramen (arrow)

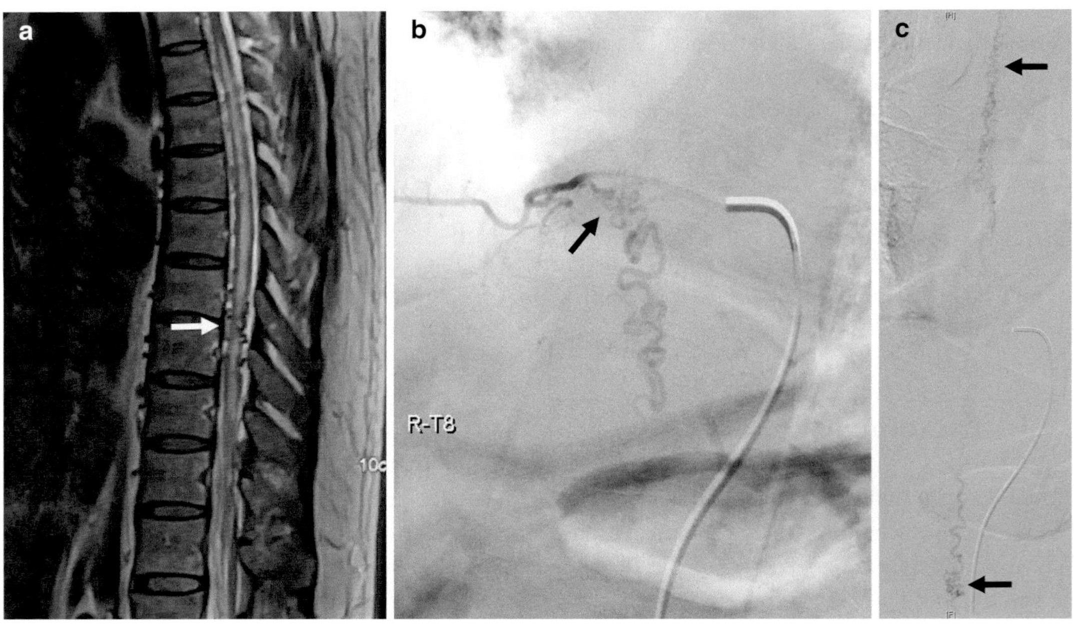

Fig. 16.2 A 44-year-old male patient presented with 2 days of weakness in both lower limbs and bowel movements. (**a**) Thoracic magnetic resonance imaging, sagittal review, revealed spinal cord edema in the thoracic region with multiple flow void signals on the surface of the spinal cord (arrow). (**b**) Right T8 segmental artery angiography revealed a dural arteriovenous fistula (arrow). (**c**) Late phase of angiography showed that the venous drainage affected the entire length of the spinal cord (arrows)

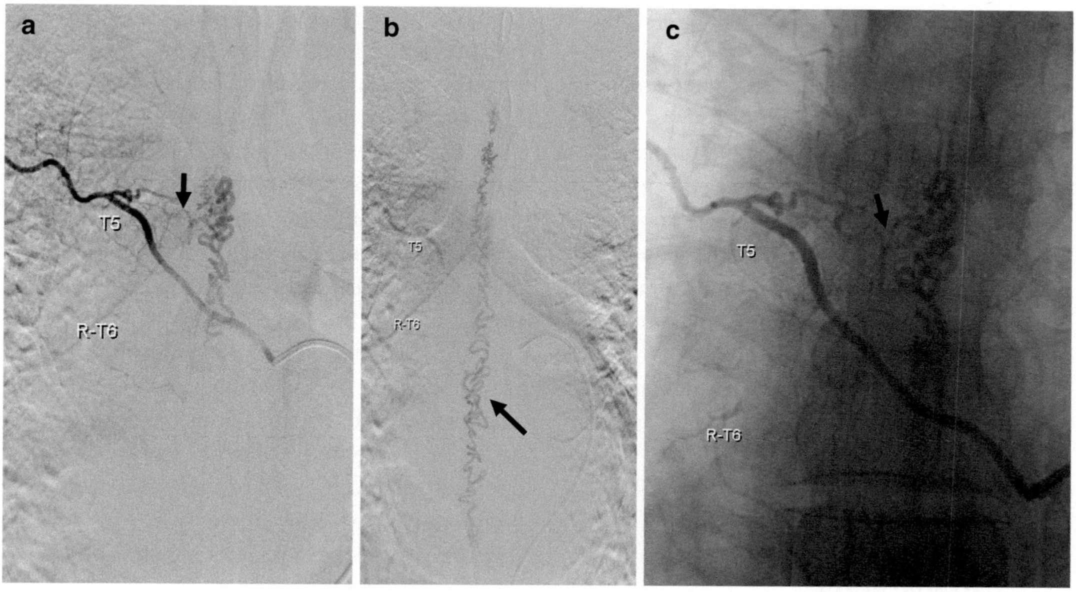

Fig. 16.3 A 49-year-old male patient presented with weakness in both lower limbs for 20 days. (**a**) Right T6 segmental artery angiography revealed a dural arteriovenous fistula (arrow). (**b**) Late phase of angiography showed that the venous drainage affected the entire length of the thoracic spinal cord (arrow). (**c**) The non-subtractive image showed that the fistula was located in the intervertebral foramen (arrow)

occupying effect. These lesions are usually sensitive to endovascular therapy.

The exposure of epidural fistula behind the midline allows direct surgical occlusion and relief of local compression. The entrance point of dural fistula is rarely located in the ventral part of the dural or far from the level of blood supply to the nerve root artery.

Intradural dorsal arteriovenous fistula (AVF) is treated by occlusion of the root pulp artery that supplies blood, because the root pulp artery arterializes the coronary venous plexus when it enters the dural nerve root cuff. These fistulas may be supplied by single or multiple feeding arteries.

The intradural ventral arteriovenous fistula is located on the ventral side of the spinal cord and is supplied by the anterior spinal artery. These lesions are further classified according to the size of the vascular shunt. The increase of arteriovenous fistula size and blood flow can lead to blood theft and spinal cord compression, thus showing more significant clinical symptoms. Although the anterior or anterolateral approach is necessary for full exposure, the posterolateral approach is most suitable for ventrolateral lesions. Embolization has a high risk due to the involvement of the anterior spinal artery, but it is likely to be suitable for large lesions with complex vascular structures and multiple pedicle feeding arteries.

Arteriovenous malformations may be accompanied by acute myelitis, progressive myelopathy, radiculopathy, or pain. They are divided into epidural-intradural, intramedullary, and spinal conic arteriovenous malformations. Epidural-intradural arteriovenous malformations are not common. They were previously described as variant, immature, or type III arteriovenous malformations. Giant lesions are not limited to tissue boundaries but can involve the neural structure, bone, and soft tissue of the involved plane. Multidisciplinary treatment is necessary, and surgery is needed to remove the space-occupying effect of the nerve root and spinal cord.

Although the lesion can be removed completely, it can cause obvious disability. Therefore, the purpose of treatment is to decompress neurons, stabilize locally, and block the blood supply of diseased neurons through multidisciplinary methods.

Intramedullary arteriovenous malformations are composed of feeding arteries, draining veins, and a focus similar to intracranial arteriovenous malformations. They may be supplied by multiple branches of the anterior spinal artery and the posterior spinal artery.

There are typical related aneurysms. The lesions may be concentrated or diffuse.

Although the arteriovenous malformations of the spinal conus are mainly located outside the medulla and on the pia mater and are supplied by the anterior and posterior arteries of the spinal cord, the lesions may have intramedullary components. Surgical resection is the main treatment of spinal arteriovenous malformations, but the long-term effects of reflex therapy and embolization are not clear.

16.2 Surgical Details and Preoperative Preparation

Preoperative imaging examination of spinal cord arteriovenous malformations should include MRI and angiography. Enhanced MRA of the spinal cord may distinguish the feeding arteries of the nerve roots, including the anterior spinal artery and the arteries at the lumbar enlargement. The focus characteristics (concentration or diffusion) of simple intramedullary arteriovenous malformations should be paid attention to. Intramedullary arteriovenous malformations were successfully cured by embolization, but the focus of treatment is still surgical removal of the lesions. For extradural and epidural arteriovenous malformations, we should consider the intradural malformations. The scope of progress and space-occupying effect. Complex and multi-pedicled lesions should be embolized before surgery, especially for the feeding artery in front of the lesion, which complicates surgical removal from the posterolateral pathway. However, this method is likely to be limited by the relationship between the feeding artery and the anterior spinal artery. Preoperative arterial embolization should be carried out under neuroelectrophysiological monitoring, and the induction test is helpful to understand the relationship between the feeding artery and the blood supply of the spinal cord.

Multimodal neuroelectrophysiological monitoring, including somatosensory evoked and motor evoked potentials, and indocyanine green angiography are usually used. Before the appearance of intraoperative indocyanine green angiography, intraoperative arteriography is usually used, and if angiography is needed during the operation, the puncture of the femoral ductus arteriosus should be prepared before the body position. Intraoperative microscopes with high magnification and illumination, straight and curved microscissors, and anti-adhesion bipolar electrocoagulation are essential (Figs. 16.4 and 16.5).

Most arteriovenous malformations are treated with posterior median laminoplasty or posterolateral approach. For ventral intramedullary arteriovenous malformations, anterior or anterolateral approach can be used. X-ray and C-arm fluoroscopy may help to locate, especially for chest lesions. Large area exposure makes the operation of arteriovenous malformations easier. The dura mater is opened from the midline, and its edge is suspended with 4–0 nylon thread, and the absorbable gelatin sponge is placed above the open dura mater to prevent blood flow to the surgical field. After the lesions were fully exposed, indocyanine green angi-

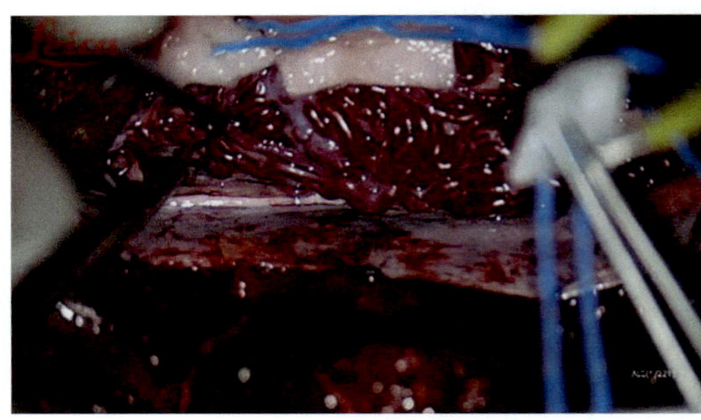

Fig. 16.4 Spinal arteriovenous malformation under microscope

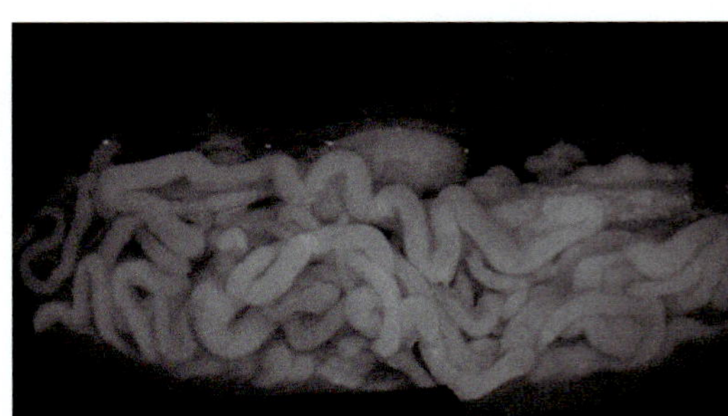

Fig. 16.5 Intraoperative indocyanine green fluorescence imaging of spinal arteriovenous malformation

ography was performed to identify the feeding arteries, draining veins, and perforating vessels. For the concentrated intramedullary lesions affecting the surface of the pia mater, the operation can be completely removed. For intramedullary dilated diffuse lesions, pial meningectomy is often used to block the blood supply and limit the injury to the spinal cord. [2] Then burn the remaining blood vessels on the surface of the pia mater.

The importance of careful sharp separation and extensive use of bipolar coagulation should not be overstated. It is very important to dissect the blood vessels from the pia mater and spinal cord in the process of separating the feeding arteries, especially in the pia mater resection, which can facilitate bipolar electrocoagulation and sharp separation of blood vessels. The failure of complete separation may limit the electrocoagulation around the blood vessels and lead to bleeding during the separation of blood vessels, resulting in blood flow into the spinal cord and increasing the risk of postoperative complications.

Lesions of the conus medullaris are usually characterized by large swollen venous structures, which are usually treated by combined endovascular and posterior median approach microsurgery. Great care should be taken to protect the branches of the anterior and posterior arteries of the spinal cord during the operation, as they may supply blood to the lesions in the spinal cord.

Indocyanine green angiography was used to verify the complete resection and the opening of other channels after resection. Motor evoked potentials were reexamined after resection of the lesions. Carefully stop the bleeding during the operation, and then use 6–0 polypropylene suture to close the dura mater to prevent cerebrospinal fluid leakage.

16.3 Prognosis and Postoperative Management

Postoperative spinal cord angiography is very necessary, and the patient is allowed to sit up on the first day after lying flat for one night. Blood pressure should be strictly controlled 24 hours after operation, and steroids should not be used as routine medication after operation.

For patients with symptoms due to compression, vascular theft, and venous hypertension, we expect a slow and steady functional recovery. The sharp decline of motor function after operation is due to the injury of the anterior spinal artery or lumbar inflated artery during operation. Somatosensory evoked potentials may not change and therefore do not indicate injury. The disappearance of the motor evoked potential response signal is due to the injury of the anterior spinal artery, which usually occurs within a few minutes of the injury, and the signal will not be transmitted back. The acute deterioration of the disease after operation should be vigilant against postoperative bleeding. MR should be performed immediately to determine the lesion, and then surgery is needed to remove the hematoma.

Because of the risk of recurrence, patients should be followed up after operation. Recurrence should be suspected in patients with new neurological deterioration and no improvement in symptoms after treatment.

16.4 Summary

The overall diagnosis and treatment of spinal cord arteriovenous malformations require high clinical work. How to cure the spinal cord arteriovenous malformations without damaging the neurological function is the ultimate pursuit of every clinician. With the continuous improvement of medical technology and examination methods, more and more children get good treatment.

References

1. Spetzler RF, Detwiler PW, Riina HA, Porter RW. Modified classification of spinal cord vascular lesions. J Neurosurg. 2002;96(2 Suppl):145–56.
2. Velat GJ, Chang SW, Abla AA, Albuquerque FC, McDougall CG, Spetzler RF. Microsurgical management of glomus spinal arteriovenous malformations: pial resection technique: clinical article. J Neurosurg Spine. 2012;16(6):523–31.

Intramedullary Spinal Cord Cavernous Malformations: Clinical Features and Surgical Management

17

Rajab Al-Ghanem, Eskandar Yagui, and José Manuel Galicia

Abstract

Cavernous malformations (CMs) are thin dilated capillary-type, sinusoidal low-flow vascular malformations, without intervening neural tissue, which are prone to repeated hemorrhage and growth over time. Intramedullary spinal CMs (ISCMs) constitute a rare pathology, accounting for 5–12% of all intraspinal vascular malformations. Intramedullary spinal cord cavernous malformations tend to be clinically progressive. The incidence of initial intramedullary hemorrhage is estimated to be 2.1% patient/year, increasing to 66% in those with a previous history of hemorrhage. The annual hemorrhage and rehemorrhage rates in children are higher than in adults.

It has become a reasonable consensus on early microsurgical resection, usually within 3 months, as the primary option in symptomatic patients of SCCMs that can provide good outcomes, in spite of the existing potential risk of operative neurological complication. Continuous multimodal intraoperative neurophysiological monitoring (IONM) of somatosensory evoked potentials (SSEP), motor-evoked potentials (MEP), and D-wave recording is essential to reduce the risk of surgery-related deficits by providing real-time feedback about the degree of spinal cord manipulation. An individualized surgical approach to achieve complete resection in carefully selected symptomatic patients is required to prevent further neurological decline from rebleeding.

Keywords

Intramedullary hemorrhage · Natural history Risk factors · Surgical approach · Cavernous malformations of the spinal cord · Cavernous angioma · Vascular disorders

17.1 Introduction

Cavernous malformations (CMs) or cavernous angiomas are low-flow vascular lesions of the central nervous system prone to symptomatic hemorrhage. Cerebral CMs are estimated to be present in approximately 0.5% of the population [1, 2]. Usually, they are characterized by a relatively benign clinical course, staying asymptomatic in many patients. Most lesions are found intracranially within (more than two-thirds of cases) the supratentorial compartment, followed by infratentorial CM where usually the CM will be found in the brainstem. Intramedullary spinal CMs (ISCMs), by contrast, constitute a rare pathology, accounting for 5–12% of all intraspinal vascular malformations [3]. Pediatric

R. Al-Ghanem (✉) · E. Yagui · J. M. Galicia
Department of Neurosurgery, University Hospital of Jaén, Jaén, Spain

X. Lv (ed.), *Endovascular and Neurovascular Surgery for Spinal Vascular Malformations*,
https://doi.org/10.1007/978-981-97-4661-3_17

ISCCMs are much more rare, representing 1% of all intramedullary lesions [4, 5]. Compared with their intracranial counterparts, ISCCMs are more aggressive because the narrow spinal cavity contributes to a low tolerance for space-occupying lesions. With the advent of high-resolution MRI, these lesions are being more commonly detected in the general population, but overall prevalence still remains low. Given their overall rarity, in contrast to cerebral CMs, data on natural history, prognosis, and outcomes following surgical or conservative management are limited for ISCMs and exist mostly in the form of case series and cohort studies.

The location of the ISCM is usually in the cervical and thoracic spinal cord according to the literature, with conus CM or lumbar CM being a very rare entity. Previous literature described thoracic as being the most common (46%) and then cervical (38%), cervicothoracic (8%), and conus being the least common (8%) [4, 5].

Spinal CMs are increasingly being diagnosed by magnetic resonance imaging (MRI) in patients with varying spinal cord-related symptoms or pain syndromes. Spinal CMs can occur along the neuraxis and are predominantly located intramedullary. However, exophytic growth and extradural CMs are reported as well. While there is often gliotic and hemosiderin-stained neural parenchyma around the lesion, there is no normal nervous tissue within the lesion itself, thus facilitating surgical resection.

These lesions pose a strategic neurosurgical dilemma. A small but significant risk of devastating hemorrhage and spinal cord injury exists, but the natural history, which is not yet clearly defined, must be weighed against the risks of surgical treatment. In selected cases, surgical excision reliably prevents progressive neurological decline with acceptable rates of morbidity and mortality.

17.2 Pathogenesis of Cavernous Malformations

Cavernous malformations (CMs) are thin dilated capillary-type, sinusoidal low-flow vascular malformations, without intervening neural tissue, which are prone to repeated hemorrhage and growth over time. Cerebral cavernous malformations (CCMs) occur with a prevalence of about 0.4–0.6% in the general population. About 80% of CCMs are sporadic, solitary, and often closely associated with a developmental venous anomaly, and about 20% of CCMs are familial/syndromic, although estimating risks is complicated by incomplete penetrance and variable presentation even within families. Heterozygous germline loss-of-function mutations can occur in one of three genes (CCM1 or KRIT1, CCM2 or malcaverin, and CCM3 or programmed cell death 10 (PDCD10)) with an autosomal dominant transmission that lead to familial CCM syndrome, causing multifocal lesions throughout the brain and spinal cord. Spinal cord cavernous malformations (SCCMs) are less common than CCMs and have been considered rare. Studies of patients with familial cerebral cavernous malformations suggested a prevalence of spinal cord cavernous malformations of 20–42% [6, 7]. Mabray et al. established the prevalence of the spinal cord cavernous malformations in the familial population CCM1 at around 70% and support the idea that this condition is a progressive systemic disease that affects the entire central nervous system [8].

The functions of these genes continue to be investigated; all are involved in signaling networks responsible for the maintenance of junctional integrity between neighboring vascular endothelial cells. The lesion is histologically identical in association with all genotypes, characterized by grossly dilated vascular spaces (known as "caverns") lined by a single layer of endothelium, lacking mature vessel wall angioarchitecture, and manifesting features of chronic hemorrhage in adjacent neuroglial parenchyma. The gross appearance of the lesion has been likened to a mulberry.

Familial lesions have been shown to harbor biallelic mutations in endothelial cells (ECs) lining the pathological vascular channels. This observation is consistent with a Knudsonian two-hit mechanism that involves a homozygous loss of function in the lesion endothelium, while all cells in the body are heterozygous for the inherited gene. The inherited mutation is an inherited risk, but not sufficient for CCM genesis. It is hypothesized that a "second hit" or somatic mutation is required for malformation development and, consistent with this, a second mutation has been described in cases where somatic tissue is tested.

Lesions surgically resected from sporadic cases lacking inherited germline mutations harbor somatic mutations of the same three *CCM* genes. This indicates identical molecular mechanisms related to *CCM* gene loss of function in both familial and sporadic lesions.

Histologically, identical cavernous angioma lesions arise in the brain after irradiation, which is not surprising in view of the propensity of radiation to cause somatic mutations. Vascular hyperpermeability in the irradiated brain may also play a role, as may radiation-induced hemorrhagic microangiopathy—both described in the spectrum of pathology leading to radionecrosis.

Genetic testing of familial cases that should include direct sequencing and deletion analysis of CCM1–3 results in a mutation detection rate of at least 75% of all cases with multiple CCMs, with approximately 53–65% of cases due to mutations in CCM1, 20% in CCM2, and 10–16% in CCM3. The majority of mutations in CCM1–3 are loss of function mutations including nonsense, frameshift, and splice site, leading to a premature stop codon and an unstable mRNA. Larger deletion and duplications of multiple exons and the entire gene have been recognized.

Clinical severity is highly variable, but CCM1 gene mutations may cause the least severe clinical course, and PDCD10 (CCM3) mutations are associated with more severe disease manifestations. CCM3 mutation carriers have a greater chance of spontaneous mutation, an increased CCM burden, and a younger mean age of presentation, which is often associated with clinical hemorrhage. There is also a significant association with other manifestations including skin CCMs, scoliosis, spinal cord cavernous malformations, cognitive disability, and benign brain tumor including meningioma, vestibular schwannoma, and astrocytoma. Genotype does not entirely explain CCM clinical variability; investigation of possible genetic and environment modifiers is currently underway [6].

Spinal cord cavernous malformations (SCCMs) are less common than CCMs and have been considered rare, with relatively less attention in the CCM literature and most reported cases being sporadic nonfamilial SCCMs. A 2009 report on a single Italian family with familial CCM found SCCMs in 5 of 12 patients (41.7%), 2 of which were discovered clinically and 3 of which were discovered with screening MR imaging (3 of 6 screened patients had SCCMs). An additional 2017 report on 13 patients with familial CCM found upper SCCMs in 3 patients (23.1%).

Findings from in vitro and in vivo studies may provide insight into CCM pathogenesis and indicate molecular mechanisms as potential therapeutic targets. These studies report dysregulated cellular pathways shared between CCM, cardiovascular diseases, and cancer. CCM1, CCM2, and CCM3 are components of the CCM complex, while CCM3 is peculiarly included into the STRIPAK (striatin-interacting phosphatase and kinase) complex. Loss of CCM proteins is associated with a disruption of such complexes and activates signaling pathways in brain endothelial cells, eventually leading to lesion formation. Blocking these dysregulated pathways with targeted inhibitors has proven therapeutic efficacy in animal models and requires further investigation. Moreover, several pathologic features of CCM overlap with those observed in cardiovascular diseases and cancer, namely, autophagy, angiogenesis, inflammation, and oxidative stress. These commonalities support the feasibility of drug repurposing (statins, atorvastatin). In this perspective, two pioneering and ongoing clinical trials are evaluating the efficacy of statins to control CCM progression [2, 9].

17.3 Pathology

The caverns resemble well-circumscribed, multilobulated, mulberry-like structures (Fig. 17.3C). CM is similar for morphology to a "cauliflower," with protrusions extending variably into the surrounding parenchyma with resultant "pockets" of gliotic, but normal, cord in between the protrusions of the CM.

Histologically, cavernous malformations of the spine cord are identical to those of the brain [6]. Grossly, they have a mulberry-like appearance, are stained with hemosiderin, and contain various blood products that may be thrombosed or in liquid form. Most lesions are associated with cryptic venous malformations that are identified intraoperatively. Calcifications within spinal CMs are rare. Microscopically, they are composed of dilated thin-walled sinusoidal vascular channels that contain endothelial cells and an adventitial layer, but they are devoid of a medial layer. The surrounding tissue can be stained with hemosiderin and is gliotic in reaction to the blood products. The absence of intervening neural tissue and the presence of surrounding gliosis make CMs, even in eloquent areas such as the spinal cord, more amenable to resection. Due to space-occupying growth, recurrent micro-bleeding or significant hemorrhage (in respect of the available space) spinal CMs can lead to severe neurological deteriorations, such as progressive myelopathy and right up to paraplegia, unlike their intracranial counterparts. Based on histological findings, it has been suggested that repetitive hemorrhage or thrombosis within ICs is responsible for gradual enlargement leading to stepwise deterioration. These episodes repeat over months or even years [10].

17.4 Epidemiology and Natural History

Cavernous malformations can cause devastating neurological injury secondary to acute overt hemorrhage events, repetitive episodes of intralesional microhemorrhages, and mass effects, especially in the spinal cord. Optimal management of ISCCMs requires a comprehensive understanding of the natural history. Cavernous malformations (CMs) constitute 5–10% of the vascular malformations that occur in the CNS and mostly occupy the intracranial compartment. Abundant data with large cohorts estimating the natural course of cavernous malformations of the brain exist. They describe a rather benign course of the disease depending on CCM location and occurrence of intracerebral hemorrhage (ICH), which is estimated to be around 20% over 5 years. Unfortunately, this is not the case for ISCCMs, in which an intramedullary hemorrhage (IMH) is often associated with severe neurological deficits such as paraplegia. Compared with their intracranial counterparts, ISCCMs are more aggressive because the narrow spinal cavity contributes to a low tolerance for space-occupying lesions [11].

The initial onset of symptoms of CMs is usually between the third and fourth decades of life. The mean patient age was 39.1 years (range 2–80 years). The male-to-female ratio was 1.1:1. The spinal level of the cavernous malformation was cervical in 240 (38%) patients, cervicothoracic in 15 (2.4%), thoracic in 349 (55.2%), thoracolumbar in 4 (0.6%), lumbar in 13 (2.1%), and conus medullaris in 11 (1.7%) [12].

The prevalence of cavernous ISCCM is believed to be underestimated, and large epidemiological studies are missing compared with cerebral cavernous malformations (CCMs).

Notably, clinical trials investigating patients with ISCCMs and risk factors leading to IMH are rare and usually limited to small patient cohorts, short follow-up periods, and mainly surgical outcome. Additionally, because it is believed that cavernous SCMs have a high rate of bleeding, a correct estimation of IMH and rehemorrhage during follow up, as well the neurological impact after such events, could thoroughly affect current treatment strategies.

Spinal cord cavernous malformations (SCCMs) are uncommon spinal cord lesions, comprising 5% of intramedullary lesions and 5–12% of all spinal vascular malformations. However, a recent multicenter study from Japan has reported that among the 1033 intramedullary spinal cord tumor cases, 160 were cavernous malformations, i.e., surgical removal of ISCCMs was performed in 15.4% of total intramedullary tumor surgeries [13].

According to previous studies, the annual risk of first hemorrhage varies from 1.7% to 10% per year [11]. Such different values might be attributed to the variable definitions of hemorrhage across the literature. A meta-analysis estimated that the rate of hemorrhage was approximately

2.1% per year; however, the risk of rebleeding will increase up to 66% [14]. The 5-year cumulative hemorrhage risk was calculated to be 35.1–41.3%, and the risk of recurrent hemorrhage for patients with IMH at presentation was 55.69% [11, 15]. Moreover, prior hemorrhage and pediatric patients were independent predictors of subsequent hemorrhage, and subsequent hemorrhage events were independent risk factors for worsening of neurological function in the long-term follow-up. Outcomes were better for those who underwent resection than for those who underwent conservative management for ISCCMs, where 11.3% of cases in conservative management presented exacerbation of neurological function suggesting the natural history of SCCMs totally seems to be progressive deterioration over time. It has been reported that 50% of untreated patients with spinal vascular malformations presenting any functional impairment in the lower limbs at follow-up finally developed severe locomotor disability within 3 years after the onset of weakness.

According to Ren J. et al., the annual bleeding risk and rebleeding risk of ISCCMs were higher in affected children than in affected adults [4]. The annual hemorrhagic risk in pediatric patients was 8.2% per patient/year.

After the initial hemorrhage events, the annual overt rehemorrhage risk increased to 30.7% per patient/year. In adult patients, the respective rates were 2.8% and 7.4% [4].

17.5 Clinical Presentation

The initial onset of symptoms of CMs is usually between the third and fourth decades of life [12]. Clinically, the manifestation of ICs is highly variable and nonspecific. Patients have a varied presentation ranging from asymptomatic with incidentally detected lesions to acute onset, acute on chronic, and chronic progressive myelopathy. On account of the nonspecific symptomatology, the median duration of symptoms is relatively long-lasting, typically for 29 months preceding the final diagnosis. Most patients suffer from sensory and motor deficits. These deficits affect about two-thirds of individuals with ISCCMs. Intramedullary cavernomas may manifest by variable sensory deficits such as radicular and central pain, hyperesthesia or dysesthesia, paresthesia (even episodic), thermosensory deficit, allodynia, central neuropathic itch, and rarely hypothermia of extremities. Motor deficit usually develops below the level of IC; nevertheless, curious ascending flaccid paraplegia over several weeks has been also reported. Autonomic disorders are seen less frequently, occurring in approximately one-third of patients [16–20]. Interestingly, Liang et al. diagnosed sphincter dysfunction in 68 patients (71%) out of their 96 patients with IC [21]. A relatively large retrospective meta-analysis of 632 patients by Badhiwala et al. showed that only the minority of patients have no symptoms (1%) or present with respiratory distress (0.5%) [12].

The clinical course prior to presentation was classified into five types as described by Ogilvy et al. [10, 22]: (1) type A, discrete episodes of neurological deterioration with varying degrees of recovery between episodes; (2) type B, slow progression of neurological decline; (3) type C, acute onset of symptoms with rapid decline; (4) type D, acute onset of mild symptoms with subsequent gradual decline lasting weeks to months; and (5) type E, asymptomatic incidentally detected lesions.

The variable clinical course follows three different patterns—acute, stepwise, and slow progressive neurological deterioration. It is supposed that acute neurological decline is caused by bleeding into the cord parenchyma or into the wall of the cavernoma itself. Patients with acute intramedullary hemorrhage present with sudden onset with a rapid decline over hours even days [20, 21].

The next possible pathophysiological mechanism of acute neurological worsening is thrombosis of hyalinized vascular channels. Rarely, intramedullary cavernous malformation is associated with subarachnoid hemorrhage presenting with prominent lower or upper back pain. At last, there is the course of slow progressive neurological decline without improvement. This is supposed to be due to the hyalinization and thickening of vascular walls or gradual thrombosis. McCormick et al. proposed that neurotoxicity of hemosiderin deposits and compromised surrounding microcirculation may be another pathophysiological mechanism responsible for this course [23].

Acute and stepwise neurological decline was tracked in 45% and slow progressive in 55% of patients. It has been reported that the onset of symptoms may be associated with minor trauma, strenuous activity, or pregnancy. A modified McCormick scale, Frankel scale, or ASIA score is usually used for objective pre- and postoperative scoring of patient's clinical status [24–26].

17.6 Diagnosis

Cavernous malformations must remain in the differential diagnosis of intradural intramedullary lesions; while angiographically occult, these are increasingly recognized now due to the widespread availability of MRI. The imaging characteristics of CMs in the brain and spinal cord are nearly pathognomonic. If a patient's age, history, and presentation are compatible, an intramedullary CM can be diagnosed on magnetic resonance (MR) images with confidence, which can facilitate subsequent management decisions. Hemorrhage, widening of the spine, and rarely calcification can be nonspecifically appreciated on computed tomography (CT) scans. Due to its low blood flow feature, intramedullary cavernous malformations are usually occult with digital subtraction angiography. MRI remains the gold standard imaging modality [27–29].

On MRI, cavernous malformations are typically described as multilobulated, heterogeneous lesions with features of hemorrhage, including a "popcorn" appearance, T2-weighted (T2w) hypointense hemosiderin rim, and internal blood-fluid levels. On T1- and T2-weighted MR images, the characteristic lesion appears heterogeneous because of blood products of various ages. Hemosiderin deposition creates a typical rim of low-intensity signal on T1- and T2-weighted MR images (Fig. 17.3a). Gadolinium enhancement (Fig. 17.2a and b) is seldom present unless the lesion is associated with a resolving intramedullary hematoma. On gradient-echo sequences, the presence of hemosiderin within the lesion results in the artifact of "blooming." Based on the signal characteristics, SCMs were also classified according to Zabramski's criteria previously described for CCMs [22]. Thus, a SCM was considered type I (subacute hemorrhage) if it was hyperintense on T1w and hypo−/hyperintense on T2w with an incomplete or absent T2w hypointense rim. It was considered type II ("classic") if it was heterogeneous on both T1w and T2w with complete/near-complete T2w hypointense rim. It was considered type III (chronic hemorrhage) if it was isointense/hypointense on T1w and T2w with varying extent of T2w hypointense rim. It was considered type IV (punctate hemorrhage) if it was not well seen on T1w and T2w but showed prominent blooming on gradient echo images. SCMs were considered unclassifiable if they did not fit into any of these types. According to Panda et al., the classically described popcorn morphology and internal blood-fluid levels were seen in a minority of SCMs, 22% and 4%, respectively. A T2w hypointense rim was seen in 37%. Meanwhile, adjacent intramedullary hemorrhage was a common imaging feature, observed in 58%, often eccentric and bidirectional, a potential key clue [28].

The presence of flow voids on MR images, however, may warrant spinal angiography to rule out the presence of an associated high-flow vascular lesion such as an arteriovenous malformation.

17.7 Treatment

17.7.1 Surgical Resection: Indications, Timing, and Risks

Decision-making with spinal cord cavernous malformations (SCCMs) should be based on comprehensive knowledge of the natural history of this pathology and expected outcome after surgical treatment. Currently, complete surgical removal of intramedullary cavernous malformations remains the only curative treatment option in symptomatic patients with intramedullary cavernomas. Prolonged observation of symptomatic lesions is likely to lead to progressive clinical decline with resulting poorer patient outcomes.

The major aim of surgical treatment is total excision of the tumor and prevention of postoperative deterioration of motor paresis, especially ambulatory ability. Meticulous presurgical planning is essential to achieve the best possible result. And more advanced surgical techniques including neuromonitoring, which assist complete and safe resection, can provide more aggressive surgical indication and early surgical timing. Recent introduction of intraoperative neurophysiological monitoring (IONM) has contributed to prevention of postoperative neurological deterioration [30].

Contrary to arteriovenous malformations, which are characterized by arterial feeders and draining veins of large caliber, cavernomas cannot be treated by embolization, and to our knowledge, there are no data in the literature on treatment of intramedullary cavernous malformations by radiosurgery.

The appropriate therapy strategy (conservative or surgical) for those with mild symptoms or asymptomatic incidentally diagnosed patients remains controversial [25, 31].

An intramedullary spinal cord tumor is relatively rare, but the increasing use of MRI is resulting in incidental detection of these tumors in asymptomatic patients, thus increasing the number of cases. In a study comparing outcomes of conservative and surgically treated patients, 23 of 27 patients in the conservative group reported satisfying results, but 1 patient died of respiratory failure that resulted from lesion bleeding [32]. In Li et al. series, most of the patients showed symptoms of at least mild dysesthesia or numbness. Currently, there are insufficient data to choose therapy strategies for asymptomatic SCM.

Meta-analysis reports indicate favorable neurologic outcomes for patients who underwent surgery compared with those who underwent clinical observation. Recent study data showed that the surgical management gives a marginal superiority over clinical observation in patients with an acute onset of neurologic deterioration. In the long term, surgical treatment resulted in an improved neurological status in 36.9% of the patients; in 55.8%, it remained stable; and in 7.3%, it deteriorated compared to the preoperative state. In the conservative cohort, 21.7% improved, 69.6% remained stable, and 8.7% deteriorated [33].

Early surgery is generally recommended for symptomatic SCCMs, and reports have indicated the surgical timing within 3 months provides an improved outcome [12, 33–35].

On the other hand, emergent operation includes some problems because conditions of the spinal cord are not ordinarily suitable for intramedullary perilesional dissection especially in acute phase after hemorrhage. Zevgaridis et al. [36] recommended that 4–6 weeks after hemorrhage seems to be the optimal timing if lesion is in critical areas. In this phase, lesion removal becomes easier by a glial scar formation and hematomas in resolution with minimal damage to the spinal cord.

Imagama et al. [37] also suggested SCCM resection after hemorrhage should be conducted after primary and secondary damage to the spinal cord are reduced as much as possible. They concluded surgery may be postponed after maximum motor recovery if patients have preoperative paresis.

In a recent study, predictors of unfavorable outcome were multiple bleeding events, surgery >3 months after intramedullary hemorrhage, ventral localization of the cavernoma in the ventral part of the spinal cord and incomplete SCM resection, and incomplete resection [35]. Patients with deep-seated lesions might be at higher risk for postoperative deficits, and the indication for surgery should be carefully considered.

17.7.2 Intraoperative Neurophysiological Monitoring (IONM)

The inherent risk for neurological deterioration in intramedullary SCCM surgery demands for the utilization of IONM modalities. Due to their different biology, the resection of vascular lesions, like ISCCM or hemangioblastomas, has to be considered separately from resection of infiltrating intramedullary tumor lesions. Compared to infiltrating lesions, where complete resection is sometimes not possible, ISCCMs often show a clear dissection plane [13]. Moreover, resection of ISCCM should aim for complete removal whenever possible, as incomplete removal does not appear to eliminate the risk of rebleeding. Microsurgical tumor resection should be performed under ultrasound guidance and continuous multimodal IONM of somatosensory-evoked potentials (SSEP), motor-evoked potentials (MEP), and D-wave recording. Recording from segmental target muscles for all relevant myotomes simultaneously ensured that all pertinent motor tracts/fibers were monitored [38, 39].

In case of MEP deterioration, warnings were issued and—if possible—stimulation intensity increased.

After patient positioning, baseline recordings of SSEP and MEP are obtained. SSEP and MEP were continuously recorded in an alternating fashion throughout surgery.

Electrophysiological data were continuously analyzed by a neurophysiologist trained in IONM.

All procedures were performed with total intravenous anesthesia, avoiding the application of muscle relaxants despite for intubation purposes.

Any reduction of SSEP amplitude and/or an increase of SSEP latency as well as decrement in MEP amplitude, especially during or immediately after surgical manipulation, should be immediately issued to the surgical team and checked for relevance excluding technical (e.g., dislocation of electrodes, technical artifact) and anesthesiologic (e.g., lowering of blood pressure or body temperature, change of intravenous anesthesia management, or addition of volatile anesthetics) causes and temporary surgical reasons (e.g., irrigation with cold saline solution). In circumstances of IONM changes, the most recent surgical steps were reconsidered, and immediate corrective actions were stepwise initiated, i.e., modification of the surgical technique with temporary halted resection, reduction of traction on the tumor or surrounding tissue, irrigation with warm saline solution, application of high-dose dexamethasone, and/or continuation of resection at distant sites. The corrective measures are easily recalled by the acronym TIP (time, irrigation, pressure/papaverine) [38].

D-wave monitoring improves monitoring of the corticospinal tract during spinal cord surgery and has proven to be the best surrogate for long-term outcome [39].

Rather than predicting a neurological deficit, IONM should be aimed to warn the surgeon of an impending neurological deficit, which can be aided by surrogacy analysis that takes reversible IONM changes into account and evaluates their effect on clinical outcome. Termination of resection might be considered if corrective maneuvers are not followed by recovery of MEP and further MEP deterioration occurs during careful resumption of resection outbalancing gains and risks of a subtotal resection versus a potentially severe and permanent postoperative deficit. The operation was interrupted, and the operative field is filled with warm saline if a 70% decrease in amplitude was detected as an alarm point of spinal cord damage. The operation could be resumed when the waveform recovered.

17.7.3 Surgical Approaches

A thorough understanding of the spinal cord microanatomy is essential for the surgeons to accomplish successful surgery. As neurosurgeons, we should train in microsurgical techniques so that we can remove tumors without damaging the spinal cord function when there is a surgical dissection plane.

Differences in the locations of ISCCMs and their preoperative symptoms support the importance of taking an individualized surgical approach. Surgical approaches have to be planned and performed on a case-by-case basis after considering the proximity of the ISCCM to the pial surface, its location in the horizontal plane, and preoperative neurological symptoms.

The spinal cord is a highly eloquent tissue similar to that of the brainstem, where only a subtle hemorrhage may lead to significant neurological decline.

As there are multiple surgical approaches available, the neurosurgeon should pick out the most appropriate one in advance of the surgery. Intramedullary cavernous malformations may be located superficially or deep-seated, anteriorly, laterally, or posteriorly. Notwithstanding the variety of approaches to the spinal cord, the posterior approach is the most frequently elected [29, 40, 41].

It is of great advantage that the posterior approach provides extensive exposure of the spinal cord, it is relatively safe, and furthermore, it is an approach which all neurosurgeons are familiar with. Nevertheless, posterior approach cannot be used for every. Especially in the case of ventrally or ventrolaterally located intramedullary cavernous malformation, the posterior approach would lead to extensive myelotomy or stretch of the spinal cord while rotated. In such cases, other surgical routes should be also considered: an anterior, anterolateral, transthoracic, or posterolateral approach. These approaches are technically advanced, providing a decreased exposure of the operating field, which is limiting during all stages of the procedure including watertight suture of the dura.

Based on this anatomical fact, the use of a two-point method is advocated to find the safest entry point, along with careful microsurgical resection under high magnification. The two-point method is using a line drawn on an axial MRI scan connecting the center of intramedullary cavernous malformation with the most superficial part of the IC in regard to the pial surface or the non-eloquent entry zone. There are three recommended non-eloquent entry zones in the spinal cord—dorsal root entry zone (DREZ), dorsal median sulcus, and lateral entry zone. The lateral entry zone is located between the ventral and dorsal nerve roots. Since there is a ballooning effect due to hemosiderin deposits, T2-weighted images tend to overstate the real lesion, and therefore, the T1-weighted sequence is more appropriate for estimation of the relation between IMCMs and pial surface. For the majority of intramedullary cavernomas, a posterior approach is the most suitable. For ventrolateral lesions approached through a posterior laminectomy, it is important to avoid excessive “twisting” of the cord during exposure, which may compromise flow through the delicate arterial network. Even if the CM comes close to the lateral portion of the spinal cord, simple division of the dentate ligament allows the small additional degree of gentle cord rotation to afford better exposure. In case of a purely intramedullary CM, intraoperative ultrasound imaging is a reliable method to confirm the localization of the lesion.

There are three possibilities for bone removal—laminectomy, laminoplasty, and hemilaminectomy.

Several authors have reported progressive spinal deformity following laminectomy and laminoplasty.

The locations of the lesions were identified by the preoperative MRI and intraoperative ultrasound imaging, which were very useful for the deep lesions. For superficial lesions, myelotomy was performed through the abnormal surface. Approaches across the safe entry zone (i.e., trans-safe entry zone) were used for embedded lesions. For dorsally or centrally located deep lesions, a traditional posterior midline myelotomy was performed through the dorsal median sulcus. For ventrolaterally located deep lesions, a new surgical approach called the ADREZotomy (anterior to dorsal root entry zone) has been recently described as a novel safe corridor [40]. Lateral myelotomy between the ventral and dorsal nerve roots and dorsal root entry zone myelotomy (DREZotomy, equivalent to the posterolateral sulcus approach) were performed only in select patients due to the relatively high risk of worsened neurological conditions (Fig. 17.1).

As mentioned above, the spinal cord is a highly eloquent tissue, and the surrounding hemosiderin-stained tissue should not be resected. Surgical resection of intramedullary CMs can be performed safely using a meticulous microsurgical technique [24]. These lesions do not usually bleed during resection when manipulation of cord tissue is minimized and resection is performed in the correct layer. If an associated venous malformation is observed, it should be preserved because it provides venous drainage to normal spinal cord tissue [42]. Coagulation or

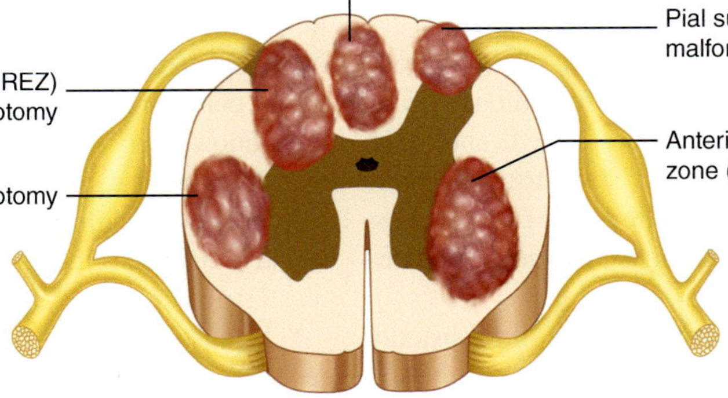

Fig. 17.1 An illustration of the spinal cord demonstrating the main myelotomies used for access to spinal cord cavernous malformations (CMs) [29, 40]. Because spinal CMs are typically located posteriorly in the midline, posterolaterally, or laterally within the spinal cord, myelotomies are made in the posterior midline, at the dorsal root entry zone, or laterally between the ventral and dorsal nerve roots, utilizing the superficial discoloration of the hemorrhage to enter the cord substance, dentate detethering and cord rotation to access a ventral lesion, and the goal of nidus localization in a multisegment spinal cord hemorrhage. Arrows show the approach to posterior or posterolateral lesions through the dorsal median sulcus (between the left and right dorsal columns) or the dorsal root entry zone, respectively. For laterally located lesions, additional bony removal and gentle retraction of the spinal cord with the dentate ligament can provide access to the lateral aspect of the cord for a myelotomy midway between the ventral and dorsal nerve roots, on the ventral side of the dentate ligament. The anterior to dorsal root entry zone (ADREZ) myelotomy adds a safe corridor to surgical approaches for ventrolateral deep lesions

accidental injury of the vein may result in infarction and edema, leaving the patient with significant neurological deficits. Surrounding hemosiderin-stained tissue should not be resected, as this significantly raises the risk of postoperative neurological dysfunction and has no discernible benefit for the patient. Identification and preservation of the gliotic plane appears important in order to minimize neurological morbidity; the use of neurophysiologic monitoring and intraoperative ultrasound can facilitate removal.

Besides postoperative worsening due to the simple manipulation of the cord, other short-term complications include cerebrospinal fluid leak and infection, while long-term complications include spinal cord tethering, vertebral canal stenosis, and kyphotic deformity. In order to prevent postsurgical tethered cord syndrome, we feel it is important to preserve the arachnoid membrane (Fig. 17.3d) and reapproximate it using dedicated sutures in the closure phase. Some surgeons recommend reapproximating with micro-sutures also the pial edges after resection of the lesion.

In cavernous malformations, we could expect dissecting margins between the lesions and the normal spinal cord, making complete resection a reasonable approach. If there is no plane, making the difficult decision to discontinue the surgical resection is crucial. Currently, spinal cord monitoring is mandatory when performing intramedullary tumor surgery. Sensory deficits and transient worsening of preoperative symptoms can be observed in the postoperative period, and patients must be prepared for a variable period of postsurgical inpatient rehabilitation [42].

17.7.4 Illustrative Cases

Case 1

A 47-year-old male. Acute clinical course with paraparesis. Intramedullary cavernous malformation of the conus with subacute evolving hematoma. A complete excision was achieved. At 5 years' follow-up, the patient holds improvement (Fig. 17.2).

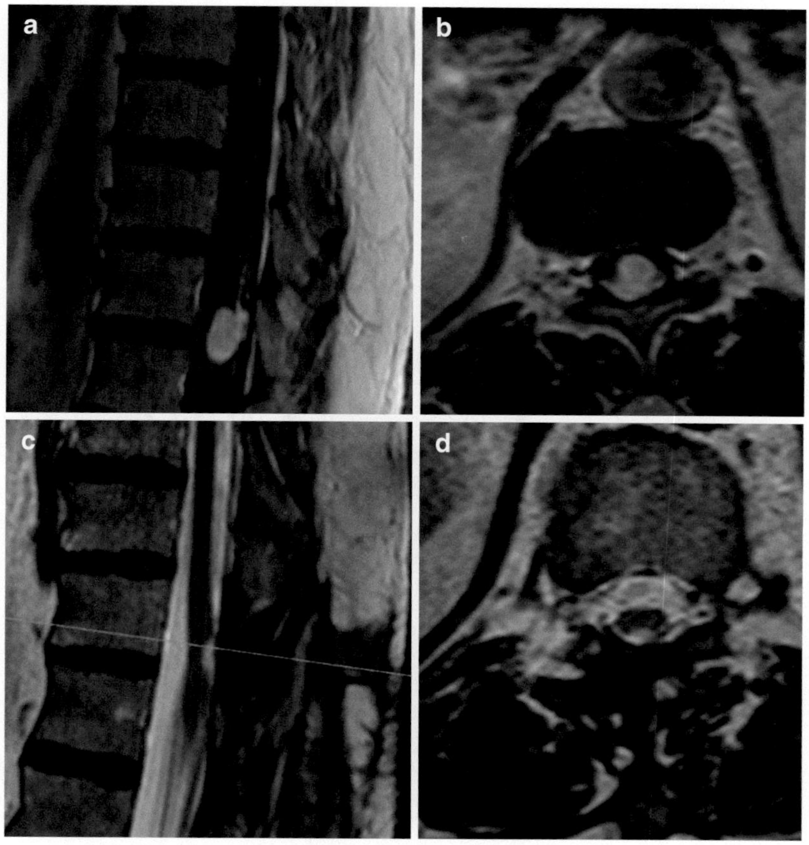

Fig. 17.2 Case 1. (**a**) Sagittal and (**b**) axial T1w contrast-enhanced MRI of evolving conus medullaris hematoma. (**c**) Sagittal and (**d**) axial T1w MRI at 5 years' follow-up after complete excision of the intramedullary cavernous malformation

Case 2

A 51-year-old female. At initial conservative follow-up, the patient had progressive clinical course, with severe burning pain and motor and sensory deficits. Stepwise deterioration and gait instability followed. Complete excision was achieved via lateral myelotomy. After surgical excision of the SCCM, the patient experienced neurological improvement and pain remission (Fig. 17.3).

17.7.5 Outcomes

Recent study data show improved outcomes [24, 32, 34, 35]. The main reason may be related to the progress of neurosurgery, such as advanced minimally invasive surgical techniques, microneurosurgical skills, and the intraoperative neurophysiological monitoring (e.g., SSEP and MEP) in spinal cord operation, which assist complete and safe excision can provide more aggressive surgical indication and early surgical timing enables less surgical injury.

According to current knowledge, the final postoperative outcome is dependent on prehospital symptoms and preoperative clinical status, MR findings, and the chosen therapeutic option. It is claimed that the length of symptoms is an important factor predicting postsurgical recovery. Patients having symptoms of less than 3 months were found to have better postsurgical outcomes. Zevgaridis et al. [36] reported improvement in 76% of patients with symptom duration less than 3 years and only in 52% of patients with longer-lasting symptomatology.

Similarly, patients with acute or stepwise clinical course are prone to benefit more significantly from surgery when compared to those with progressive neurological decline. It is a general

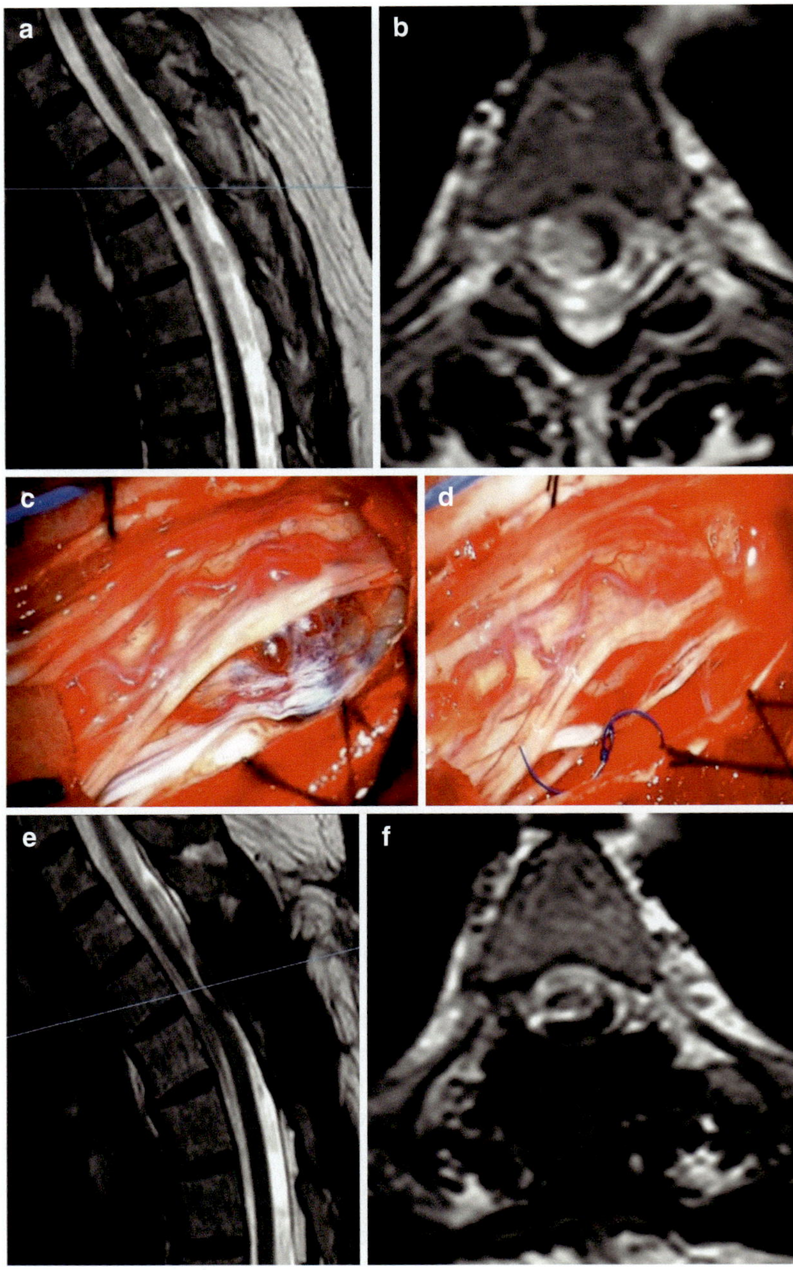

Fig. 17.3 Case 2. (**a**) Sagittal and (**b**) axial T2w MRI of thoracic intramedullary cavernous malformations. Hemosiderin rim may be appreciated. (**c**) and (**d**) Intramedullary cavernoma mulberry-like appearance and arachnoidal layer reapproximation. (**e**) Sagittal and (**f**) axial MRI at 1-year follow-up

agreement that patients with motor deficits have the highest possibility of postsurgical improvement reaching up to 86%. Interestingly, several studies pointed out that sensory deficit, pain (radicular or central), and bladder dysfunction often do not favor a full recovery following the surgery. It has been repeatedly claimed that those presenting with a purely sensory deficit are associated with a slower and less complete recovery.

Park et al. [43] performed total removal of IC in 14 patients and reported that only 7% of patients with preoperative sensory deficit recovered completely by the final postoperative follow-up (compared to a 46% rate of complete recovery in a group of patients with the preoperative motor deficit). Currently, there are ambiguous data regarding relief of pain following the surgery. Kharkar et al. [44] operated on four patients with both pain and weakness. They detected complete pain resolution in one patient only, and the others had limited or no improvement. In a series of 23 patients presenting with pain by Kim et al., 78% had improvement of pain immediately following the surgery, but only 52% reported pain relief lasting over a year. On the contrary, Deutsch et al. [20] surgically treated five patients with predominant complaints about pain. According to their results, all patients had some degree of pain resolution. Kivelev et al. [3] reported a 90% rate of radicular pain relief after surgical removal. Only one patient (10%) developed permanent painful allodynia in her hand. Data about the recovery of bladder function are scarce and heterogeneous.

Several studies have reported improvement of sphincter function following surgery. On the other hand, Kivelev et al. [3] reported no significant improvement of bladder dysfunction in any of five patients undergoing intramedullary CM resection.

As previously mentioned, asymptomatic patients are diagnosed rarely (1%), and data about their natural course are limited. Goyal et al. [22] treated 85 patients, initial conservative management was offered to 64 patients, and 16 patients incurred a hemorrhage on follow-up, leading to an annual hemorrhage rate of 5.5%, which is on the higher end of the spectrum of hemorrhage rates reported in the literature, ranging from 1.4% to 6.8%. While 64 patients were managed conservatively following initial presentation, 21 underwent immediate surgical resection. There were 16 patients (25%) who experienced a hemorrhage on follow-up, 11 (69%) of whom subsequently underwent surgical resection, bringing the total number of patients treated surgically to 32. Symptomatic patients and those with a prior history of hemorrhage had significantly higher annual hemorrhage rates, 9.5% and 9.7%, respectively. In contrast, the annual risk for hemorrhage was lower for the 22 asymptomatic patients with lesions detected incidentally (0.8%). Nowadays, watchful follow-up is the standard proposed course of action for asymptomatic patients, and some authors recommend operating on asymptomatic patients with proven growth in time.

Surgery is generally accepted as the primary treatment option and still the only curative treatment [26, 45–47]. Gross total resection is the most important factor in eliminating the risk of a new hemorrhage in the future. It is achieved in 94% [12]. The transient worsening of patients immediately following the surgery is seen in 24–50%, and the majority resolves during the first 3 months. Long-term clinical worsening is seen in about 12% of patients after intramedullary CM removal.

In a meta-analysis of 396 patients, most of the patients (66.6%) underwent microsurgical resection, and only 33.4% underwent conservative management, as 41.1% and 19.4%, respectively, presented with hemorrhage, reflecting the general practice among neurosurgeons of microsurgical management of these lesions when patients are symptomatic [31].

Our series show similar results to the published data. Retrospective data analysis was performed in 17 patients with histologically diagnosed intramedullary cavernous malformations. All patients were treated with laminectomy and microsurgical resection of the malformations.

There were nine males and eight females (mean age 43 years) harboring symptomatic intramedullary cavernous malformations. The most common neurological deficits were sensory (76%), followed by a motor (65%) and less commonly bladder dysfunction (35%). Pain was present in 53%. Most frequently, patients presented with acute (47%), fewer with slow progressive (35%), and least frequently with stepwise neurological decline (23%). The annual retrospective hemorrhage rate was 2.7% per patient/year. All cavernous malformations were completely resected under neurophysiological monitoring with somatosensory and motor evoked potentials. Nine of 17 patients (65%) experienced the improvement of the neurological state; in 6 (35%), clinical features remained unchanged; and 2 patients (12%) deteriorated during the follow-up period. There was a transient worsening of preoperative (especially sensory) symptoms immediately following the surgery in two patients (18%), and all resolves during the first 3 months requiring a variable period of postsurgical inpatient rehabilitation that may be necessary. The most frequent complication was CSF fistula (12%).

17.8 Discussion

To date, the available data for patients with SCCM are still insufficient due to the low incidence of SCCMs. The current debate focuses on two points: the natural history of SCCMs and conservative vs. surgical management. Bleeding rates of ISCCM are believed to be high and can result in considerable neurological impairment due to the rather small space of the spinal cavity and the high number of functional fiber tracts; hemorrhage-associated functional impairment is more frequent in spinal lesions than in brain lesions, which may simultaneously imply that "silent" hemorrhages are less frequent. Regarding SCCM treatment, an increasing number of studies do exist. However, only a paucity of studies have tried to address the impact of hemorrhagic events in the spine, making appropriate treatment guidelines difficult. In addition, the guidelines that exist are usually limited to observational studies, meta-analyses, small cohorts, short follow-up periods, and postsurgery studies.

It has been suggested that the high rate of bleeding and rebleed mandates active treatment in most cases. The current consensus is that operative treatment of symptomatic lesions can provide good outcomes and will at least halt neurological deterioration in the majority of cases. Recommendations for management must take into account the patient's symptoms, evidence of progression, the risk of further hemorrhages, size and accessibility of the lesion, and the risks of surgery [24, 26, 47–50]. Although the annualized hemorrhagic risk may seem acceptable at 3.9% (1.6–6.8%) with conservative management, this is still a lifelong risk that may expose younger patients to a high accumulative hemorrhagic risk [32]. However, the annual rate of hemorrhage of symptomatic patients is 9.5–17.6%, and the annual risk for hemorrhage of asymptomatic patients is 0.8% [22]. In the pediatric intramedullary spinal cord malformations, the annual hemorrhage rate (8.2% per patient/year) and rehemorrhage rate were higher than in adults with up to 30.7% for rebleed if not treated [4]. These authors suggest that although the conservative management may be an option in patients at high surgical risk, these patients should be closely monitored because of persistent hemorrhagic risk. It is important to understand the natural history of this pathology and tailor the treatment appropriately.

In a recent multicenter prospective cohort, the multivariable logistic regression analysis showed that the predictors for unfavorable neurological outcome in postoperative patients with ISCCMs were symptom duration ≥26 months, lesion size ≤5 mm, complete intramedullary (deep location in contrast to exophytic growth), subarachnoid hemorrhage, Frankel grade B, and Frankel grade C [15].

Regarding risk factors for poor functional improvement after surgery, a worse neurological status prior to surgery, a larger lesion size, and preoperative unstable gait were identified as predictive factors that affected surgical outcomes.

Delayed complications were the result of incomplete resection [42]. The resultant hemorrhage required re-exploration, which led to tethering of the spinal cord. Most patients who underwent resection, however, had improved neurologically at long-term follow-up.

A recent meta-analysis comparing surgical and conservative treatment long-term outcomes of intramedullary spinal cord cavernous malformations (ISCCMs) found that surgical treatment resulted in an improved neurological status in 36.9% of the patients; in 55.8%, it remained stable; and in 7.3%, it deteriorated compared to the preoperative state. In the conservative cohort, 21.7% improved, 69.6% remained stable, and 8.7% deteriorated [33]. Solitary lesions, duration of preoperative symptoms less than 3 months, and postoperative symptom improvement were prognostic predictors of a favorable long-term outcome. Based on these data, whenever feasible, symptomatic patients with ISCCMs are recommended to undergo surgery, preferably within 3 months from symptom onset, which may lead to better clinical outcomes.

Gross total resection is the only certain prevention of rebleeding but implies immediate (e.g., infection, deep vein thrombosis, and cerebrospinal fluid leakage) or late (e.g., kyphosis, tethered cord, stenosis, SCM rebleed, and subsequent surgery) risks. For this reason, conservative and surgical approaches must be well balanced against each other, and the final decision should be made on a case-by-case basis in experienced neurovascular centers. Recent studies contribute novel data to this rare disease and underline the value of early surgery while highlighting the need for personalized decision-making. There is an unmet need for further studies, especially prospective multicenter studies with a large number of patients to pool data on natural history and outcomes that may provide basis for more definitive evidence-based management.

17.9 Conclusions

Intramedullary spinal CMs (ISCMs) constitute a rare pathology, accounting for 5–12% of all intraspinal vascular malformations. Intramedullary spinal cord cavernous malformations tend to be clinically progressive. The incidence of initial intramedullary hemorrhage is estimated to be 2.1% patient/year, increasing to 66% in those with a previous history of hemorrhage.

Complete and safe surgical resection assisted by continuous multimodal intraoperative neurophysiological monitoring of SSEP, MEP, and D-wave is generally accepted as the primary treatment option and still the only curative treatment. An individualized surgical approach to achieve complete resection in carefully selected symptomatic patients is required to prevent further neurological decline from rebleeding.

However, the evidence is mainly based on cohort studies, and one has to acknowledge the selection bias introduced by such a study design. In that respect, the treating neurosurgeon should always try to tailor treatment to each patient's individual needs by weighing the risk of surgery against the risk of irreversible neurological deficits. Further research is required to better understand the short- and long-term risks and benefits of surgery.

References

1. Akers A, Al-Shahi Salman R, et al. Synopsis of guidelines for the clinical management of cerebral cavernous malformations: consensus recommendations based on systematic literature review by the Angioma Alliance scientific advisory board clinical experts panel. Neurosurgery. 2017;80(5):665–80.
2. Dammann P, Santos AN, Wan XY, Zhu Y, Sure U. Cavernous malformations: updates in surgical management and biology. Neurosurg Clin N Am. 2022;33(4):449–60.
3. Kivelev J, Laakso A, Niemelä M, Hernesniemi J. A proposed grading system of brain and spinal cavernomas. Neurosurgery. 2011;69(4):807–14.
4. Ren J, Hong T, Zeng G, et al. Characteristics and long-term outcome of 20 children with intramedullary spinal cord cavernous malformations. Neurosurgery. 2020;86(6):817–24; discussion 524–7
5. Khalatbari MR, Hamidi M, Moharamzad Y. Pediatric intramedullary cavernous malformation of the conus medullaris: case report and review of the literature. Childs Nerv Syst. 2011;27(3):507–11.
6. Awad IA, MD, Polster SP. Cavernous angiomas: deconstructing a neurosurgical disease. J Neurosurg. 2019;131:1–13.
7. Al-Shahi Salman R, Kitchen N, Thomson J, et al. Top ten research priorities for brain and spine cavernous malformations. Lancet Neurol. 2016;15(4):354–5.
8. Mabray MC, Starcevich J, Hallstrom J, et al. High prevalence of spinal cord cavernous malformations in the familial cerebral cavernous malformations type 1 cohort. AJNR Am J Neuroradiol. 2020;41(6):1126–30.
9. Chohan MO, Marchiò S, Morrison LA, et al. Emerging pharmacologic targets in cerebral cavernous malformation and potential strategies to alter the natural history of a difficult disease: a review. JAMA Neurol. 2019;76(4):492–500.
10. Ogilvy CS, Louis DN, Ojemann RG. Intramedullary cavernous angiomas of the spinal cord: clinical presentation, pathological features, and surgical management. Neurosurgery. 1992;31(2):219–30.
11. Santos AN, Rauschenbach L, Darkwah Oppong M, et al. Natural course of untreated spinal cord cav-

ernous malformations: a follow-up study within the initial 5 years after diagnosis. J Neurosurg Spine. 2021;36(6):1030–4.
12. Badhiwala JH, Farrokhyar F, Alhazzani W, et al. Surgical outcomes and natural history of intramedullary spinal cord cavernous malformations: a single-center series and meta-analysis of individual patient data: clinic article. J Neurosurg Spine. 2014;21(4):662–76.
13. Endo T, Inoue T, Mizuno M, et al. Current trends in the surgical management of intramedullary tumors: a multicenter study of 1,033 patients by the Neurospinal Society of Japan. Neurospine. 2022;19:441–52.
14. Sandalcioglu IE, Wiedemayer H, Gasser T, et al. Intramedullary spinal cord cavernous malformations: clinical features and risk of hemorrhage. Neurosurg Rev. 2003;26:253–6.
15. Ren J, Jiang N, Bian L, et al. Natural history of spinal cord cavernous malformations: a multicenter cohort study. Neurosurgery. 2022;90:390–8.
16. Lu DC, Lawton MT. Clinical presentation and surgical management of intramedullary spinal cord cavernous malformations. Neurosurg Focus. 2010;29(3):E12.
17. Gross BA, Du R, Popp AJ, Day AL. Intramedullary spinal cord cavernous malformations. Neurosurg Focus. 2010 Sep;29(3):E14.
18. Kim LJ, Klopfenstein JD, Zabramski JM, Sonntag VK, Spetzler RF. Analysis of pain resolution after surgical resection of intramedullary spinal cord cavernous malformations. Neurosurgery. 2006;58(1):106–11; discussion 106–11.
19. Ardeshiri A, Özkan N, Chen B, et al. A retrospective and consecutive analysis of the epidemiology and management of spinal cavernomas over the last 20 years in a single center. Neurosurg Rev. 2016;39(2):269–76.
20. Deutsch H, Jallo GI, Faktorovich A, Epstein F. Spinal intramedullary cavernoma: clinical presentation and surgical outcome. J Neurosurg. 2000;93(1 Suppl):65–70.
21. Liang JT, Bao YH, Zhang HQ, Huo LR, Wang ZY, Ling F. Management and prognosis of symptomatic patients with intramedullary spinal cord cavernoma: clinical article. J Neurosurg Spine. 2011;15(4):447–56.
22. Goyal A, Rinaldo L, Alkhataybeh R, et al. Clinical presentation, natural history and outcomes of intramedullary spinal cord cavernous malformations. J Neurol Neurosurg Psychiatry. 2019;90(6):695–703.
23. McCormick PC, Michelsen WJ, Post KD, Carmel PW, Stein BM. Cavernous malformations of the spinal cord. Neurosurgery. 1988;23(4):459–63.
24. Bian LG, Bertalanffy H, Sun QF, Shen JK. Intramedullary cavernous malformations: clinical features and surgical technique via hemilaminectomy. Clin Neurol Neurosurg. 2009;111:511–7.
25. Li J, Chen G, Gu S, et al. Surgical outcomes of spinal cord intramedullary cavernous malformation: a retrospective study of 83 patients in a single center over a 12-year period. World Neurosurg. 2018;118:e105–14.
26. Liu T, Wang L, Zhang S, et al. Prediction of outcomes for symptomatic spinal cavernous malformation surgery: a multicenter prospective clinical study. Eur Spine J. 2023;32(4):1326–33.
27. Chabert E, Morandi X, Carney MP, Riffaud L, Louail C, Carsin-Nicol B. Intramedullary cavernous malformations. J Neuroradiol. 1999;26(4):262–8.
28. Panda A, Diehn FE, Kim DK, Bydon M, Goyal A, Benson JC, Carr CM, Rinaldo L, Flemming KD, Lanzino G. Spinal cord cavernous malformations: MRI commonly shows adjacent intramedullary hemorrhage. J Neuroimaging. 2020 Sep;30(5):690–6.
29. Mitha AP, Turner JD, Spetzler RF. Surgical approaches to intramedullary cavernous malformations of the spinal cord. Neurosurgery. 2011 Jun;68(2 Suppl Operative):317-24:discussion 324.
30. Maslehaty H, Barth H, Petridis AK, Doukas A, Mehdorn HM. Symptomatic spinal cavernous malformations: indication for microsurgical treatment and outcome. Eur Spine J. 2011;20(10):1765–70.
31. Fotakopoulos G, Kivelev J, Andrade-Barazarte H, Tjahjadi M, Goehre F, Hernesniemi J. Outcome in patients with spinal cavernomas presenting with symptoms due to mass effect and/or hemorrhage: conservative versus surgical management: meta-analysis of direct comparison of approach-related complications. World Neurosurg. 2021;152:6–18.
32. Zhang L, Yang W, Jia W, Kong D, Yang J, Wang G, et al. Comparison of outcome between surgical and conservative management of symptomatic spinal cord cavernous malformations. Neurosurgery. 2016;78:552–61.
33. Asimakidou E, Meszaros LT, Anestis DM, Tsitsopoulos PP. A systematic review on the outcome of intramedullary spinal cord cavernous malformations. Eur Spine J. 2022;31(11):3119–29.
34. Kurokawa R, Endo T, Takami T, et al. Acceptance of early surgery for treatment of spinal cord cavernous malformation in contemporary Japan. Neurospine. 2023;20:587–94.
35. Rauschenbach L, Santos AN, Engel A, et al. Functional neurological outcome of spinal cavernous malformation surgery. Eur Spine J. 2023;32(5):1714–20.
36. Zevgaridis D, Medele RJ, Hamburger C, et al. Cavernous haemangiomas of the spinal cord. A review of 117 cases. Acta Neurochir. 1999;141:237–45.
37. Imagama S, Ito Z, Ando K, et al. Optimal timing of surgery for intramedullary cavernous hemangioma of the spinal cord in relation to preoperative motor paresis, disease duration, and tumor volume and location. Global Spine J. 2017;7:246–53.
38. Deletis V, Sala F. Intraoperative neurophysiological monitoring of the spinal cord during spinal cord and spine surgery: a review focus on the corticospinal tracts. Clin Neurophysiol. 2008;119(2):248–64.
39. Niedermeyer S, Szelenyi SC, Tonn JC, Siller S. Intramedullary spinal cord cavernous malformations—association between intraoperative neurophysiological monitoring changes and neurological outcome. Acta Neurochir. 2022;164(10):2595–604.

40. Ren J, He C, Hong T, et al. Anterior to dorsal root entry zone myelotomy (ADREZotomy): a new surgical approach for the treatment of ventrolateral deep intramedullary spinal cord cavernous malformations. Spine (Phila Pa 1976). 2018;43(17):E1024–32.
41. Ren J, Hong T, He C, et al. Surgical approaches and long-term outcomes of intramedullary spinal cord cavernous malformations: a single-center consecutive series of 219 patients. J Neurosurg Spine. 2019;31:123–32.
42. Vishteh AG, Sankhla S, Anson JA, Zabramski JM, Spetzler RF. Surgical resection of intramedullary spinal cord cavernous malformations: delayed complications, long-term outcomes, and association with cryptic venous malformations. Neurosurgery. 1997;41(5):1094–100.
43. Park SB, Jahng TA, Chung CK. The clinical outcomes after complete surgical resection of intramedullary cavernous angiomas: changes in motor and sensory symptoms. Spinal Cord. 2009;47:128–33.
44. Kharkar S, et al. The natural history of conservatively managed symptomatic intramedullary spinal cord cavernomas. Neurosurgery. 2007;60(5):865–72. Discussion 865–72.
45. Mitha AP, Turner JD, Abla AA, Vishteh AG, Spetzler RF. Outcomes following resection of intramedullary spinal cord cavernous malformations: a 25-year experience. J Neurosurg Spine. 2011;14:605–11.
46. Azad TD, Veeravagu A, Li A, Zhang M, Madhugiri V. Steinberg GK (2018) long-term effectiveness of gross-total resection for symptomatic spinal cord cavernous malformations. Neurosurgery. 2018;1(83):1201–8.
47. Ohnishi YI, Nakajima N, Takenaka T, et al. Conservative and surgical management of spinal cord cavernous malformations. World Neurosurg X. 2019;5:100066.
48. Reitz M, Burkhardt T, Vettorazzi E, et al. Intramedullary spinal cavernoma: clinical presentation, microsurgical approach, and long-term outcome in a cohort of 48 patients. Neurosurg Focus. 2015:39(2):E19.
49. Nagoshi N, Tsuji O, Nakashima D, et al. Clinical outcomes and prognostic factors for cavernous hemangiomas of the spinal cord: a retrospective cohort study. J Neurosurg Spine. 2019;31(2):271–8.
50. Liu T, Li K, Wang Y, et al. Treatment strategies and prognostic factors for spinal cavernous malformation: a single-center retrospective cohort study. J Neurosurg Spine. 2021;35(6):824–33.

18 Spinal Cavernoma

Arunkumar Sekar and A. R. Prabhu Raj

Abstract

Cavernous malformations of the central nervous system (CNS), particularly spinal cavernomas, are rare vascular pathologies with a prevalence of 0.4–0.6%. While MRI has significantly increased detection, evidence on the natural history and outcomes of spinal cavernomas remains limited. The mean age of presentation is 39.1 years. Clinical manifestations include a mix of motor, sensory, and autonomic deficits, and 92% of reported cases underwent surgical intervention, potentially overestimating severity. Hemorrhage rates range from 1.4% to 6.8%, with higher rates in symptomatic and about 0.8% in asymptomatic cases. Pathologically, spinal cavernomas resemble those in the brain, displaying slow-flow, non-shunting malformations. MRI is the preferred diagnostic tool, revealing characteristic "popcorn-like" mixed signals. Surgical removal is the primary curative option, demanding meticulous planning due to the spinal cord's eloquence. Outcome studies predominantly involve surgical cases, with reported neurological recovery depending on initial presentation and timing of surgery. Pediatric cases exhibit a higher rehemorrhage rate, emphasizing the need for early intervention. In the absence of a clear role for conservative management, surgery within 3 months of symptom onset is recommended for symptomatic cases. Factors such as acute presentation, motor symptoms, and superficial lesions correlate with better surgical outcomes. Conversely, deep-seated, asymptomatic, or mildly symptomatic lesions may be safely managed conservatively. Overall, despite challenges, surgical resection remains the preferred treatment for spinal cavernomas, with nuances depending on various clinical and radiological factors.

Keywords

Spinal cavernomas · Cavernous malformation of the spine · Intramedullary spinal tumors Vascular lesions of the spine

18.1 Introduction

Cavernous malformations of the CNS are a rare group of low-flow vascular pathologies with a reported prevalence of 0.4–0.6% in general population [1]. Cavernous malformations of the spinal cord as a group account for 5–12% of all spinal

A. Sekar (✉)
Department of Neurosurgery, AIIMS, Bhubaneswar, India
e-mail: neurosurg_arun@aiimsbhubaneswar.edu.in

A. R. P. Raj
Department of Neurosurgery, NIMHANS, Bangalore, India

X. Lv (ed.), *Endovascular and Neurovascular Surgery for Spinal Vascular Malformations*,
https://doi.org/10.1007/978-981-97-4661-3_18

vascular abnormalities. Although they can be asymptomatic, they can present with motor or sensory symptoms leading to permanent neurological deficits. In comparison to their cranial counterpart, spinal cavernomas have an overall lack of evidence regarding the natural history, prognosis, and outcomes [2].

18.2 Epidemiology

Since the first reported case in 1903 for the next eight decades, only 19 cases were available in literature including autopsy studies. With the advent of MRI in the mid-1980s, there is an exponential increase in the number of cases reported. Most of them were surgical case reports and small series [3]. Only recently studies with larger cohort of patients have enhanced our understanding of this pathology. The mean age of presentation is 39.1 years but with age range as wide as 2–80 years. There is a slight male predilection in the distribution with a ratio of 1.20:1 (male to female). They have a distribution throughout the spinal column with thoracic region (60.2%) being the most common location in the spinal cord followed by cervical (38.0%) and lumbar in 1.8%. Although older reviews have a higher incidence of positive family history and concomitant intracranial lesions, a more recent study estimated it to be lower, about 4.4% with a positive family history and 6.6% with concomitant intracranial lesions [4]. Familial systemic cavernous malformations like Klippel-Trenaunay-Weber syndrome or Cobb syndrome can rarely present with associated spinal cavernomas [5].

18.3 Clinical Presentation

Although with the advent of advanced imaging of spinal cord there is an increase in cases reported, most of them were evaluated for symptoms, and hence, almost 92% of the reported cases were treated surgically [4]. This overestimates the severity of presentation in spinal cavernomas as many of them can be asymptomatic or incidental findings. Clinical presentation is usually a mix of motor, sensory, and autonomic deficits. About 60.5% have motor symptoms, 57.8% have sensory symptoms, and 33.8% have pain and 23.6% present with bladder and bowel dysfunction; rarely reports of respiratory distress can also be noted. Only 0.9% of them are asymptomatic; however, this could be due to the selection bias in reported literature [6].

These clinical presentations can be present in various combinations in different patterns. Most commonly patients present with a slowly progressive clinical course. Oglivy et al. categorized the symptomatology into five different patterns: a relapsing-remitting course with varying degrees of recovery, a slowly progressive decline, acute onset with rapid or gradual decline, and patients with only sudden onset back pain without any neurological deficits [7]. A recent meta-analysis has shown that about 60.3% of cases present with progressive deficits and 39.7% had an acute/stepwise pattern of progression [8].

18.4 Natural History

Only 10% of the cases published in literature are managed medically. As the reported literature is predominantly surgically managed, there is some difficulty in predicting the natural history as to the hemorrhage rate and change in neurological status without surgery. Studies measure the hemorrhage rate for spinal cavernous malformations that ranges from 1.4% to 6.8%, and two recent meta-analyses estimate it to be around 2.1% per year [9, 10]. However, it should be noted that most studies consider cavernomas as congenital lesions. Hemorrhage rates, however, don't predict the natural course of the disease once symptomatic. Symptomatic patients and those with acute hemorrhage have a higher annual hemorrhage rate of about 9% approximately. Asymptomatic patients have an annual rehemorrhage rate of 0.8%. This considerably lower rehemorrhage rate may be due to the lack of associated developmental venous anomalies as in deep-seated intracranial cavernomas [11].

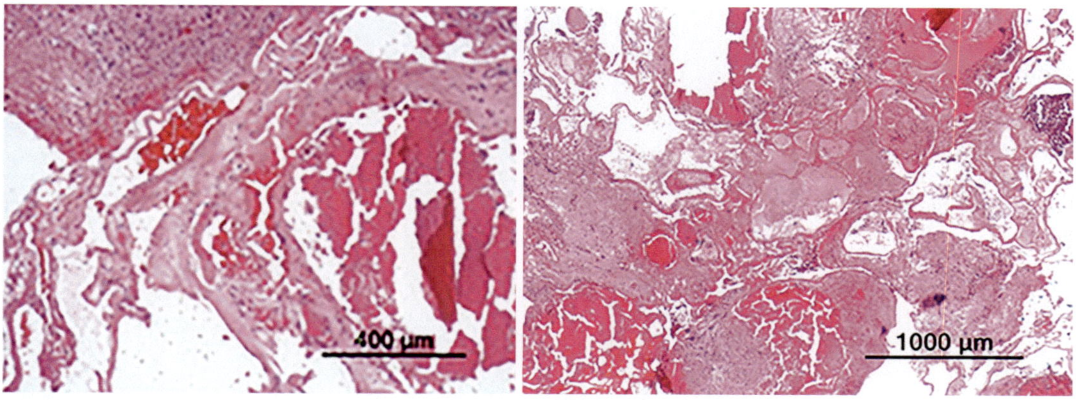

Fig. 18.1 Hematoxylin and eosin staining of a cavernoma with a single layer of endothelium without any intervening CNS tissue packed with blood cells. There are areas of calcification and hyalinzation. Usually there are areas of hemosiderin deposition

18.5 Pathology

On gross examination, cavernomas of the spinal cord is not different from that of brain cavernoma. They are well-demarcated, lobulated, soft, and bluish or reddish-brown mulberry-shaped vascular lesion without intervening spinal tissue (Fig. 18.1). There is absence of mural elements of mature vasculature. Hemodynamically, they are slow-flow, non-shunting vascular malformations. Due to this low-flow hemodynamics, they tend to have intralesional thrombosis, calcifications, and recanalization, which lead to accumulation of hemosiderin-laden macrophages in and around the lesion. The lesion is mostly considered congenital but has been discovered following radiation also.

18.6 Radiology

The average size of a spinal cavernoma is measured about 9.2 mm spanning not more than two vertebral levels. Magnetic resonance imaging is the preferred modality to detect spinal cavernomas. MRI shows heterogeneous signal intensity on both T1- and T2-weighted images. Spinal cavernomas can be classified based on MR imaging findings into four categories [12]: type 1, subacute hemorrhage (Fig. 18.3), hyperintense on T1 and hyper- or hypointense on T2; type 2, mixed subacute and chronic (popcorn lesion) (Fig. 18.2), reticulated heterointense on T1 and reticulated heterointense with dark rim on T2; type 3, chronic, iso- or hypointense on T1 and hypointense with dark rim on T2; and type 4 (Fig. 18.4), small punctate hypointensity on gradient recalled echo (GRE) T2. This is due to the blood products in its various stages of degradation due to thrombosis and hemorrhage. This gives a typical "popcorn-like" mixed signal [13]. A recent intralesional bleeding presents hyperintense on T1-weighted images due to presence of methemoglobin. Hemosiderin rim around the lesion presents a well-circumscribed hypointense rim on T2-weighted imaging. Small lesions may not have these characteristics. There is no contrast enhancement. Due to the absence of direct arterial feeding, conventional angiography is not useful in diagnosing [12].

One of the close differential diagnoses is a hemorrhagic ependymoma, in which 22–33% of cases have a T2-weighted dark rim, which is termed as a "cap sign." Jeon et al. observed that eccentric axial location, small size, absence of edema, and minimal contrast enhancement suggest a cavernoma than an ependymoma [14].

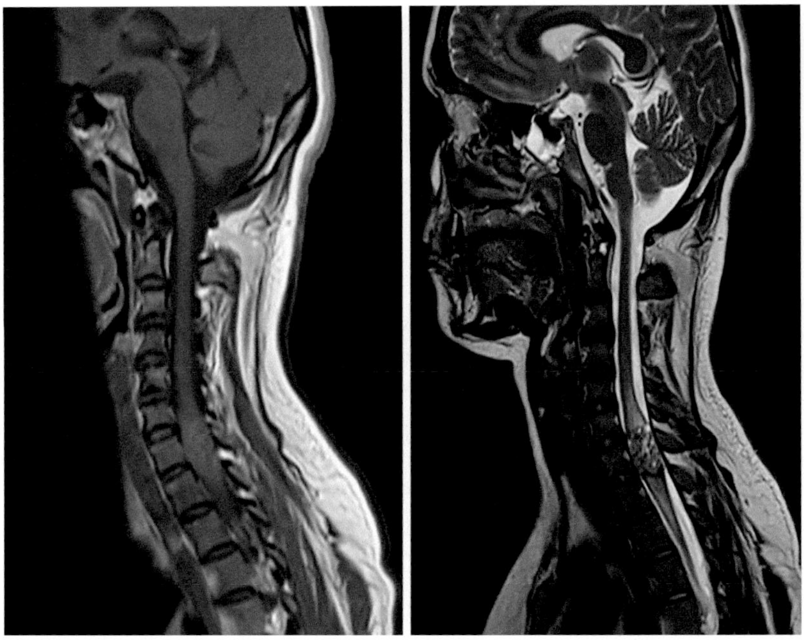

Fig. 18.2 MR imaging of the cervical spine showing T1 and T2 heterointense with reticulated appearance and dark T2 rim. Type 2 cavernoma with mixed subacute and chronic bleed

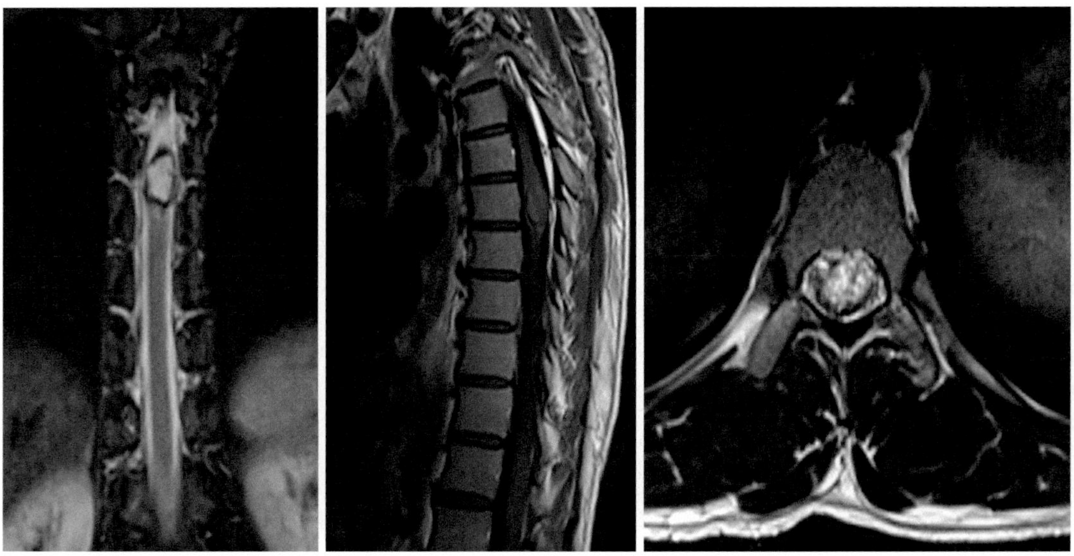

Fig. 18.3 MR imaging showing T1 isointense and T2 hyperintense with dark T2 rim. Type 3 cavernoma with subacute bleed type 1 variant in the mid-thoracic spine

18.7 Management

Surgical removal of cavernoma is currently the only curative treatment option [11]. However, like the brainstem, the spinal cord is a highly eloquent region, and hence, meticulous presurgical planning is required. The two-point method is done by a line drawn on an axial MRI connecting the center of the lesion with the most surfacing part of the lesion in the non-eloquent pial surface. In the spinal cord, there are three recommended non-eloquent pial entry zones: dorsal root entry zone (DREZ), dorsal median sulcus, and lateral [15]. Depending on the entry zone, the approach is planned. The most commonly advocated approach is the midline posterior approach. However, anterior, anterolateral, posterolateral, and transthoracic approaches were used in select cases [16].

For majority of spinal cavernomas, a standard midline posterior approach is the most commonly used. Surgical steps that involve laminectomy, laminoplasty, or hemilaminectomy are used depending on the location and the number of levels [13]. We prefer laminoplasty when the lesion involves multiple levels, and routine wide laminectomy is done in most cases. We routinely use intraoperative ultrasound to localize the lesion and confirm the adequacy of the laminectomy. Once the dura and the arachnoid leaflets are opened, retracted and secured. The spinal cord is inspected for any discoloration, dilated vessels in case of superficially located cavernomas. In case of deep-seated ones, there still may be surrounding hemosiderin deposition and localized cord fullness. Intraoperative ultrasound becomes very useful in these cases in planning the myelotomy. The posterior median sulcus myelotomy is done. Localizing this in a distorted anatomy may be slightly difficult, but usually the posterior median sulcal vein or a septum identifies the structure reliably. Once identified, the tumor is removed piecemeal using standard microsurgical techniques (Fig. 18.4).

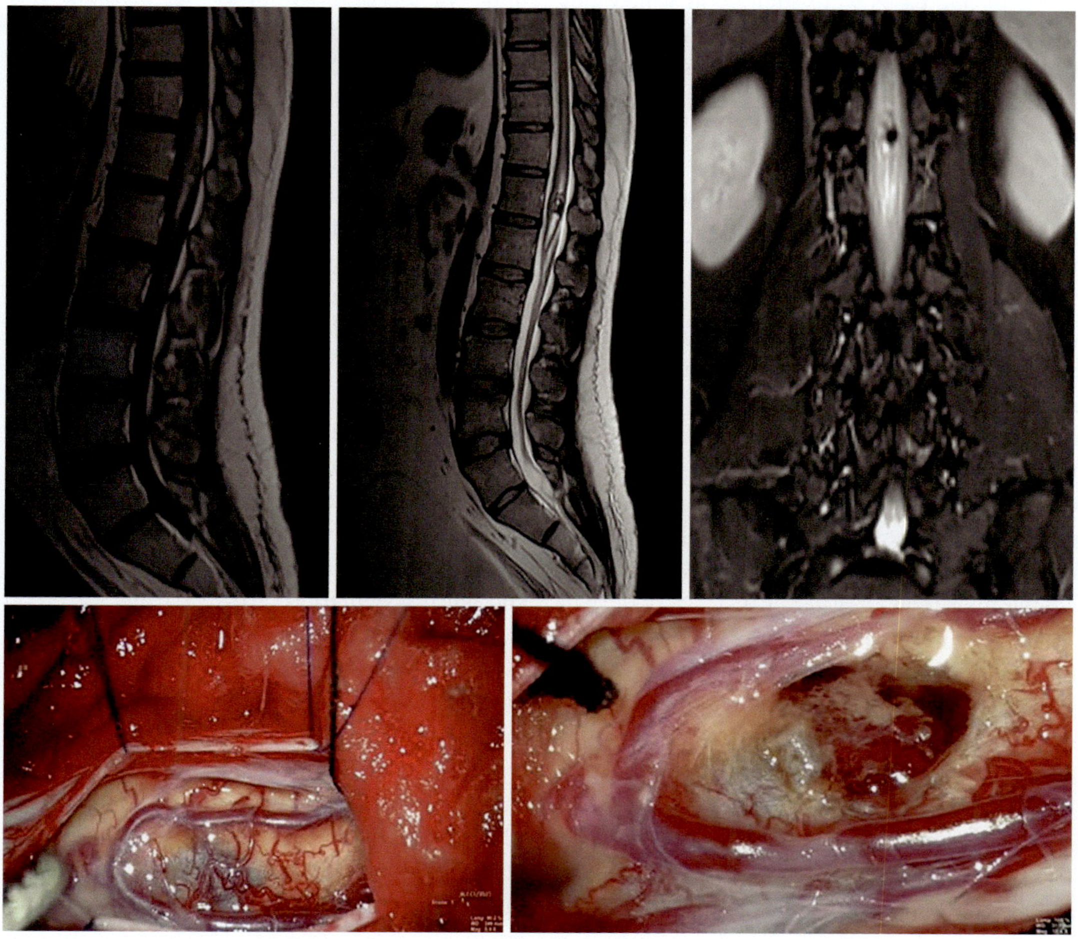

Fig. 18.4 Deep-seated type 4 conus cavernoma with recent bleed in a child managed initially with conservative management and later underwent surgery. Intra-op bluish discoloration and eccentric location with a large posterior medial sulcal vein. Post-op resection cavity noted with preserved venous anatomy

18.8 Outcome

The reported literature has cases that predominantly underwent surgical resection (92.3%), and in most of the cases, the surgical outcome depends on the initial presentation. Most of the systematic reviews and case series support surgical intervention for symptomatic cases with good accessibility. Data available from studies suggests a neurological recovery reduces with each hemorrhage event. Although surgical intervention is established as a curative modality, the timing of surgery, surgical corridor, management approach to deep-seated lesions, and other factors like symptom severity and outcome of each symptom are not established well [11].

In one of the earliest reviews by Gross et al., a group of 352 cases were studied, in which they had suggested a treatment paradigm suggesting surgical intervention of exophytic lesions. Deep-seated lesions were suggested to be managed conservatively unless the disease is progressive or recurrent with initial severe symptoms. Surgical techniques and intraoperative neuromonitoring have improved the outcomes since then [3].

In a recently published meta-analysis by Fotakopoulos et al., which comprised major series of spinal cavernomas in the past two decades, it was found that motor recovery is superior in cases of acute neurological deterioration. Acute presentation has a better functional outcome when compared to progressive stepwise deterioration. As far as bladder dysfunction is concerned, surgical and conservative group has similar long-term recovery [17].

Rauschenbach et al. in their study looked for functional outcome of surgical intervention for spinal cavernous malformations and found that multiple bleeding, deep location, and incomplete resection are associated with poorer outcomes. Early surgery within 3 months of the initial bleeding presentation had a better outcome [8].

Zhang et al. studied 111 cases of spinal cavernomas and found that surgical removal of symptomatic spinal cavernomas can avoid further deterioration and have overall better long-term outcome. Among them, cervical location demonstrated a shorter duration of symptoms, acute pattern, and larger lesion size compared to other locations. Thoracic and lumbar location had predominant motor complaints and aggressive course. These locations need early surgical resection than other locations. Preoperative neurological status and immediate improvement after surgery are positive indicators for better long-term outcome [18]. Another study by Azad et al. supporting this view also suggested patients with poor neurological status at presentation should not be ruled out of surgery as they found better improvement in this group of patients [19].

Li et al., in their series of 80 patients, found that surgical intervention within 3 months of onset of symptoms showed better improvement than all other predictive factors. They had used modified McCormick score to measure this improvement [20].

In a meta-analysis by Bhadiwala et al., they found that 90% underwent surgical treatment and 10% conservative management. Among the patients who underwent conservative management, 30% improved, 58% were stable, and 11% declined in neurological status. This was poorer in comparison to patients managed with surgical resection in whom 51% improved, 38% were stable, and 11% declined in neurological status. The outcomes of patients, who were observed with conservative management beyond 5 years, were even less favorable suggesting a progressive disease and hence needs surgical treatment. Among the clinical presentation, acute presentation and presence of motor symptoms had better outcomes than chronic progressive presentation and sensory symptoms [10].

Ren et al. in their study identified that pediatric spinal cavernomas account for 5.6% of spinal vascular lesion in children. Majority is sporadic in nature. Misdiagnosis is common due to the rarity of the lesion. In this age group, annual hemorrhage rate is higher than the adult counterparts. There is an 8.2%/year rate of hemorrhage and 30.7%/year rate of rehemorrhage in children. Surgical resection gives a good functional recovery in almost 50% of cases. Due to the aggressive nature and higher rehemorrhage rate, early surgical intervention is recommended in children as rebleeds usually leave a permanent neurological deficit. In their series including adult patients, they found the cervical location had a better outcome. In patients with lesion in thoracolumbar region with preoperative mild symptoms and deep-seated lesions, they suggested discretion during surgical intervention [21, 22].

Kim et al. analyzed the clinical outcome of conservative management in spinal cavernomas, divided the patients into four categories based on clinical presentation, and found that patients who are asymptomatic or with only pain without neurological deficits on conservative treatment remained without any rebleeds and pain had improved in a group of patients. Among the patients with only sensory deficits, improvement of sensory symptoms post-surgery is doubtful, but motor symptoms have a better chance of recovery. However, patients with sensory or motor symptoms have higher chances of rebleeding as compared to asymptomatic or patients with only pain. Hence surgery should be offered in these groups of cases. This study has significant selection bias and a very small sample size [23]. Liang et al. suggested observation for ventrally located, small, and deep-seated lesions, but the sample size was small. These cases would require long-term rigorous follow-up [24]. In a retrospective review of spinal cavernomas managed conservatively by Kharkar et al. [25], nine of ten patients remained the same or improved at a mean follow-up of 80 months. The risk of profuse hemorrhage in spinal cavernoma ranges between 1.4% and 4.5% per patient per year, increasing to 66% per patient per year in patients with a previous history of hemorrhage [26, 27]. The same has been suggested by other studies addressing the issue of role of conservative management in treatment of spinal cavernomas [6, 25, 28].

Park et al. reviewed 14 patients who underwent surgical intervention and found motor symptoms to improve better after surgical resection. Sensory symptoms remained the same on mean long-term follow-up of up to 55 months. They have also observed posterolateral and deep-seated approach to have a poorer surgical outcome [29].

In a study by Mitha AP et al. [30], they found that the resection of intramedullary spinal cord cavernomas can be achieved with good long-term outcomes. They found that during immediate postoperative period, 55% of the patient had Frankel grade D and 21% had Frankel grade E clinical outcome, whereas none of the patients in the study was found to have Frankel grade A. On long-term follow-up, 23% patients showed improved Frankel grade, and long-term outcome was better in spinal cavernomas less than 1 cm. Fifty-one (64%) of 80 patients had symptoms of pain at the time of their presentation. In most cases, this pain was described as a burning dysesthesia. On long-term follow-up, 56% patients had an improvement in pain compared to their pre-op period. They found that the complete surgical excision of symptomatic intramedullary spinal cavernomas will decrease pain as well as prevents decline in neurological function.

In a study by Deutsch et al. [31] on the surgical outcome, it was noted that 50% of the patient who were with chronic symptoms had transient decline in their neurological function that necessitated physiotherapy. On long-term follow-up, 50% patients regained their preoperative strength, and 44% patients had improved motor strength compared with their preoperative function [31]. In pediatric intramedullary tumors, they found that 10% of intramedullary spinal cavernoma occurs in pediatric population in the cervical region. Unlike adults, they have an acute presentation, and surgical excision will result in good functional outcome.

In a multicenter retrospective study by Labauge et al. [32], long-term follow-up data (mean 7.3 years) were available for 37 patients and demonstrated clinical improvement in 54%, no change in 16%, and clinical worsening in 30%. Jallo GI et al. [33] found that among 26 patients of spinal cavernoma, 50% worsened immediately after surgery. At a mean follow-up of 4.5 years, only 8% were worse, 46% were stable, and 46% reported improvement compared with their preoperative functional status. In their study, however, long-term follow-up was subjective and described without the use of an established neurological or functional grading system.

Their review on literature about surgical resection of spinal cavernoma showed a stable functional outcome in 61%, improvement in functional outcome in 31%, and worse functional outcome in 8% of patients.

Bian LG and their associates [34] on their retrospective study on 16 patients on spinal cavernomas who underwent hemilaminectomy and excision of cavernoma showed 75% clinical improvement, and 25% were stable based on Frankel grade during the mean follow-up period of 23.1 months.

In a study by Kim LJ et al. [35], they postulated that due to low tolerance of the medulla to a mass lesion, patients frequently present with progressive focal sensorimotor deficits often combined with intensive radicular or central pain. After surgical excision, 52% of patients showed improvement in their preoperative pain symptoms at a mean follow-up of 44.5 months.

In a study by Kivelev J et al. [36], after surgical resection of spinal cavernomas in the immediate postoperative period, 57% showed improvement of symptoms, 14% remained the same, and 29% had worsening of symptoms. At the time of discharge, 71% had improvement of neurological status, and 21% had worsening of symptoms or some new deficits. Hemorrhage occurred in seven patients (50%) before surgery. One patient had symptomatic rebleeding after 14 years of observation who was intact after the first hemorrhage, which was treated conservatively, but his condition was deteriorated acutely due to rehemorrhage, indicating a need to surgically remove the lesion. Ten (71%) of the 14 patients suffered from radicular pain before surgery. During follow-up, nine (90%) of these ten patients showed significant pain relief.

18.9 Conclusion

In summary, surgical resection of the cavernoma has a higher proportion of reported cases; hence, the role of conservative management is not clearly delineated. However, with the available literature, it is clear that surgery is the preferred curative treatment. In symptomatic cases, early surgery less than 3 months is recommended. Acute symptoms, motor symptoms, and superficial lesions have better surgical outcome as compared to chronic progressive pathology, sensory pathology, pain, and deep-seated lesions. Children have an aggressive course, and rebleed chances are higher than adults; hence, aggressive surgical treatment is recommended. As such, cervical location has better outcome than thoracolumbar location. Lesions, which are deep-seated, asymptomatic, or mildly symptomatic, without any previous features of bleed and small size can be safely conservatively managed.

References

1. Clark AJ, Wang DD, Lawton MT. Spinal cavernous malformations. Handb Clin Neurol. 2017;143:303–8.
2. Lu DC, Lawton MT. Clinical presentation and surgical management of intramedullary spinal cord cavernous malformations. Neurosurg Focus. 2010;29(3):E12.
3. Gross BA, Du R, Popp AJ, Day AL. Intramedullary spinal cord cavernous malformations. Neurosurg Focus. 2010;29(3):E14.
4. Asimakidou E, Meszaros LT, Anestis DM, Tsitsopoulos PP. A systematic review on the outcome of intramedullary spinal cord cavernous malformations. Eur Spine J. 2022;31(11):3119–29.
5. Matsui Y, Mineharu Y, Satow T, Takebe N, Takeuchi E, Saiki M. Coexistence of multiple cavernous angiomas in the spinal cord and skin: a unique case of cobb syndrome. J Neurosurg Spine. 2014;20(2):142–7.
6. Goyal A, Rinaldo L, Alkhataybeh R, Kerezoudis P, Alvi MA, Flemming KD, et al. Clinical presentation, natural history and outcomes of intramedullary spinal cord cavernous malformations. J Neurol Neurosurg Psychiatry. 2019;90(6):695–703.
7. Ogilvy CS, Louis DN, Ojemann RG. Intramedullary cavernous angiomas of the spinal cord: clinical presentation, pathological features, and surgical management. Neurosurgery. 1992;31(2):219–29; discussion 229-230.
8. Rauschenbach L, Santos AN, Engel A, Olbrich A, Benet A, Li Y, et al. Functional neurological outcome of spinal cavernous malformation surgery. Eur Spine J. 2023;32(5):1714–20.
9. Otten M, Mccormick P. Chapter 22 - natural history of spinal cavernous malformations. In: Spetzler RF, Moon K, Almefty RO, editors. Handbook of clinical neurology. Elsevier; 2017. p. 233–9; Arteriovenous and Cavernous Malformations; vol. 143. https://www.sciencedirect.com/science/article/pii/B9780444636409000229.

10. Badhiwala JH, Farrokhyar F, Alhazzani W, Yarascavitch B, Aref M, Algird A, et al. Surgical outcomes and natural history of intramedullary spinal cord cavernous malformations: a single-center series and meta-analysis of individual patient data: clinical article. SPI. 2014;21(4):662–76.
11. Svoboda N, Beneš V, Bradáč O. Spinal cavernous malformations. In: Bradáč O, Beneš V, editors. Cavernomas of the CNS: basic science to clinical practice [internet]. Cham: Springer International Publishing; 2020. p. 215–37. https://doi.org/10.1007/978-3-030-49406-3_14.
12. Da Ros V, Picchi E, Ferrazzoli V, Schirinzi T, Sabuzi F, Grillo P, et al. Spinal vascular lesions: anatomy, imaging techniques and treatment. Eur J Radiol Open. 2021;8:100369.
13. Reitz M, Burkhardt T, Vettorazzi E, Raimund F, Fritzsche E, Schmidt NO, et al. Intramedullary spinal cavernoma: clinical presentation, microsurgical approach, and long-term outcome in a cohort of 48 patients. Neurosurg Focus. 2015;39(2):E19.
14. Jeon I, Jung WS, Suh SH, Chung TS, Cho YE, Ahn SJ. MR imaging features that distinguish spinal cavernous angioma from hemorrhagic ependymoma and serial MRI changes in cavernous angioma. J Neuro-Oncol. 2016;130(1):229–36.
15. Crispino M, Vecchioni S, Galli G, Olivetti L. Spinal intradural extramedullary haemangioma: MRI and neurosurgical findings. Acta Neurochir. 2005;147(11):1195–8. discussion 1198
16. Brotchi J. Intrinsic spinal cord tumor resection. Neurosurgery. 2002;50(5):1059–63.
17. Fotakopoulos G, Kivelev J, Andrade-Barazarte H, Tjahjadi M, Goehre F, Hernesniemi J. Outcome in patients with spinal cavernomas presenting with symptoms due to mass effect and/or hemorrhage: conservative versus surgical management: meta-analysis of direct comparison of approach-related complications. World Neurosurg. 2021;152:6–18.
18. Zhang L, Yu X, Qiao G, Shang A. Long-term surgical outcomes and prognostic factors of adult symptomatic spinal cord cavernous malformations. J Clin Neurosci. 2021;90:171–7.
19. Azad TD, Veeravagu A, Li A, Zhang M, Madhugiri V, Steinberg GK. Long-term effectiveness of gross-total resection for symptomatic spinal cord cavernous malformations. Neurosurgery. 2018;83(6):1201–8.
20. Li J, Chen G, Gu S, Liu X, Shou J, Gu W, et al. Surgical outcomes of spinal cord intramedullary cavernous malformation: a retrospective study of 83 patients in a single center over a 12-year period. World Neurosurg. 2018;118:e105–14.
21. Ren J, Hong T, Zeng G, He C, Li X, Ma Y, et al. Characteristics and long-term outcome of 20 children with intramedullary spinal cord cavernous malformations. Neurosurgery. 2020;86(6):817.
22. Ren J, Hong T, He C, Li X, Ma Y, Yu J, et al. Surgical approaches and long-term outcomes of intramedullary spinal cord cavernous malformations: a single-center consecutive series of 219 patients. J Neurosurg Spine. 2019;31(1):123–32.
23. Kim KM, Chung CK, Huh W, Lee WJ, Park SB, Kim CH, et al. Clinical outcomes of conservative management of spinal cord cavernous angiomas. Acta Neurochir. 2013;155(7):1209–14.
24. Tao LJ, Hai BY, Qi ZH, Rong HL, Yu WZ, Ling F. Management and prognosis of symptomatic patients with intramedullary spinal cord cavernoma: clinical article. J Neurosurg Spine. 2011;15(4):447–56.
25. Kharkar S, Shuck J, Conway J, Rigamonti D. The natural history of conservatively managed symptomatic intramedullary spinal cord cavernomas. Neurosurgery. 2007;60(5):865.
26. Zevgaridis D, Medele RJ, Hamburger C, Steiger HJ, Reulen HJ. Cavernous haemangiomas of the spinal cord. A review of 117 cases. Acta Neurochir. 1999;141(3):237–45.
27. Sandalcioglu IE, Wiedemayer H, Gasser T, Asgari S, Engelhorn T, Stolke D. Intramedullary spinal cord cavernous malformations: clinical features and risk of hemorrhage. Neurosurg Rev. 2003;26(4):253–6.
28. Steiger HJ, Turowski B, Hänggi D. Prognostic factors for the outcome of surgical and conservative treatment of symptomatic spinal cord cavernous malformations: a review of a series of 20 patients. Neurosurg Focus. 2010;29(3):E13.
29. Park SB, Jahng TA, Chung CK. The clinical outcomes after complete surgical resection of intramedullary cavernous angiomas: changes in motor and sensory symptoms. Spinal Cord. 2009;47(2):128–33.
30. Mitha AP, Turner JD, Abla AA, Vishteh AG, Spetzler RF. Outcomes following resection of intramedullary spinal cord cavernous malformations: a 25-year experience. J Neurosurg Spine. 2011;14(5):605–11.
31. Deutsch H, Jallo GI, Faktorovich A, Epstein F. Spinal intramedullary cavernoma: clinical presentation and surgical outcome. J Neurosurg Spine. 2000;93(1):65–70.
32. Labauge P, Bouly S, Parker F, Gallas S, Emery E, Loiseau H, et al. Outcome in 53 patients with spinal cord cavernomas. Surg Neurol. 2008;70(2):176–81.
33. Jallo GI, Freed D, Zareck M, Epstein F, Kothbauer KF. Clinical presentation and optimal management for intramedullary cavernous malformations. Neurosurg Focus. 2006;21(1):e10.
34. Bian LG, Bertalanffy H, Sun QF, Shen JK. Intramedullary cavernous malformations: clinical features and surgical technique via hemilaminectomy. Clin Neurol Neurosurg. 2009;111(6):511–7.
35. Kim LJ, Klopfenstein JD, Zabramski JM, Sonntag VKH, Spetzler RF. Analysis of pain resolution after surgical resection of intramedullary spinal cord cavernous malformations. Neurosurgery. 2006;58(1):106.
36. Kivelev J, Niemelä M, Hernesniemi J. Outcome after microsurgery in 14 patients with spinal cavernomas and review of the literature: clinical article. J Neurosurg Spine. 2010;13(4):524–34.

MIX
Papier aus verantwortungsvollen Quellen
Paper from responsible sources
FSC® C105338

If you have any concerns about our products,
you can contact us on
ProductSafety@springernature.com

In case Publisher is established outside the EU,
the EU authorized representative is:
Springer Nature Customer Service Center GmbH
Europaplatz 3, 69115 Heidelberg, Germany

Printed by Libri Plureos GmbH
in Hamburg, Germany